High Dependency Nursing Care

Level 2 (highly dependent) patients are nursed in a variety of clinical areas. *High Dependency Nursing Care* has been written for pre-qualified and post-qualified students undertaking modules and placements to prepare them for nursing the acutely ill and for nurses caring for these patients. Written by a team of nurses experienced in providing, supporting and developing high dependency care, it discusses practical issues and explores the current evidence base for clinical practice.

This essential textbook covers the context of care with chapters on fundamental aspects such as sleep, nutrition, pain management and stress. It goes on to look at the main causes of critical illness and the treatments often given, as well as the skills necessary for monitoring patients. Completely updated throughout, this second edition also includes new chapters on infection control, heart failure, tissue removal and transferring the sicker patient.

High Dependency Nursing Care is:

- Comprehensive: it covers all the key areas of knowledge needed.
- User-friendly: it includes learning outcomes, time out exercises, implications for practice, up-to-date references and details of useful websites.
- Clearly written: by a team of experienced nurses.
- Practically based: clinical scenarios provide stimulating discussion and revision topics.

Tina Moore is a Senior Lecturer in Acute and High Dependency Care at Middlesex University, London.

Philip Woodrow is a Practice Development Nurse in Critical Care at the East Kent Hospitals University NHS Trust, where he delivers a six-day course for ward staff caring for level 2 (highly dependent) patients. He is also the author of *Intensive Care Nursing: A Framework for Practice*, 2nd edition (Routledge, 2006).

High Dependency Nursing Care

Observation, intervention and support for level 2 patients

Second edition

Tina Moore and Philip Woodrow

with

Noirin Egan, Debbie Higgs, Sheila O'Sullivan, Mary Tilki and Lisa Tupper

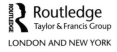

Routledge
Taylor & Francis Group

LONDON AND NEW YORK

First edition published 2004
by Routledge

This edition published 2009
by Routledge
2 Park Square, Milton Park, Abingdon, Oxon OX14 4RN

Simultaneously published in the USA and Canada
by Routledge
270 Madison Ave, New York, NY 10016

Routledge is an imprint of the Taylor and Francis Group, an informa business

© 2004, 2009 Tina Moore and Philip Woodrow

Typeset in Sabon by Wearset Ltd, Boldon, Tyne and Wear
Printed and bound in Great Britain by TJ International Ltd, Padstow, Cornwall

British Library Cataloguing in Publication Data
A catalogue record for this book is available from the British Library

Library of Congress Cataloging in Publication Data
Moore, Tina, 1962–
High dependency nursing care : observation, intervention, and support for level 2 patients / Tina
Moore, Philip Woodrow. – 2nd ed.
p. ; cm.
Rev. ed. of: High dependency nursing care / edited by Tina Moore and Philip Woodrow. 2004.
Includes bibliographical references and index.
1. Intensive care nursing–Textbooks. I. Woodrow, Philip, 1957 Sept. 4- II. High dependency
nursing care. III. Title.
[DNLM: 1. Critical Illness–nursing. 2. Critical Care–methods. 3. Nursing Process. WY 154
M824h 2009]
RT120.I5H55 2009
616.02'8–dc22   2008054217

ISBN10: 0-415-46794-2 (hbk)
ISBN10: 0-415-46795-0 (pbk)
ISBN10: 0-203-87588-5 (ebk)

ISBN13: 978-0-415-46794-0 (hbk)
ISBN13: 978-0-415-46795-7 (pbk)
ISBN13: 978-0-203-87588-9 (ebk)

For Vincent, Charlene and Calvin
T.M.
For Laura and Michael
P.W.

Contents

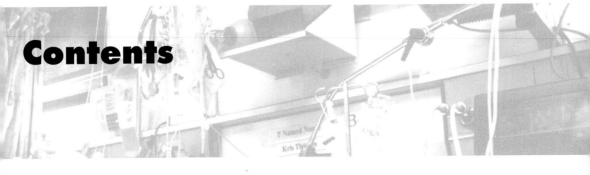

Part 1: Contexts for care

Figures

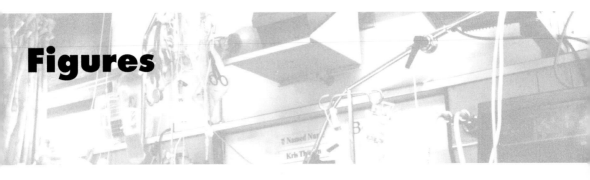

Tables

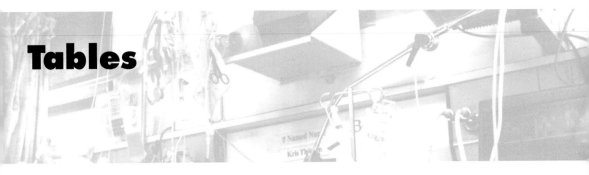

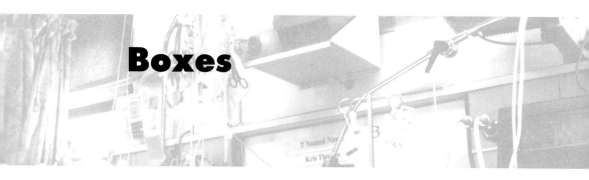

Boxes

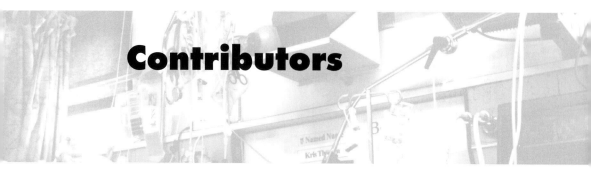

Contributors

Noirin Egan is a Clinical Nurse Specialist in Cardiology, working in the Rapid Access Chest Pain Clinic. She was previously a ward manager of a coronary care and high dependency unit.

Debbie Higgs is a Consultant Nurse in Critical Care at East Kent Hospitals University NHS Trust.

Sheila O'Sullivan is currently the Acting Assistant Director of Nursing at Whipps Cross University Hospital NHS Trust.

Mary Tilki is Principal Lecturer/Programme Leader in the School of Health and Social Sciences, Middlesex University with considerable experience in intensive care and high dependency care. Her publications include *Transcultural Education and Care, Older People from Minority Ethnic Groups* and *The Health of Irish People in Britain*.

Lisa Tupper RGN, BSc (Hons) is an experienced gynaecology nurse and student sonographer at East Kent Hospitals University NHS Trust.

Preface to the second edition

This text is for nurses caring for acutely ill adults. Many aspects may also be applicable for sick children, but unless children are specifically stated, readers caring for children should check paediatric sources.

In revising this book, we started with two main aims:

- to focus on ward care;
- to update evidence and practice.

The first edition was developed at a time when high dependency units were encouraged, so that was the focus of the first edition. While some high dependency units have opened, more high dependency patients are cared for in general medical/surgical/other wards. This second edition, therefore, focuses on higher dependency patients in ward environments – level 2 patients (DOH, 2000a). This is explained further in the opening chapter. To update evidence and practice, all chapters have been thoroughly revised, and some new chapters added. We aimed to minimise references predating the first edition, but in many chapters had to use more pre-2004 evidence than originally hoped – although much has been published in the intervening years, we considered disappointingly little new evidence to be useful for nurses in everyday clinical practice. While upheavals faced by the NHS (Mandelstam, 2007) could explain limited progress in the UK, it does not explain similar lack of progress from international literature and evidence. However, there have been a number of important guidelines and reports published, of which the most important is probably NICE (2007), which identified significant avoidable morbidity and mortality in acute hospitals. Unlike most other healthcare professions, nurses are in the vicinity of in-patients throughout their stay, and so are best placed to identify problems and initiate action. This book aims to help nurses fulfil this important role.

In the UK, and many other countries, there has been increasing emphasis on safety issues. Coincidentally at the time when the Internet has facilitated access to information, this has contributed to development of national guidelines. Many have been cited in this book, but readers can find useful information on websites such as those for the

- National Institute for Clinical Excellence;
- National Patient Safety Agency;
- Department of Health;
- Scottish Intercollegiate Guidelines Network;

as well as special interest groups (such as the British Thoracic Society). Similar bodies exist in many countries. Acknowledging our international readership, we have used 'hospitals' rather than 'Trusts'.

A good basis for care is whether, in the event of illness, we would wish ourselves or our loved ones to be cared for in our hospitals. We hope this book helps you to deliver the quality of care to your patients that you would wish for yourselves.

Thank you to everyone who has helped in the production of this book: guest authors and Jane Fallows, and to the many people 'behind the scenes' who have contributed so much – Sarah Coulling (Chapter 10), Bryony Johnson (Chapter 7), Janet Smith (Chapter 35), Grace McInnes and the team at Routledge, and especially to Jane Roe and John Albarran for their continuing and consistently valuable reviews and advice.

T.M.
P.W.

A special thank you to Iván Abraján MD, Alvarez-Tostado MD and Marcelo Basave MD; Hospiten Cancún, México, whose tireless commitment, dedication and humane approach during my own need for critical care made it possible for the production of this second edition.

T.M.
December 2008

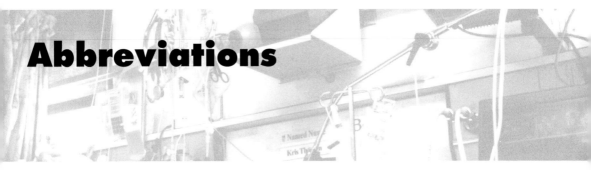

Abbreviations

AECOPD	acute exacerbation of chronic obstructive pulmonary disease
AKI	acute kidney injury (previously called acute renal failure)
ATN	acute tubular necrosis
ATP	adenosine triphosphate, produced in cells and used by cells for energy
AVPU	Alert – Verbal – Pain – Unresponsive
β-hCG	beta-human chorionic gonadotrophin hormone
CPAP	continuous positive airway pressure
CVC	central venous catheter
CVP	central venous pressure
FBC	full blood count
GCS	Glasgow Coma Scale
LDL	low-density lipoprotein
LFTs	liver function tests
LTOT	long-term oxygen therapy
MAP	mean arterial pressure
MEWS	Modified Early Warning Score
OHSS	Ovarian Hyperstimulation Syndrome
PID	pelvic inflammatory disease
SG	specific gravity
STI	sexually transmitted infection
SVR	systemic vascular resistance
TC	total cholesterol
U+Es	urea + electrolytes (biochemistry blood test)

Part 1

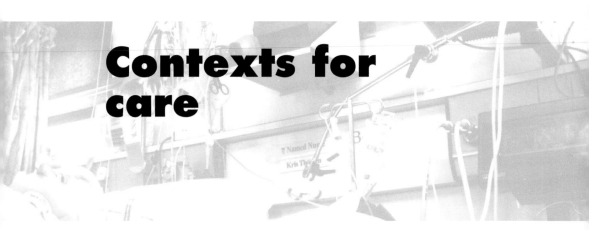

Contexts for care

Chapter 1

Comprehensive critical care

Tina Moore

Contents

Learning outcomes

After reading this chapter you will be able to:

■ demonstrate knowledge of the changes occurring within critical care;
■ understand the principles of high dependency nursing;
■ appreciate the role of advocacy and the critically ill patient.

Fundamental knowledge

Patient-centred care (Chapter 2); ethics (Chapter 3); rehabilitation (Chapter 36).

Introduction

The philosophy of high dependency unit (HDU) nursing pervades this book. This particular chapter will provide a summary/overview of the principles of high dependency nursing.

Time out 1.1

1 Think back to when you first cared for acutely/critically ill patients. What do you consider to be the main aspects of care?

2 Now write down the approaches to care you have been involved in today.

3 Have you noticed any changes in the way these patients are cared for?

4 If so, why do you think these changes have occurred?

The discontent regarding Intensive Care Unit (ICU) provision occurred during the 1990s, highlighting the failings of critical care services. Recently, healthcare professionals have seen many great changes in the way critical care is delivered. Today, there is a more consistent approach in the organisation of critical care services, achieved through the strategic document *Comprehensive Critical Care* (DOH, 2000a). This strategy led to a revision of critical care services and produced a complete process of care for the critically ill and focused on the level of care needed by individual patients and their families at any point during their illness. There is now a pro-active approach using a 'whole systems' approach which attends to the needs of those at risk of critical illness as well as those who are critically ill. *Comprehensive Critical Care* strategy is emerging as a uniform standard throughout the NHS, regardless of location or speciality, i.e. 'no walls' philosophy. It is now viewed as a new speciality based on the severity of illness that is focusing on the needs of the patient, central to the service provided.

While there has been significant improvement in caring for acutely/critically ill patients there are many improvements still to be done. There is still the possibility that patients who are, or become, acutely unwell may receive suboptimal care (NICE, 2007a). This is possibly due to unrecognised deterioration, lack of knowledge to interpret indications of clinical deterioration, lack of rapid intervention or indeed gross underfunding to provide adequate resources, including staff. In response the National Institute for Health and Clinical Excellence (NICE) has produced guidance and recommendations on a number of areas affecting the acutely ill adult in hospital. These include: physiological observations, physiological track and trigger, recognition of deterioration and transfer.

Nature of high dependency nursing

HDUs have been developed as a result of failure of hospitals to address the increased demand for intensive care services. In many hospitals there are no designated HDUs but instead they have 'HDU bed areas' within the ward. The term 'critical care' is used as a global term that covers a diverse set of services (DOH, 2000a), including both intensive care and high dependency care. Both units are now merging to become one managed Critical Care Unit. These units may be specialised, e.g. surgical, neurology, cardiac and hepatic.

Intensive (level 3) care provides detailed observation and treatment for patients with potential recoverable conditions, involving multiple organ failure or requiring mechanical ventilation. High dependency (level 2) care supplies an intermediate level of care between the ICU and the general wards, involving patients with single system failure (not respiratory). HDUs can be used as a 'step-up' facility (patient requiring greater monitoring, support and supervision than is available on a general ward). This may prevent the need for admission to the ICU. Alternatively, HDU care may provide a 'step-down' facility for patients no longer requiring ICU services but are not well enough to be discharged to the wards, with the lack of HDU beds, many of these patients are on general wards.

The categories of patients requiring HDU care are explained in Box 1.1. These patients will require continuous or intermittent (but regular) observation, care and intervention. Nurses provide highly specialised, technological care to the very ill patient, therefore, skill mix should be determined upon the needs of the patient and levels of dependency rather than determined by numbers of beds (DOH, 2000a).

It is clear that some patients may not benefit from HDU nursing because they are 'too sick to benefit' (extremely poor prognosis or a level 3 patient) or 'too well to benefit'. Box 1.1 provides a non-exhaustive list of those patients who would benefit from HDU admission.

Box 1.1 Examples of patients requiring HDU provision

- Patients requiring level 2 type care
- Patients requiring single organ support, e.g. non-invasive ventilation (excluding artificial mechanical ventilation), high-risk surgical patients, patients with major uncorrected physiological abnormalities
- Patients requiring more detailed observation/monitoring
- Patients who no longer need intensive care but are not well enough for a general ward

---

Characteristics of high dependency nursing

The distinguishing features of intensive care, high dependency care and ward care can be determined through the intensity of nursing input (namely, the amount of time spent with any one patient) in delivering both the nursing and medical plan of care. Nursing intensity will vary depending upon the patient's condition, for example, weaning patients from non-invasive ventilation may require more intensity than patients who are fully sedated or unconscious. The recommended nurse–patient ratios are ICU 1:1 (ICS, 1997), HDU 1:2 (Garfield *et al.*, 2000); on the wards no ratio has been agreed, but staff should determine the degree of nursing intensity by the amount of monitoring and nursing intervention required. *Comprehensive Critical Care* recommends flexible use of staff with a move away from the use of rigid ratios to determine nurse staffing for patients requiring level 2 and 3 care to the use of more flexible systems of assessing nursing workload (DOH, 2000a). The expert group suggests tools such as the System Of Patient

Related Activity (SOPRA). The RCN has provided guidance for nursing staff in critical care. It is a cautious document and is non-committed in terms of providing ratios. It supports the concept of flexibility and provides factors that should be considered when determining staffing levels (RCN, 2003b). In practice, the general view is that of comprehensive critical care.

Nonetheless, the RCN's guidance could be manipulated into expecting minimal and potentially unsafe nurse–patient ratios. Flexibility could become a 'slippery slope' potentially affecting quality of patient and safety. The British Association for Critical Care Nursing rightly voiced concerns relating to the pressure of working with less than desirable nurse–patient ratios and subsequent inability to cope with demands (Pilcher and Odell, 2000). Currently, this debate appears dormant.

There is also no recognition of 'invisible' work, such as continuous observation. Patient allocation should be based on skill mix and competency within the nursing ratio, enabling those observations to be understood, analysed and acted upon 24 hours per day.

Critical care nurses (registered) should have the right knowledge, skills and competence to meet the needs of the critically ill patient without direct supervision (RCN, 2003b). Critical care skills (which acute care nurses should possess) are not only important in providing appropriate and safe nursing care but should also aid the prevention of critical illness. Constant observation of the vulnerable critically ill is imperative. This involves assimilation, interpretation and evaluation of patients' physical and psychological status.

Nurses caring for acutely ill patients need to be able to:

- collect the data, interpret information and act appropriately;
- ask for physiological parameters (desired outcomes) to be set (NCEPOD, 2007), e.g. BP, heart rate, respiratory rate from the Medical team;
- make decisions quickly, accurately and often independently, based on patient cues;
- be attentive to the minute detail of patient care for prolonged periods of time;
- be pro-active and make predictions and prevent complications; make prompt and skilled intervention in the event of sudden deterioration (RCN, 2003b);
- have a specialist body of knowledge pertinent to the care of critically ill patients and promote competent care;
- respond quickly and effectively in a variety of emergency situations;
- be an effective team member;
- work efficiently within a potentially stressful environment;
- deliver holistic care including family and significant others.

Advocacy

Time out 1.2

1 Write down your definition of advocacy, highlighting the key words. Now compare your views with a dictionary definition.
2 Consider how you advocate for the patients within your care.
3 Compare your actions to the words previously highlighted. Is there any difference?

The term 'advocacy' has become a dormant 'buzzword' that has been linked with concepts of morality, ethics, autonomy and patient empowerment (Snowball, 1996). The interpretation of advocacy can vary among healthcare professionals. Baldwin (2003) has, through a concept analysis, highlighted that in most cases where nurses act as advocates for patients, they do so by attempting to influence a third party on behalf of their clients. For example, a patient who lives alone deteriorates, prognosis is poor and he wishes to die in peace and with dignity. Nurses would advocate the patient's point of view to all concerned within the delivery of care. However, this may change with the introduction of the Mental Capacity Act (2005), where the patient has a right to appoint their own advocate.

Within acute care many of the patients are dependent/semi-dependent. This puts a demand on the nurse to shoulder the role of advocate. Reservations about the suitability of the healthcare professionals to act as patient advocate have been expressed (Mental Capacity Act, 2005). Patients are now able to choose their advocate, which does not automatically mean nurses. Within acute care there may be no alternative as the majority of patients are in no position to choose their advocate, a situation that may change once the patient's condition improves. The patient could, in advance, identify their advocate (Mental Capacity Act, 2005), which the relatives should enforce, but may be challenging if there is only one qualified nurse on duty.

There is a moral duty to protect patients' rights and autonomy; it may be difficult for nurses to advocate for the patients they do not know (due to severity of illness, reduced consciousness/unconsciousness). Once healthcare interventions have been adapted to meet the special needs of the patient, the nurse's role should be to articulate the patient's needs within the multidisciplinary team, creating patient-centred approaches to care. However, in reality this may be seen as a lower priority for nurses with the focus on surviving the shift, exposing patients to as few risks as feasibly possible.

The advocacy role of the nurse has been hindered by little practical guidance offered on how this role should be interpreted in clinical practice. Empirical evidence is sparse and a few individuals ground theories in anecdotal accounts (Hewitt, 2002). A small-scale study conducted by Lindahl and Sandman (1998) highlighted the following themes within the role of an advocate:

- building a caring relationship;
- being committed to the patient;
- empowering the patient (shifting of appropriate power);
- being a moral agent;
- creating a trusting atmosphere conducive to recovery.

Advocacy should be viewed as a temporary role. In order to promote the nurse's advocacy role, they need to be willing to hand over power and control to the patient (Chapter 36); this can be achieved through nurses' education in theory and practice. An aim of promoting the advocacy role is that the patient's autonomy is secured. Literature addressing nursing ethics also notes that patient advocacy is supported by the principle of autonomy because the nurse is obliged to enable patients to be self-determining. A therapeutic nurse–patient relationship should secure a patient's freedom and self-determination. Nurses have a role in promoting and protecting a patient's rights to be involved in decision-making and informed consent.

Implications for practice

- Assessment of a patient is dependent upon his or her care needs, and not location.
- Nurses need to be willing to take on the responsibility for advocacy (or indeed relinquish it) and also releasing control.
- Nurses should actively be involved in constantly enhancing the quality of care provision.
- Acute care nurses need sound generic knowledge and skill together with acute/critical care knowledge and skill.

Summary

Nursing the critically/acutely ill patient is not restricted to traditional ICUs and HDUs and, therefore, ward staff will need to expand their level of expertise to be able to care for these patients effectively and efficiently. Care is not just physiologically orientated, but should be holistic, acknowledging psychological, emotional and social influences.

Bibliography

Key reading

DOH document (2000a).
Mental Capacity Act (2005) – provides detailed information regarding the acutely ill patient's rights and the implications of ignoring patient's autonomy.
NCEPOD (2007) – offers comprehensive guidance for the emergency admission of acutely ill adults, particularly to the ward care areas.

Chapter 2

Patient-centred care

Tina Moore

Contents

Learning outcomes

After reading this chapter you will be able to:

- appreciate the possible impact of modern technology on patient care;
- recognise characteristics of dehumanisation;
- understand the importance of delivering appropriate, sensitive care to patients requiring high dependency care.

Introduction

The noisy, unfamiliar environment together with machinery, medical jargon, loss of day–night cycle and painful invasive procedures characteristic of high dependency care areas are associated with a high incidence of psychological trauma and sleep deprivation (Cuthbertson *et al.*, 2004). This type of environment can appear hostile and even threatening to patients.

The development and spread of modern technology within acute care areas offer highly sophisticated machines that provide further continual and accurate monitoring and in some cases assisting in the diagnostic process. Consequently, technology has become one of the major determinants that shape the delivery of acute/high dependency care. As the task of technology develops, nurses should minimise its potentially conflicting demands and increase the demands of humanity.

Therefore, this chapter identifies problems associated with influences on the delivery of patient-centred care, e.g. the use of technology, particularly those relating to humanity, patient acuity and disruption/noise, some of which are discussed in more detail in other related chapters. Suggestions will be offered enabling nurses to create and maintain a balance between delivering a humanistic approach to care and the demands incurred by modern machinery.

There is an abundance of literature expressing concern over the patient's environment, including the use of technology.

Time out 2.1

Identify barriers (actual and potential) to the delivery or patient-centred care within your area of practice.

Intrusion of technology?

While the aim for the use of technology is to minimise errors, the nature of high dependency/acute care necessitates the initial prioritisations of physical needs but in doing so a number of human needs, particularly psychological and social, may be compromised.

Despite the fact that the use of technology can promote feelings of security for nurses (Almerud *et al.*, 2008), it can be viewed as having an intrusive and imposing presence. Its dominance may cause experiences of care to be invisible. As a result, the concept of inhumanity has been linked to this type of nursing. Technology is part of the problem and part of the solution (Nadzam and Mackles, 2001) and will have good effects if used appropriately and bad effects if misused or abused. But within high technological environments the patient and equipment meld, forming one unit (Almerud *et al.*, 2008).

Current developments indicate that in the future, within the acute care setting, there will be an increase in the use of modern machinery. Technology has the potential to create a barrier to human interactions, inducing dehumanisation (technological romanticism). Families may be reluctant to touch loved ones who are connected to machines. This often results from the fear of upsetting equipment and causing possible malfunctions and alarms being triggered. Patients who are confined or restricted by and dependent on equipment may remind family members of the loss of control that they have, not only over their loved ones but also over their own fate, leading to feelings of vulnerability and helplessness.

Owing to the possible demands of technology, nurses may become distracted from being involved in the personal emotional care and forget that among the machinery there is a person who is a precious and significant part of family life.

Technical optimists suggest that technology is not necessarily opposed to humanised care, but can indeed specifically and deliberately be engaged in the service of humanising it (Barnard, 2004). Hence, technology is seen as a means to an end. Some patients (and family) are reassured by the presence of technology.

Scientific knowledge is the basis of medicine and technology, as well as being associated with the dehumanisation, depersonalisation and objectification of patients. Dehumanisation can be associated with depriving patients of their individuality, subjectivity and dignity as human beings. Dehumanisation can also prevent nurses from their mission to care (Sandelowski, 2000; Barnard, 2004). Technology is an integral part of nursing care provision but it should be used to compliment and support nursing monitoring and interventions not to be overpowered by it.

There is concern that life-sustaining technology has greatly expanded the possibilities of medical intervention at the end of life. However, these technologies may have outpaced development of good judgement concerning their appropriate use.

Factors that contribute to dehumanisation include:

- inconsistent philosophies about patient care delivery and decision-making (e.g. paternalism versus patient autonomy);
- personal and professional value conflicts (e.g. prolonging life, care versus cure);
- poor communication pattern (e.g. one-way communication, missing patient cues);
- unresolved ethical dilemmas (e.g. withholding information, failure to respect patient autonomy);
- increased technology (e.g. clinical information systems, extra monitoring equipment);
- shortages of human and material resources (e.g. shortage of technical support, poor patient:nurse ratios)
- inadequate support systems for staff delivering care (e.g. lack of clinical supervision, performance reviews and staff development plans);
- lack of professional skill in the various dimensions of humane care (e.g. patient consent, advocacy);
- inadequate administrative support (e.g. nurses having to answer telephone rather than delivering care);
- the physical design of the unit environment (e.g. bed-space small, difficulty in reaching the patient).

(Harvey, 1992)

Time out 2.2

From the barriers identified in Time out 2.1, suggest strategies to provide patient-centred care.

Humanism

Anecdotal observations indicate that there as been a slow shift away from the illness-cure model towards a more holistic, individualised and person-centred approach within high dependency/acute care areas. However, there are some practices that remain within the positivist paradigm.

Humanism refers to any system or model of thought or action in which human interest, value and dignity predominate. It reflects a philosophy that emphasises an individual's uniqueness and freedom to choose a particular course of action (providing they are able). This is grounded in the idea that as individuals, we are the only ones who can know our own perceptions; we are, therefore, the best experts on ourselves. If patients are unable to achieve this self-knowledge (and many of them are not), then the family should be involved in the delivery of care, including clinical decision-making (if they are able/willing, or indeed, if it is appropriate). As the patient's advocate, nurses will need to embark upon a sensitive approach to delivering care in accordance with their perceptions of the patient's needs.

Humanism as a philosophy appears to offer a basis of care beyond the disease orientation of practice. The concept has many guises and challenges. Humanistic care requires the nurse to have emotional intelligence that constantly questions themselves and seeks awareness of them and others but most importantly they must always be genuine, sincere and transparent in dealing with others. Nurses should strive continually to foster a culture of humanness and should be constantly encouraging and supervising their personal growth.

Humanism demands attitudes and actions that demonstrate interest in, and respect of, the patient and that address the patient's concerns and values. These are, generally, related to the patient's psychological, social and spiritual domains (Branch *et al.*, 2001). It has been recognised that such approaches are inherently vague, offering little by way of guidance to the nurse practitioner (Branch *et al.*, 2001).

Some writers advocate that the humanistic approach is well suited to addressing the needs of a culturally diverse population, facilitating transcultural nursing practice capable of offering culturally sensitive healthcare (see Chapter 5).

Watson (2007) provides the links between the concepts of humanism and care. Caring is viewed as the moral ideal of nursing, where there is utmost concern for human dignity and preservation of humanity. Fostering humane care for patients and their families cannot occur unless the environment also treats caregivers humanely. Humane care recognises the uniqueness of each patient and strives to provide a holistic approach to caring. The provision of care within a humanistic framework should be dynamic, individualised and also requires the involvement of the patient (where possible).

Principles of humanism suggest that:

- each individual is unique and has specific needs, values and beliefs;
- individuals are the source of expertise and authority regarding their own unique needs;

- preservation of the patient and their family's autonomy;
- respect for privacy;
- participation in clinical decision-making as far as the patient's condition allows;
- the patient's safety should not be compromised.

(Harvey, 1992)

The centrality of the nurse–patient relationship, based on such tenets as empathy, genuineness, mutual respect and joint participation has been recognised and taught as the basis for a more human approach to nursing care. However, there are inherent difficulties associated with defining and operationalising humanism and its components such as compassion, empathy, caring, integrity and respect.

Individualised care is a key element of nursing, being an important component of both high-quality care and patient satisfaction. Nurses have constant contact with hospitalised patients and because of this close relationship have the potential for the greatest influence over the delivery of individualised care. It is important to recognise that the patient's perceptions of the care actually received represent their reality. No amount of preparation or imagination can come close to the real experiences of the patient, therefore, it is crucial that nurses listen very carefully to the patient and try and understand the lived experiences from the patient's perception and their realities. Whilst it is tempting for nurses to interpret the patient's experiences they should avoid doing so as this may lead to misconceptions.

Patient-centred care requires the nurse to have a number of qualities: tactful, accessible, approachable, sensitive, open, honest, sincere and caring attitudes. There is a concern with meeting human needs and answering human problems, recognising the existence of moral dilemmas and focus on a supportive positive atmosphere and exchange of ideas.

Optimising patient care through a humanistic framework

The relationship between technology and care is paradoxical, holding in tension the objective values of science and the subjective values of human well-being (Cooper, 1993). Patients and their families see nurses as the interface between themselves and the technology (McConnell, 1998). Despite being constantly monitored and observed, patients felt invisible as people, reduced to the status of organs, objects and diagnosis (Almerud et al., 2007).

Nurses who are effective in their care delivery will know how to interact with technology and with people. They will understand the principles behind the technology they use in order to be able to recognise and respond to patient needs, particularly when a problem develops, or a patient condition changes. For instance, if a patient is having arterial blood pressure monitoring and a flattened waveform occurs, there is a need to look beyond the equipment and at the patient, search for other indicators to support the technological findings. Nurses must be able to solve problems and think critically. Care has been described as a moral imperative for nurses, relying on empirical, aesthetic, ethical, personal (Carper, 1978) and professional/legal knowing.

Nurses should continually assess the patient and the effect that the environment has or may have on the patient and take appropriate action to minimise this effect, e.g. if a patient is to have non-invasive ventilation (NIV) the nurse should explain (using simple language) the equipment and enable as much movement as possible, perhaps even allowing the patient to sit out of bed. Nurses are in a unique position, as people who have special knowledge and skills about others and their responses to illness and as a result should be able to make sense of the patient's human experience. While many nurses try, they cannot totally appreciate the patient's perspective until they themselves have had the experience. The technology and the humanity of care pose a challenge to nurses within the high dependency/acute care areas. With each recounting of a caring experience by nurses (possibly through reflective practice) care becomes more visible and valued.

Optimising the human experience includes:

- being there
- sharing
- supporting
- involving
- interpreting
- advocating.

(Andrew, 1998)

The concept of 'being there' as described by Watson (1999) and Ashworth (1990) goes beyond the physically present and involves connectedness in a holistic way, i.e. being empathetic and emotionally/psychologically available. However, it is necessary to give a sense of space and time to both the patient and the family members. The notion of presence requires the nurse to recognise that simply being with a patient (mentally as well as physically) can be therapeutic in itself and, therefore, the nurse is seen as a therapeutic tool (Watson, 2007). In order to achieve this, it is vital that nurses are self-aware and in touch with their own values and beliefs.

The 'humanistic nurse' will be able to, once having deconstructed professionalism and humanism into their key elements and building blocks, resynthesise these components and processes into an integrated whole and can sense the individual uniqueness of a patient and adjust treatment accordingly (Swick, 2007).

Communication – i.e. precise wording; tone; pacing and inflection of the voice; timing of the message and body language; use of therapeutic touch; ability to be flexible, creative and constantly sensitive to the patient feedback – are all characteristics of humane care.

'Mindful' nursing practice

Putting the acutely ill first entails a thorough appreciation of their special needs, including their psychological well-being. This also means that nurses must do their best to decrease and allay fears and anxiety, rather than only treat symptoms and disease. Sometimes, deciding with uncertainty what the best care is for the patient is difficult and complicated, unsure of which option(s) is the best. Family members are often in a poor position to make good choices, they are often exhausted, irritable, shattered or despondent.

Therefore, 'mindful' practice requires mentoring and guidance and recognition of one's limitations and areas of competence and is an individual and subjective process (Kissoon, 2005).

Box 2.1 Characteristics of 'mindful practice'

- Active observation of oneself, the patient and the problem
- Peripheral vision
- Pre-attentive processing
- Critical curiosity
- Courage to see the work as it is rather than as one would have it be
- Willingness to examine and set aside categories and prejudices
- Adoption of a beginner's mind
- Humility to tolerate awareness of one's area of incompetence
- Connection between the knower and the known
- Compassion based on insight
- Presence

(Epstein, 1999)

The goal for mindful practice is a compassionate informed action using a wide array of data, making correct decisions, understanding the patient and relieving suffering (Epstein, 1999).

Implications for practice

- Nurses should continually assess the patient and family for the effect technology may have on them.
- The delivery of safe, efficient and effective care needs to be balanced with sensitive, caring approaches.
- The concept of humanism should be integral to the provision of care.
- Nurses need to be self-aware before they can embark upon the delivery of humanistic care.

Summary

Nursing consists of interaction between unique individuals with unique experiences and it always takes place within unique situations. Nurses need to function effectively within a patient-driven system in which nurses can care for patients and their families in a holistic fashion. That challenge gives a clear mandate for controlling the patient's environment; it must function efficiently and invisibly so nurses can spend less time staring at monitors and writing in charts and more time interacting directly with patients and families (McConnell, 1998). Technology should be utilised to allow just that, releasing more time for nurses to provide emotional, psychological and sociological care. Hence, technology should be used to help nurses to care in an efficient and effective manner.

Nursing is both an art and a science and, therefore, it is in nursing's best interest to be conversant with changes for its own survival but not at the expense of humane caring. Technology has to be integrated into everyday practices. For that reason, nurses must retain the caring humanistic qualities that have threaded through the profession as well as the evidence-based practice. It is important not to lose sight of the foundations of caring as identified by the seminal work of Roach (1987) identifying the five 'C's of professional caring:

- compassion
- competence
- confidence
- commitment
- conscience.

There is a need to integrate care and technology to the extent where technology does not impede care but enhances it. Nurses must be competent in managing the technology, even though technological competence does not necessarily have an easy relationship with the response of care.

Clinical scenario

Anna Cummings, 46 years old, is behaving in an agitated manner, she looks anxious and in pain. Cardiovascularly, she has a tachycardia of 148 bpm, her BP is 150/100 mmHg and she is sweaty. One of her ECG electrodes becomes disconnected and the monitor alarms repeatedly. Noise from the alarm further upsets Anna. When the nurse approaches, Anna apologises profusely for setting off the monitor alarm.

1   How should the nurse respond? (Analyse the tensions between caring and technology.)

2   How could the nurse implement 'mindful practice' for Anna?

3   Analyse why Anna felt she was the cause of the equipment alarming (consider the nurse's behaviour – non-verbal, observing and touching equipment more than the patient).

Bibliography

Further reading

Almerud, S., Alapack, R.J., Fridlund, B., Ekebergh, M. (2007) Of vigilance and invisibility: being a patient in technological intense environments. *Nursing in Critical Care* 13 (3): 151–158.

Almerud, S., Alapack, R.J., Fridlund, B., Ekebergh, M. (2008) Beleaguered by technology: care in technologically intense environments. *Nursing Philosophy* 9: 55–61.

Both articles present a philosophical view about the use of technology. Not only are they interesting to read, they also highlight concerns about the use of technology and provide some strategic direction. Certainly these are thought-provoking articles.

Chapter 3

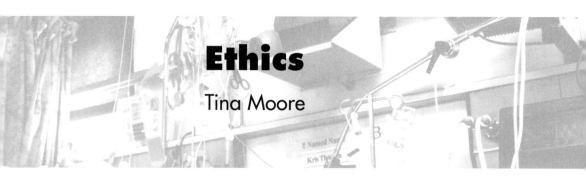

Ethics

Tina Moore

Contents

Learning outcomes

After reading this chapter you will be able to:

- demonstrate an understanding of the need to be aware of the ethical issues and their importance in clinical practice as a guidance for care delivery;
- identify actual and potential ethical situations relating to the acutely/critically ill patient and suggest strategies for resolution/coping;
- develop an awareness of one's own beliefs and values during exposure to clinical situations;
- apply ethical principles as a guide in the provision/ framework of care;
- describe and discuss the stages of ethical decision-making.

Introduction

Acute care can involve highly specialised and complicated care planning, including ethical decision-making on a daily basis. Conflicts can arise from situations involving withholding/withdrawing treatment; deciding when the burdens of further therapeutic measures outweigh the benefits; allocation of limited resources. Arguably, technological advances in healthcare have developed at a rate faster than society is able to cope with ethically.

Many of the acutely ill patients are unable to act completely autonomously and, therefore, rely on healthcare professionals (particularly nurses) to make decisions for them. Consequently, there is a risk of initial decisions being made, mainly in relation to patients' ailments and not necessarily in their best interest. healthcare professionals may think they are making decisions in the best interest of patients, but sometimes this is not the case. Clinical decisions, whether by patient or nurse, may not be generally acceptable and thus can create a sense of uneasiness and possible resentment.

Due to its complexity ethical decision-making is not an easy process. However, nurses must develop a clear understanding of ethical considerations in order to ensure that the care they provide is morally and legally acceptable. While some ethical issues have been discussed in Chapters 1, 2 and later in Chapter 39, this particular chapter will create an opportunity for nurses to examine their own values and beliefs in relation to nursing the acutely ill. The intention is not to provide answers (this would be considered morally wrong), but to create an awareness/wider understanding of some of the fundamental issues faced by nurses within the acute care setting.

Time out 3.1

1 Write down your understanding of the term ethics. Now compare your understanding with a dictionary definition.
2 How do you think ethics relates to healthcare?
3 Make a list of ethical 'ground rules' you consider appropriate for nurses.

Nature of ethics

To appreciate ethical dilemmas, the meaning of ethics and its relationship to practice needs to be examined. The term 'ethics', derived from the Greek word 'ethos' relates to the philosophical study of the moral values of human conduct, including rules and principles that govern it (how we behave). In essence ethics is the practical application of moral philosophy.

Ethics integrates influencing themes:

■ Legal – what *must* be done. (This is debatable; as the law could be seen to be unethical. This could be interpreted to justify actions of a number of regimes/ actions as being ethical.)

- Practical – what *can* be done.
- Ethical – what *should* be done.

> **Time out 3.2**
>
> 1 Explain your understanding of the differences between right and wrong.
> 2 Think of a situation that you have been involved in where ethical issues emerged. List the aspects that you considered to be right and wrong within the situation. Was there a clear distinction between the two?
> 3 Now make another list, this time (if you can) from the perspective of others involved in the situation. Did you have similar/same values/views, or were there differences/conflicts?
> 4 Read the following section and try to determine (from the perspective of established theories) the values/views in relation to right and wrong.

Determination of exactly what is right from wrong is very difficult (what may be seen to be right for one person could be wrong for another). Ethical values directly relate to beliefs concerning what is right and proper, as opposed to what is effective or desirable. A clinical decision to withdraw treatment may be viewed the most effective way to reduce prolongation of life, but might be wrong in relation to quality of life (e.g. effects of dehydration). Nurses may face situations where the patient's belief of what is right conflicts with their own beliefs, e.g. a Jehovah's Witness refusing life-saving blood replacement. Nurses should not force their own beliefs and values onto the patient, but should try to recognise and understand the perspective of others.

Ethical theories

Some knowledge of these theories is necessary for nurses to deal with the ethical problems they have to face. Three main ethical theories exist (Beauchamp and Childress, 2008).

Consequentialism

This involves the ethical merit of an act that is best determined by the consequence (outcome) it produces, i.e. 'the ends can justify the means'. Actions are deemed right and good when they produce benefit; pleasure/happiness or prevent harm; pain/unhappiness. The action is judged on the consequences. The decision-maker is required to consider and predict the likely consequences of the contemplated action (weighing the good the act will produce against the harm it may cause). The motivation of the person involved in the action is not considered important.

Consider the case of Miss B (B v Secretary for Health, March 2002) who had sarcoma of her C2 (cervical vertebrae) and as a result was paralysed from the neck down and ventilated. She was fully conscious and deemed to be of a competent mind. Prognosis was extremely poor. She decided to take legal action to have all treatment stopped, including ventilatory support, and in doing so would end her life. In balance, life on the ventilator was seen as living but was a living torture. She wanted to die with dignity and thus ending her life was good in comparison to the harm she suffered. This scenario clearly illustrates the consequences of freedom from suffering (evil) and being allowed to die with more dignity (benefits). Freedom from pain is another such example.

Utilitarianism (a form of consequentialism) would state that as the majority was opposed to turning off the ventilator, then the patient should remain on it. The problem with this theory is the potential for injustice to occur to minorities in order to provide the greatest benefit for the majority. Hence, minority rights are imposed upon.

Duty-based (deontological)

This theory believes that people have an absolute duty to do the right thing under all circumstances, and what is 'right' has nothing to do with the actual consequences produced or avoided. The Code: Standards of Conduct, Performance and Ethics for Nurses and Midwives (NMC, 2008) reflects a deontological perspective. Unlike utilitarianism, the person's motives are crucial in determining the moral worth of their actions. There are fundamental rules that must be followed, whatever the consequences. Concepts such as 'duty' and 'obligation' are central to this theory.

The foundation of morality is the ability to act rationally (a rational being is free to act out of principle and to refrain from acting out of impulse or the desire for pleasure), but is debatable as to whether an individual whose beliefs and values that are in direct contradiction to those of deontological beliefs and values are deemed irrational.

This theory is shared by most healthcare professionals who believe they have a duty to preserve life (the act of life is sacrosanct) – but not always at all costs. Conflicts can and do arise between the duties of healthcare professionals and respect for the autonomy of the patient, e.g. patients who want to end their lives and the healthcare professionals who want to save it.

Rights-based theory

Autonomy is a central concept within this theory. It demands a respect for individual rights and these rights are seen as justified claims that the individual (or groups) can make upon others. The Human Rights Act (1998) sets out the articles of the European Convention of Human Rights. These reflect 'negative' (liberty) rights. While the 'right to life' is mentioned, there is an omission of 'right to die' despite there being attempts in the past to use some of the articles to end life by withdrawal of treatment.

Rights are equal and must be universally applied. One person's right can impinge on the rights of another. Prioritisation of individual rights may be difficult, if not impossible to achieve. However, the patient's rights and the rights of others may be in conflict, e.g. the right to refuse treatment versus the right to give safe and competent care.

Ethical principles

Ethical principles cannot address all situations but may help to clarify some of the issues involved. All have significant implications for nurses as they provide moral frameworks. There are four main ethical principles (Beauchamp and Childress, 2008):

- autonomy;
- beneficence – actions are intended to benefit and prevent harm;
- nonmaleficence – the obligation not to inflict harm intentionally and not to engage in actions that risk harming others (could be argued as impossible within healthcare);
- justice and fairness – treating everyone equally.

Beneficence, justice, autonomy, veracity (truthfulness) and respect for persons are characteristics that all nurses must have in order to be ethical (Beauchamp and Childress, 2008). Beneficence and nonmaleficence are not absolute principles and may at times come into conflict with each other, e.g. a patient may be complaining of considerable pain and require analgesia (via injection), but while the administration is viewed as beneficial, the injection will cause harm (skin puncture), or a patient with hypoxia requiring oxygen treatment and requires regular arterial blood gas analysis – arterial puncture is very painful.

   The principle-based approach to problem solving has been criticised as too abstract to be helpful in reality due to its complex nature (Edwards, 1996). It also provides little guidance on the every-day nursing issues, particularly in relation to the standards of care that should be provided. Edwards (1996) advocates an alternative, i.e. situational ethics, which determines the decision-making processes to be distinctive to each situation. Nurses should view each situation as unique and consider other influencing factors (e.g. patient prognosis and quality of life). Each moral problem should be regarded positively.

Autonomy

This principle of autonomy is the dominant ethical principle in Western cultures and is grounded ultimately in the integrity of the person and in his/her ability to make decisions. The action of an autonomous person is intentional, taken with understanding and without controlling influences that determine actions. Autonomy is to do with self-determination rather than other determination (Rady *et al.*, 2008).

   Patients with decision-making capacity have the right to make decisions about the course of their treatment (reflected in the Mental Capacity Act (2005)) or to delegate their autonomy to a family member/significant other. Patients now have the option to appoint a lasting poser of attorney to act as an independent advocate. Please see Chapter 41 for discussions regarding consent.

The limits of autonomy are not defined in demanding ineffective or inappropriate treatment (Doig *et al.*, 2006), where care could be reduced to 'everything possible' versus 'everything reasonable'.

While it is acknowledged that some patients are clearly unable to refuse to be autonomous, many do not automatically become dependent and unthinking once they become acutely/critically ill. Anecdotal observations support the notion that junior nurses may become preoccupied with pathology and medical treatment, with areas such as information giving, communication, recovery and rehabilitation possibly being neglected. Even in situations where passivity is the only option, information is vital for the purpose of consent and in some cases to enhance the patient's feelings of personal control. The principle of informed consent involves the concept of the patient's right to be adequately informed and the right to authorise or refuse medical treatment. Many patients strive to keep/exercise whatever little control they have left within hospital. To remove this control strips them of their individuality and personhood. Nurses may not appreciate the level of trust patients have in them, to the point where this trust may be abused intentionally or unintentionally.

Paternalism may be appropriate under certain conditions, particularly in the instances where patient safety is affected. Depending upon views – paternalism could be seen as an interference from one person to another making decisions against their will. Alternatively, it could be seen as someone making decisions in their best interest. Nurses should act in the best interest of the patient. In such situations, acting paternalistically is regarded as a duty: it is assumed (unless proven otherwise) that the patient desires health. However, its overuse can be sometimes contradictory to maintaining and promoting patient autonomy.

Autonomy should not be imposed. Patients need to be given the choice to execute their autonomy. It can be quite difficult to focus on the assessment of what the patient *can* do as opposed to what the patient cannot do, but it is crucial in the assistance of patient autonomy.

In the ideal situation, appropriate dependency is merely the precursor to a restoration of autonomy (Steele *et al.*, 2001). Problems develop when dependency is unnecessarily prolonged and then there is a risk that actions become paternalistic and nurses may find it difficult to separate acceptable beneficent acts from unacceptable paternalistic ones.

Nonmaleficence

While interrelated to beneficence, nonmaleficence is distinct. The core concept is primarily doing no harm. Obligations of nonmaleficence are not only obligations of not inflicting harm but also include obligations of not imposing risks of harm. Within this is included the concept of patient safety and indeed to the tort of negligence.

Nonetheless, there is a need to be clear about the boundaries of the obligation to provide benefits and avoid harm in patient care. Many issues centre on the critically ill in relation to this principle. It must be remembered that harm could be induced through omission, or lack of information – not just physical harm. It is unclear whether harm relates to situations beyond the control of nurses/ healthcare professionals, e.g. in the case of patient's condition deteriorating.

Nurses are bound by their professional code to safeguard patients and assume responsibility and accountability for nursing judgements and actions. This may be a difficult principle to adhere to as almost every nursing intervention that aims to benefit the patient results in harm, i.e. harm is an inevitable outcome of beneficence, e.g. patients who have enforced bedrest due to their condition and the need for monitoring may be at risk from the harm of complications of bedrest. Arguably, benefits and harm always need to be balanced against each other. In cases such as life-threatening interventions or if the harm inflicted is minor in comparison to the benefit, then the obligation of beneficence takes priority over the obligation of nonmaleficence (Beauchamp and Childress, 2008).

Nurses are often exposed to situations that involve complex networks of conflicting influencing factors and may find, therefore, this approach useful. However, some decisions may be more favourable to one person than another. Primarily, responsibility is to the patient (duty of care). It appears that this principle requires an experienced practitioner who is able to identify clearly the issues within a given situation.

Beneficence

This principle has been placed on a continuum with nonmaleficence. However, beneficence could be viewed as the 'moral foundation' of healthcare and relates to the moral obligation to act in a way to benefit others and in doing so, preventing harm. This principle forms part of the basic ethical code (along with nonmaleficence) for nurses (NMC, 2008). It is considered that nurses are obliged to practice in accordance with the obligations generated by this principle. Being made up of abstract concepts it is often difficult to work out exactly what is expected within this principle. In addition, obligations of beneficence can challenge obligations of respect for autonomy.

Time out 3.3

1   Consider any tension/conflict that may occur within each of these four ethical principles.
2   How can these tensions/conflicts be overcome?

Time out 3.4

Reflect on a 'difficult' situation that you have experienced.

1   Describe the main features arising from the situation.
2   Discuss how the issues were managed.
3   Describe the decision-making processes.
4   Were there any ethical concerns considered before making a decision?

Ethical decision-making

Making ethical choices is seldom straightforward, particularly when related to complex situations, for example, emergency admissions; the severity of patient illness; not having enough information to make a quality decision. Emotions sometimes influence the decision-making process (consider, for example, a patient who is repeatedly admitted following multiple overdoses and so has in the past stated that they no longer wish to live).

Many of the ethical dilemmas experienced by nurses are of an interdisciplinary nature. Nurses have numerous, and at times competing, obligations to various stakeholders with varying beliefs and values, and are often expected to balance commitments to all involved. This concept reinforces nurses' obligations to make all reasonable efforts to foresee possible consequences and take reasonable steps to avoid unjustified harm to others (The PLUS decision-making model, 2008).

Most ethical decisions have to be made in the context of professional, social and economic pressures that can sometimes challenge ethical goals and conceal or confuse the moral issues. Ethical decision-making refers to the process of evaluating and choosing among alternatives in a manner consistent with ethical principles. These ethical principles are considered ground rules of decision-making.

A conflict of values both internal (individual) and external (others) may make nurses unsure of how to act and as a result they may not take any course of action. Noticing the ethical issues and being committed to act ethically is not always enough. In complex situations, reasoning and problem-solving skills are also necessary.

When faced with an ethical issue nurses should approach the situation logically and systematically, in order to enable rational, ethically sound care. Where rationality exists, decision-making could be justified. An ethical decision-making model may help with this process. There are various models available but most follow the same sequencing. Box 3.1 offers one example.

Box 3.1 An example of an ethical decision-making model

Define the problem and describe why the decision is necessary
↓
Identify alternatives
↓
Evaluate the alternatives (positive and negative)
↓
Making the decision (with consultation)
↓
Implementing the decision
↓
Evaluating the decision

(Ethics Resource Centre, 2008)

In addition, nurses can integrate an ethical component of the following:

- *Policies* – the decision should reflect local national professional policies, procedures and guidelines.
- *Legal* – the decision should reflect the law of the land and professional law.
- *Universal* – as far as possible the decision should conform to the principles/values that the organization and individuals, including the patient, have adopted.
- *Self* – it is important to examine one's own beliefs and values in relation to the situation/decision.

(Ethics Resource Centre, 2008)

Withholding/withdrawing treatment: cardiopulmonary resuscitation (CPR)

Confusion exists over the aim of withholding and withdrawing treatment. 'Withholding' refers to never initiating a treatment; 'withdrawing' is concerned with stopping a treatment once it has been started. From a healthcare perspective, it is emotionally more difficult to withdraw than withhold, although both can accelerate death. However, it is legally and professionally acceptable to end treatment (withdraw) for sound moral reasons (BMA, 2007a). This concept is linked to nonmaleficence.

Giving priority to withholding over withdrawing treatment can lead to overtreatment in some cases, i.e. to continue a treatment that is no longer beneficial or desirable to the patient. In addition, 'do not attempt to resuscitate' (DNAR) is sometimes mistaken as 'not to treat'. DNAR means do not resuscitate; but underlying problems should still be treated in an attempt to enhance the quality of life left and reduce the patient's suffering as the patient's disease is still potentially curable, but in the event of a cardiac arrest their body is too frail to survive CPR.

Factors that should be considered when withdrawing treatment include:

- Caring for relatives and patients should take priority over inappropriate preservation of life.
- There must be consensus on the withdrawal of treatment (after considering factors including the ethical/moral/legal factors).
- The patient should be free from pain and suffering (withdrawing some treatment may have a detrimental effect in terms of suffering).
- Effective communication with the patient's family and other healthcare staff is vital.

(BMA, 2007a)

Implications for practice

- Nurses need to be aware of their own beliefs and values and how they influence the care they provide.
- The patient has a right to receive legally and morally accepted standards of care.
- Nurses should attempt to understand/appreciate the perspective of others, particularly if different from their own.
- Ethical guidelines may be useful in providing a framework for morally-guided care.
- Healthcare professionals should be involved in case conferences.

Summary

Within clinical practice, ethical dilemmas can create a complicated, messy approach to care. Ethical considerations need to be acknowledged and discussed by analysing situations through discussions and reflection, and ethical awareness is achieved.

Chapter 4

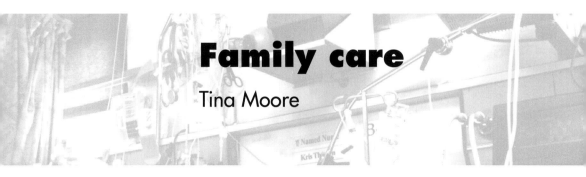

Family care

Tina Moore

Contents

Learning outcomes

After reading this chapter you will be able to:

- identify the needs of family members;
- appreciate the role of the family when caring for the acutely ill;
- critically examine current practices in relation to family care;
- acknowledge conflicts within the caring situation;
- identify the issues surrounding family-witnessed resuscitation.

Introduction

Nurses are constantly reminded to adopt a holistic perspective when performing their role. This holistic viewpoint includes considering the family members within the context of care. The importance of the role played by family members is an established one. The effects of the individual's illness constitute an important part of family life, and are closely related to the health status of its members (Keyes *et al.*, 2002; Jubb and Shanley, 2002). The family can become a significant source of information about the patient.

This chapter explores the role of the family within the context of acute care and conflicts will be identified through an exploration of the literature. Most available research relates to patient's/relatives' experiences within the intensive care environment. However, the findings can be seen to be transferable to experiences within general care areas. Nonetheless, there is a need for research data related to the needs and experiences of relatives of the acute/critically ill patient within the acute care environment.

Family nursing

Family structures in the Western world today are complicated: core family units consisting of wife, husband and children are not as common as before. New family structures have replaced these structures; these include lone parent, unmarried couples living together, children from previous relationships coming together as one unit and single-sex families.

Whatever the effects on the health of family members, acute illness is a catastrophic event that can upset the equilibrium of the family unit. Family members may display a tendency to ignore their own needs. Assessment, intervention and support must be offered to enable the family to cope with the illness of their loved ones.

There are three levels of family nursing identified:

1   individually focused family nursing;
2   interpersonal family nursing;
3   family system level nursing.

(Friedemann, 1989; Whyte, 1997)

Often within acute care environments the patient is frequently the sole focus of the nurse's attention. This may be a result of various reasons:

- The patient's safety is priority.
- Patients require a considerable amount of emotional support.
- Tension exists in promoting holistic approach to care and the nurse's legal duty of care to the patient. This duty is owed to the patient not the family.
- Lack of time prevents a focus on the family.
- Nursing acute/critically ill patients can be physically and emotionally exhausting, and leaves little time or energy for the nurse to meet the needs of the family members.

Original studies by Molter (1979) and Dyer (1997) have identified the needs of visitors (immediate family, relatives or significant others) spending time in critical care environments. These studies have been replicated many times, verifying original findings. Conclusions have identified that if family members' needs are met, they can then provide support and be a positive influence in the care of the patient.

Identifying the needs of the family

Nurses are the main resources to meet the needs of visitors on the wards (Slota *et al.*, 2003). However, family and nurses differ in their perceptions of how important needs are for visiting relatives (Quinn *et al.*, 1996; Kosco and Warren, 2000). The families' perceptions may differ according to their cultural or ethnic background.

Reasons for dissatisfaction among family members are included in Box 4.1.

Box 4.1 Reasons for dissatisfaction among family members

- Uncertainty and unanswered questions (Dreyer and Per Nortvedt, 2007)
- Lack of readily available information (Dreyer and Per Nortvedt, 2007)
- Lack of availability of a comfortable waiting room (Auerbach *et al.*, 2005)
- Lack of moral and psychological support before death (Gries *et al.*, 2008) (Gries *et al.*'s (2008) research needs to be viewed with some caution (acknowledged by the authors) as the sample was biased and results cannot be generalised.)
- Not being involved in the decision-making process
- Healthcare Professionals not being open and honest
- Feelings of frustration
- Powerlessness

(Fulbrook *et al.*, 1999)

Family needs identified include:

- to be given complete and correct information (Auerbach *et al.*, 2005; Browning and Warren, 2006);
- to be close to the patient (Engström and Söderberg, 2007);
- to be active participants in the nursing care (Engström and Söderberg, 2007);
- to feel there is hope (Leske, 1992);
- to be honestly informed (Molter, 1979);
- to be reassured that the patient is receiving the best possible care (Verhaegh *et al.*, 2005);
- to be reassured concerning the patient's future;
- to be relieved of anxiety;
- to be sure of being notified should the patient's condition deteriorate (Malacrida *et al.*, 1998);
- to be treated with empathy and compassion;
- to feel secure.

Family satisfaction is closely related to fulfilment of their needs and expectations (Fox-Wasylyshyn *et al.*, 2005). Family members tend to be more satisfied with aspects of care relating to nursing skill and competence, the respect given to the patient and pain management (Heyland *et al.*, 2002).

Wall *et al.* (2007) discovered that the families of dying patients in the ICUs were more satisfied in their experiences than were the families of ICU survivors. The reason for this could be that there were higher rates of family-centred care. Findings suggest that efforts to improve the support of ICU family members should focus not only on the family of dying patients but also those who survived. The critical care environment is complex: multiple technologies, uncertainty, high patient mortality, interdisciplinary decision-making. Similarities can be deduced within the acute care setting.

Supporting the family

Quinn *et al.* (1996) indicate that the needs of the family are often forgotten or ignored. Nurses must ensure this does not happen. Nurses should rethink the priorities within their role and consider holistic nursing care as a priority (Priestley, 1999). As nursing staff are in a position of providing 24-hour patient care, they are best placed to identify and meet family needs (Browning and Warren, 2006), and should strive towards creating an environment that is supportive to holistic practice and is family sensitive. Within this environment nurses can design and implement strategies to meet the needs of family members, but only when they have consistently assessed those needs, provided appropriate intervention and evaluated its effectiveness accurately.

Responses to family requirements are affected by the nurse's perceptions of importance, time available, environment and ability to meet those requirements (O'Malley *et al.*, 1991). By supporting the family it becomes empowered. If their stress can be reduced, this may actually reduce the stress on nurses (Dyer, 1991).

Family-centred care is a philosophical approach to provide care for patients and the family (Eriksson and Bergbon, 2007). Family-sensitive care indicates that nurses and the family must develop a rapport and respect for each other. This can be accomplished through effective communication channels; giving new information and reinforcing information already given. Family members should not be bombarded with unnecessary jargonistic information. Content should be adequate to enable them to understand what is happening and put them in a position to be able to ask questions.

Timely assessment by nurses and the implementation of appropriate interventions are essential for the functioning of a family system in crisis (Puntillo and McAdam, 2006). Family members could be encouraged to be involved in actual care delivery at a very basic level, e.g. assisting with basic hygiene needs and emptying urine bags. However, not all family members have the ability or motivation to be involved and, therefore, nurses should carefully consider and monitor their ability/desire. Some family members need to feel that they are contributing positively in some way and this involvement should not be denied. The family's interaction with supporting the patient is a way of demonstrating their love and concern and constitutes an aspect of care that only they can provide (Engström and Söderberg, 2007).

Sensitivity and discretion should be exercised, e.g. a mother of an unconscious teenage boy may not wish to be involved in the intimacy of washing her son. She may wish to respect his right to privacy. Equally, the son may not wish his mother to see his naked body. Achieving a balance between over and under involvement in therapeutic relationships may prove to be difficult. Nurses voiced concerns over balancing the care of the critically ill patients, while attempting to meet the increasing needs of family members (Farrell, 1999).

Families like to have a 'presence' within the critical care unit (Engström and Söderberg, 2007). This presence is related to 'being with' the patient, having emotional as well as a physical presence. It involves connectedness and bonding. Generally, humans have the same characteristics, so this will also represent the view of ward patient families. 'Humanistic practitioners' are emotionally involved (Watson, 2007). Nurses should act as effective role models by talking to and appropriately touching the patients, as many family members feel awkward talking to someone who is unconscious.

The family can be viewed as a social unit that has a significant effect on the patient's outcomes (Gavaghan and Carroll, 2002). Family support positively impacts on the recovery rates of critically ill patients (Dowling and Wang, 2005). They help patients to be in touch with reality and give them hope and strength with their struggle against illness (Magarey and McCutcheon, 2005).

However, as identified, supporting the family as well as the patient may prove to be stressful for some nurses. Staff need support through mechanisms such as clinical supervision, case conferences, effective practice education and training. Nurses must be aware of both their important role as a resource for meeting family needs and their responsibility to attend to those needs.

Family-sensitive care includes:

- a need for nurses and relatives to develop rapport and respect each other;
- effective communication channels with reinforcement of information;
- nurses to support family and reinforce information;
- information – talking through what is happening, giving adequate amounts of information;
- family involvement in actual care at a very basic level;
- there is potential for over- and under-involvement in therapeutic relationships;
- the concept of presence (Mills, 1999);
- supporting staff through clinical supervision, case conferences, etc. – effective practice;
- education and training must ensure that nurses are aware of both their important role as a resource for meeting visitors' needs and their responsibility to implement to research;
- nurses can design and implement strategies to assist family members in meeting their needs (Forrester et al., 1990).

It is unreliable to assume that nurses should fulfil every need for the family. Family members may not consider nurses to be the most appropriate person to fulfil specific needs for them (Quinn *et al.*, 1996). However, nurses need to identify significant needs of the family and prioritise those needs.

Patient-centredness discussed in Chapter 2 involves family-centredness as a dimension of health and quality of care (Dodek *et al.*, 2004).

Time out 4.1

1 What are your experiences in relation to a family member participating in care?
2 Consider the effects of this participation on: the patient, family member(s) and nursing staff.
3 What strategies can be adopted to enhance positive family experiences and minimise negative experiences?

Family-witnessed resuscitation

Traditionally family members have been excluded during these interventions. This has been the recipient of a long-standing debate which is both controversial and still ongoing. Please read the following section in conjunction with Chapter 6.

Box 4.2 Arguments for family-witnessed resuscitation

(Within the literature this appears mainly from the relative perspective.)

- Family finds it helpful
- Feeling of helping and supporting the patient. Also a view from the patient perspective (McMahon-Parkes *et al.*, 2008)
- Knowing that everything possible was being done (Myers, 2000)
- Help with the grieving process and the coming to terms with death (Adams *et al.*, 1994)
- Lessens feelings of guilt – more should have been done
- Coming to a closure of shared life (Hanson and Strawser, 1992)
- Reminding healthcare professionals of the patient's personhood
- Maintaining family correctness (Myers, 2000)
- Exclusion may devalue death to a clinical procedure or a failure of treatment than a unique human event that touches the lives of others (Hatchett, 1994)

> ### Box 4.3 Arguments against family-witnessed resuscitation
>
> (Within the literature this appears mainly from the healthcare professional perspective.)
>
> - Inhibits a slightly relaxed atmosphere (coping strategies of the staff), as they are always on guard
> - Fear that relatives would become disruptive and interfere with resuscitation efforts
> - Distressing for relatives (Eichorn, 1996), particularly with invasive procedures, e.g. pericardial drainage, defibrillation
> - Too cramped environment, not enough room for spectators
> - Cannot provide enough support to relatives and patient at the same time, conflict of opinions
> - Apprehensive in case something is said or done to offend relatives
> - Fears of being viewed incompetent (Schilling, 1994)
> - Breaching patient confidentiality
> - Relatives unable to cope (Higgs, 1994)
> - Hinders the grieving process
> - Relatives cannot be prepared
> - Not all patients wanted relatives to witness (McMahon-Parkes *et al.*, 2008)

Conflicts within care

When allowing family members to witness resuscitation attempts, or indeed encouraging family involvement in care, there automatically becomes a conflict between confidentiality and advocacy role of the relatives. It is suggested throughout the NMC Code (2008) that nurses should act in the capacity of an advocate for the patient, promoting and safeguarding the interests of the patient. This assumed advocacy role may come into conflict with the advocacy role of the family member. In this situation, nurses are reminded that they have a legal duty of care to the patient.

It is presumed that patients have a legitimate expectation that the information they give and information about them will be kept a secret. This is one of the fundamental principles of healthcare. Confidentiality has been described as central to preserving the human dignity of the patients. So, there is potential for breaching the patient's right to confidentiality if a family member witnesses the resuscitation.

Lack of written policy on this issue compounds these conflicts.

Supporting the family during witnessed resuscitation

- If family members request to witness resuscitation there should ideally be agreement of all concerned within the resuscitation who are comfortable with the presence of a relative.

- Briefing of relatives of the process and continuing support during the process by a trained person.
- Keeping the relatives fully informed.
- Counselling for the relatives immediately after the event.
- Relatives should be able to enter and leave when they want to and have the right to change their mind.
- Family involvement in the decision-making process.
- Pastoral care if indicated/requested.
- Professionals should react with compassion and understanding (Baskett, 1994).
- Debriefing and support for staff as many found it difficult to become emotionally detached from the relatives.

Implications for practice

- Holistic care involves caring for relatives as well as the patient.
- Nursing process approach to care delivery should extend to the family.
- Nurses should provide a sensitive, compassionate approach to family members.
- Nurses should assess the ability/motivation of family to be involved in the basic provision of care.
- Nurses (particularly junior) need support in caring for relatives.
- Discussions regarding patient-witness resuscitation need to be facilitated at a local level.

Clinical scenario

Monica Sinclair is the wife of Nigel (36 years old) who was admitted (due to lack of beds in HDU) to the acute care ward two days ago following an episode of uncontrolled blinding headaches. He is unconscious. Blood pressure is fluctuating between 100/70 mmHg to 180/110 mmHg. Monica is constantly at her husband's bedside. Occasionally other members of the family visit. She is very anxious and constantly tearful. She indicates that she is unsure of what is happening to her husband.

1   Identify Monica's needs and suggest ways of meeting those needs.

2   Consider any conflict between meeting Monica's needs and those of her husband.

Nigel's condition deteriorates and eventually he dies.

3   Evaluate the situation with Monica and suggest what type of intervention she should now receive.

Bibliography

Further reading

Although written some time ago, Fulbrook *et al.* (1999) give an insider's perspective of being a family member of someone who is critically ill. The insider's perspective is from a nurse working in critical care who then became a family member of a patient in a ICU. Findings are still pertinent today.

Chapter 5

Cultural issues

Mary Tilki

Contents

Learning outcomes

After reading this chapter you will be able to:

- understand the significance of cultural awareness both in relation to patients and colleagues from different cultures;
- demonstrate knowledge and sensitivity when caring for patients from minority ethnic groups;
- provide culturally competent nursing care for the critically ill patient.

Introduction

Acute/critical care areas in many cities are increasingly providing treatment for significant numbers of people from minority ethnic groups. Evidence from Census 2001 (National Statistics Online, 2003) shows that 7.9 per cent of the UK population are from minority ethnic groups. However, the nature of minority ethnic populations has changed, even since the 2001 census and invariably the proportion is much higher in certain areas. There is evidence of poorer health among this group with excesses of heart disease, stroke, and a high incidence of diabetes and mental ill-health (LHO, 2004). Evidence suggests that people from minority ethnic groups have difficulty accessing and are less satisfied with their GP (Kings Fund, 2006). Although referral rates for revascularisation have improved for some minority ethnic groups, rates for Bangladeshi, African and Caribbean people are still disproportionately low (APHO, 2007). Many of these problems result in crises for the individual and ultimately result in the need for acute/critical care.

The chapter is based on the Transcultural Skills Development Model (Papadopoulos *et al.*, 1998; Papadopoulos, 2006). This model proposes that the ability to care competently and safely for people of different cultures depends on practitioners being culturally aware, having knowledge of different cultures and using sensitive interpersonal skills to assess and deliver nursing care. The components of the model are used to demonstrate the meaning of cultural competence for both nurses and patients in acute areas.

Cultural awareness

There is a tendency in the UK to think of issues of race, culture and ethnicity in terms of skin colour. However, everybody is a product of their culture and ethnicity relates to the group with which they identify, or are identified with. There are many White minority ethnic groups all over Britain both as settled communities and newly arrived immigrants. British people too identify with different cultures or regional identities, with Londoners, for example, feeling different to people born in Liverpool or Glasgow.

In addition to those born abroad, increasing numbers born in the UK consider they have dual identity, identifying with the culture of parents born elsewhere as well as being British. This reflects the way in which families raise children in their own cultural heritage, often within distinct ethnic communities in Britain. The most significant growth is among people of mixed heritage who identify with the culture of one or both parents as well as their British birthplace.

Cultural labels such as 'Asian' or 'African' presume a heterogeneity which does not exist and masks the diversity of origin, religion, language or social position in these groups. Equally, it is important to remember that culture and ethnicity are dynamic, changing over time and adapting to different places and situations. They are influenced by the time, experience, birthplace and settlement, as well as differences based on gender, age, socio-economic status and education. Individuals also adhere to different aspects of culture, adopt them to differing degrees and in differing situations.

Cultural awareness can reduce the risk of ethnocentricity which predisposes the individual to view his/her own standards as the norm and to perceive those of others as less important, or in some way inferior. This can neglect issues of importance to the patient or view them as problems instead of differences. Equally, staff working in multicultural teams must recognise that overseas nurses largely espouse beliefs and practices of their homelands which may be different to Western hospital culture.

Time out 5.1

1 What is the current ethnic population profile of the area within which you work?
2 What are the particular health problems that are most commonly experienced by these populations? Speak to the patients/explore nursing medical documentation.

Cultural knowledge

Knowledge of the health profile of particular cultural groups is pertinent to nurses in acute care situations. It is beyond the remit of this chapter to discuss poverty, income and housing but acknowledges their influence in poor health and potential impact on recovery or rehabilitation (Whitehead and Dahlgren, 2006). Although some culture-specific disorders exist, people from minority ethnic groups experience the same illnesses as the rest of the population (often more excessively). The data on some groups are absent but there is evidence of high mortality from coronary heart disease in Asian and Irish people (LHO, 2004). The incidence of hypertension is particularly high among Caribbean, Asian, African and Irish people, contributing to risk levels of stroke exacerbated by high rates of diabetes in Caribbean and Asian communities. There are also high levels of mental illness among minority ethnic groups and the high incidence of attempted suicide in some groups is relevant for acute care.

In keeping with the poor health profile, there is a high use of GP services among people from minority ethnic groups but low levels of satisfaction with care (Kings Fund, 2006). Some members of minority ethnic groups are not aware of the services available to them. However, language barriers, cultural insensitivity and experiences of hostility may be more significant than lack of knowledge (Tilki, 2003). Rates of revascularisation and other surgical procedures are high among Indians and Pakistanis but lower among Bangladeshis (LHO, 2004). Institutional racism which fails to identify and treat illness early contributes to physiological crisis, which in turn creates psychological stress. Critically ill people and their relatives feel vulnerable anyway, but this is exacerbated for people from minority ethnic groups who may feel badly treated but are unable to challenge it through lack of knowledge or limited language ability.

People from many cultures hold health beliefs based on a combination of culturally shaped ideas, medical and lay messages about the causes of ill-health or ways of managing illness (Helman, 2007). However, some groups see ill-health as punishment or suffering to be endured in this life for a reward in the next. Others believe illness is caused by spirits or curses. There may, therefore, be tensions between such cultural beliefs and contemporary healthcare, but it is important that nurses understand and respect them and incorporate, where possible, into care and treatment.

Nurses must be aware of the importance of food in recovery from illness. If food or fluids are restricted this must be carefully explained to the patient and family. Every culture believes certain foods to be therapeutic or avoided in illness. In some cases this relates to ideas of hot and cold, with a 'hot' illness relying on 'cold' food and vice versa (Helman, 2007). What constitutes hot or cold does not necessarily relate to temperature or spiciness, also foods are classified differently in different cultures. The family may wish to provide culturally appropriate food, and unless inappropriate for physiological reasons they should be enabled to do so. In the absence of adequate ethnic diets in hospitals, providing familiar and palatable food is therapeutic for the patient and beneficial for the family.

There may be tensions around the balance between rest and mobility. Most people believe rest aids recovery from illness and by implication more serious illness requires more rest. The complications of bed rest invariably requires early mobilisation, but unless clearly explained, patients may perceive they are not cared for properly. Control of pyrexia may cause anxiety to people from other cultures. The natural tendency of many people is to keep warm when they have a high temperature, but nurses take active measures to cool the body. The need for specific cooling procedures must be carefully explained. Maintaining modesty is highly important and as in the case of all patients, shivering must be prevented.

Ideas about nursing differ from one culture to another. While nurses are generally valued and respected in the UK, nursing is a low-status occupation in many cultures. Patients appreciate kindness and efficiency in a nurse, but will not necessarily expect a high level of knowledge, nor the ability to make clinical decisions or to give information. They may either insist on seeing a doctor or feel disgruntled if unable to communicate with one. The gender of the nurse may be a problem and it is usually unacceptable for male nurses to care for female patients. Male patients may feel more confident when cared for by men and can be embarrassed when female nurses have to carry out intimate procedures. However, assumptions must not be made and the ability to communicate in the same language or to share in a cultural or religious background may be more important than gender differences.

Family and gender roles differ across cultures and may be misunderstood in critical care settings. The presence of a large number of visitors may be frustrating for nurses who do not understand the importance of the family in illness and hospitalisation. In many developing countries, the family provides hospital care and apart from being the only care available, there is an obligation on relatives to be present to encourage and support the patient. In the interests of safe access to all patients it is important to negotiate with the family. Clear access must be balanced against the potential for psychological distress caused by limiting visitors.

Seeking permission, making decisions, gathering or giving information are aspects of acute care which rely on the family if the patient is unable to participate. However, it is the norm in some cultures that decisions are made jointly by the family, or male relatives in particular, rather than by the individual patient. Therefore, patients may be reluctant to make a decision without reference to the wider family. It is important to respect these cultural norms, but to be alert to the fact that in some situations the patient may not be totally happy with decisions made on their behalf.

Nurses in acute care settings must understand variations in beliefs and rituals around death and dying across cultures. Groups differ about telling a patient or certain family members about the likelihood or imminence of death. Expressions of grief can range from stoicism to overt crying and wailing. Apart from differing religious observances after death, cultural practices can range from not wanting to view the body at all, to taking photographs or spending time with the dead relative. It is important to recognise that overseas nurses may find British attitudes and customs around death bizarre and may need to understand the mores of this society as well as rituals of a hospital culture.

Cultural sensitivity

Knowledge of cultural beliefs, customs and related social factors reduce the risk of cultural insensitivity. This aspect of transcultural care relies on good interpersonal skills, recognition of differing cultural norms and a commitment to respecting them. Respect is a complex phenomenon, shown in different ways ranging from correct forms of address to accepting and working with very different beliefs and values. Patients and family members respect a nurse who admits not knowing, but who asks how an individual is addressed, how a name is pronounced or for clarification of cultural conventions.

Respect is demonstrated by adhering where possible to customs about interaction between men and women, and between people of different ages. Eye contact is interpreted as a mark of respect, honesty and listening in the UK. However, in many African, Asian and other societies, respect for elders or people in authority is demonstrated by looking away. Nurses may interpret this as unwillingness to communicate, dishonesty or withdrawal.

Building trust with people who have experienced hostility or persecution is not easy, but is an essential part of nursing. It requires nurses to challenge their own stereotypes and to be sensitive about the questions they ask and in particular how they ask them. It can be enhanced when nurses take the trouble to learn a few words in the patient's language, address them by their correct title and adhere to conventions around eye contact and body language as much as possible.

This chapter only briefly considers issues of language and communication. Although a patient may have used English as a second language for many years, their ability may be impaired during serious illness. Similarly, relatives who communicate reasonably well under normal circumstances often have difficulty under stress. The importance of interpreters cannot be overstated, but it is worth remembering that a person may understand more than their level of spoken English suggests. This can both help and hinder, since they may get the gist of a conversation or simple instructions, but may have little comprehension of important information. Equally, fairly fluent spoken English can mask a low level of understanding. Continuity of care can often reduce stress, encourage non-verbal communication and increase understanding of commonly used words or gestures.

Nurses must be sensitive to the differing ways in which concern, grief and pain are expressed across cultures. Although there are geographical, generation and class differences, people in Northern and Western Europe tend to be stoical and avoid expressing physical or emotional pain openly. In contrast people from Southern and Eastern Europe, Asia and Africa express physical and emotional pain more overtly through crying, rocking and beating their chests. This can evoke anger from staff intolerant of what they see as hysteria and it can earn the disapproval of other patients or families struggling with their own pain in a stoical manner.

Respect is shown when nurses either know or attempt to find out about the patient's beliefs and values, or their adherence to particular religious codes and practices. Although it is important to recognise the differences which characterise a culture or religion, it must not be supposed that all members of a group hold the same ideas or uphold them to the same extent. Nurses must recognise the importance of religious beliefs and practices in time of distress and facilitate opportunities for support from ministers or for personal prayer.

Nurses may feel uncomfortable when a patient or family believe that illness is caused by spells, curses, spirit possession or punishment by a deity. While there may be clear evidence of pathological causation, the beliefs of the individual must not be trivialised or scorned, but accepted and understood. In many cases conventional treatment will be acceptable to a person with supernatural beliefs providing it is not incongruous with religious requirements or cultural expectations. In other cases it may mean supporting the right of the patient to decline certain aspects of treatment or care.

It is important to recognise that while it is common in Britain to be open with the patient about the nature of an illness and the prognosis, there are issues about disclosure in other cultures. Families may not want the patient to be told what the problem or prognosis is for fear of causing depression or loss of hope. In addition, some fear that in articulating the problem it may become a reality (Searight and Gafford, 2005). While these beliefs may be at odds with modern healthcare practice, a culturally congruent approach must be negotiated with the family and patient concerned.

Time out 5.2

1 Reflect on situations where a lack of understanding of the patient's culture has led to insensitive care, inaccurate assessment or misdiagnosis.
2 Consider issues/aspects that contributed to them.
3 How were these differences resolved?

Cultural competence

Culturally competent care relies on accurate assessment and diagnosis. This relies on the avoidance of stereotypes, understanding differences in language, manifestations of illness and being able to work with differing beliefs and values.

Presumptions of alcohol use among Irish people, drug abuse among Caribbean men and disbelief about experiences of persecution among refugees are just some of the stereotypes which cloud the assessment and diagnosis of people from different communities. Nurses commonly assume that people of Mediterranean, Caribbean, African or other origin have a low pain threshold and, therefore, deny or delay analgesia. They misunderstand differences in socialisation whereby people express pain more overtly. Equally, there is a danger that the stoic response of Japanese, Chinese and Northern European people to physical and emotional pain is misunderstood, especially by nurses who are more familiar with overt expressions of distress.

While critical care units use technological devices to monitor blood pressure and pulse oximetry, nurses will occasionally care for patients without such assistance. Nurses are generally unskilled in observing skin colour, detecting shock, anaemia or cyanosis in patients with black skin. Cyanosis in particular is a very late sign, and the lack of skill in observing it may mean that the condition deteriorates significantly before being noticed. It is best observed in the mouth, lips and nail-beds, as they tend to be pale or pink, even in very dark-skinned people, and readily show cyanosis.

Also, it can be difficult to identify bruising, petechiae, purpura and other lesions in black skin. Pressure sore risk tools which rely on the detection of redness are largely invalid for people with black skin. The identification of wound infection or monitoring of wound healing is equally complex. Nurses must rely more on indices such as temperature, suppuration and evidence of granulation, but must take responsibility to develop their skills with help from colleagues who are more skilled, or who have practised in other cultures.

Nurses are accountable for their own performance but also share responsibility for that of their co-workers. It is incumbent on them to challenge racist attitudes, language and practices among colleagues and patients. It is particularly important to address institutional discrimination which denies patients culturally sensitive care. Interpreting services, acceptable diet or facilities for religious observance are not added extras to be provided if funding allows. They are essential aspects of quality care and central to physical and psychological health.

Nurses must recognise the racism experienced by colleagues and confront stereotypical attitudes, unwitting prejudice and racist banter. It is particularly important to acknowledge the culture shock experienced by nurses from overseas and to support them as they become more confident in speaking English. They must challenge patients, relatives or others who racially abuse staff and support colleagues who complain of racial harassment. Rather than stereotyping and focusing on the limitations they might have, it is both caring and cost effective to capture their skills and experiences and the motivations which led them to migrate. They must take every opportunity to learn from peers who belong to other cultures and enable them to understand the cultures of this society.

Implications for practice

- Nurses must be aware of the tendency to see the patient through the perspective of the majority culture, nursing or the organisations within which they work, rather than through the patient's culture.
- There is evidence that the needs of patients from different cultures are not adequately met. This largely reflects a lack of understanding of values, beliefs, customs and practices within different cultures and a failure to learn from colleagues who may originate in those communities.
- Language is an important barrier to effective nursing care, but misunderstandings about different ways of showing respect, gender and family roles, customs relating to eye contact and touch are equally significant.
- Different expressions of emotional and physical pain coupled with stereotypical assumptions about patients from different cultures carry the risk of misdiagnosis, inappropriate assessment and endangering life.

Summary

It is important to remember that culturally competent care means high-quality care for all patients and that many aspects of such care have minimal financial costs. Even those with cost implications may be beneficial in improving diagnosis, increasing effectiveness of treatment, speeding up recovery, reducing complications and hospital stay. In addition, being able to deliver more effective care and enjoy good relationships with patients from different cultures can be a significant source of job satisfaction for nurses.

Clinical scenario

Gulten Ibrahim, a 52-year-old Turkish Cypriot Muslim woman and a recently diagnosed asthmatic, is admitted during the holy month of Ramadan with acute bronchospasm.

1   What particular cultural factors might have led to Gulten's readmission?

2   How can Gulten's cultural and religious needs be taken into account during her acute admission and in preparation for discharge?

Bibliography

Further reading

Papadopoulos *et al.* (1998), Papadopoulos (2006) and Helman (2007) are sources of information relevant to nurses working in various clinical areas. They both address conceptual issues but relate them to the care of clients from a range of different cultures.

Chapter 6

Nursing assessment

Sheila O'Sullivan

Contents

Learning outcomes

After reading this chapter you will be able to:

- understand the reasons for a comprehensive patient assessment;
- understand the need to perform a comprehensive assessment;
- review the different types of early warning systems;
- demonstrate knowledge of advanced life support algorithm.

Fundamental knowledge

Organisation of nursing care; related (to assessment) human physiology; methods of assessment; approaches to communication.

Introduction

There has been a significant change in the role of nurses over the last ten years to incorporate skills that once were not perceived within the remit of the medical profession (Cox and McGrath, 1999). Nurses are now performing more complex assessment to complement technological interventions carried out within ward environments. With this is the requirement to relate normal and abnormal physiology with the observations that are being documented to prioritise patient care. Critical care nurses, as seen in outreach teams, have performed more detailed physical assessment as part of their comprehensive role for patients. More recently education providers in the UK have incorporated physical assessment skills into programmes for post-qualified nurses.

This particular chapter is designed to complement all the chapters within this book as nursing assessment is an integral part of the overall holistic care delivery. Therefore, this chapter will provide a general, comprehensive overview of physical assessment for nurses.

Why do we perform a patient assessment?

Traditionally the role of the doctor was to carry out an assessment to establish a diagnosis, determine the course of treatment or to evaluate the effectiveness of interventions. This role has now been undertaken by many nurses, e.g. nurse prescribing.

Health assessment is the process of gathering, verifying, analysing and communicating data about a patient. The purpose is to:

- establish a data base about the patient's level of wellness;
- establish a baseline of observations to determine changes in the patient over time (Gwinnutt, 2006);
- establish past illnesses;
- determine if the patient has a problem;
- establish what impact the condition is having on the patient's independence;
- and healthcare goals (Weilitz, 2007).

Healthcare professionals are now performing comprehensive assessments that promote holistic care of patients, i.e. a collaborative approach to assessment.

Time out 6.1

Consider the type of questions you would ask patients in order to elicit information relating to the descriptive characteristics of their main symptom/associated problems.

Patient assessment

Always begin by addressing the patient formally such as Mr Smith/Ms Jones. Allow your patient to tell you how they wish to be addressed (DOH, 2007).

History taking

The nurse's goal is to focus on the patient's chief complaint and the events leading up to the current problem (O'Hanlon-Nichols, 1998). The patient's condition will determine the length and depth of interview. If the patient is unable to talk because of difficulty in breathing then nurses will need to gain information from family members, previous records and any other available documentation to confirm the information elected from your patient using closed questions. It can also be useful to provide the patient with a paper and pen.

For each symptom focus on descriptive characteristics including:

- site
- character
- quality
- quantity
- severity
- previous similar symptoms
- timing (onset, frequency, duration)
- precipitating factors or relieving factors
- other associated symptoms.

(Cox and Roper, 2005)

Past medical history

Discuss each problem separately and gain information related to how this has changed the patient's life, e.g. what was exercise tolerance in normal health compared to now. Gather information on previous investigations, procedures, illnesses and hospitalisations. For conditions where there may be a familial link determine which/if any family members have been diagnosed or treated with this condition.

Allergies

When questioning about allergies gain information as to what type of allergy and level of hypersensitivity was experienced, e.g. rash, blistering, nausea or full anaphylaxis. Include triggers or diagnosis, such as hay fever, asthma or eczema. Establish how the allergy affects the patient and what they have done to minimise the symptoms.

Psychosocial history

Ask patients about their home life, activities and key relationships, who are the immediate family and friends, as this information will be required if there is a need to talk to family members about the patient's condition (nurses should give consideration to breaches in confidentiality). Find out about the patient's occupation, has their illness kept them off work. If they have an infectious disease, discuss risk factors or recent travel abroad. Assess their normal level of activity, sleep pattern and appetite.

Current medication

Find out what medication the patient is taking and what the frequency is. Include any 'over-the-counter' medication, like antacids, histamine blockers and analgesics. Discuss if homeopathic remedies are taken, as these can contribute to symptoms.

Many nurses frequently overlook the value of the health history to get to the 'hands-on' aspect of the physical examination (McGrath and Cox, 1998). It is important to realise that to perform an accurate physical assessment nurses need to be aware of the full history of the patient's present complaint and long-standing conditions. Without this knowledge pertinent findings cannot become apparent and vital information may be lost during the assessment process.

Physical assessment

Once the health history is taken proceed to the 'hands-on' part of the assessment. Once a thorough history has been obtained the physical examination should confirm and verify the information obtained in the interview (Kessenich, 2000). It is during this, that the senses of sight, hearing, touch and smell will be used. Incorporate the data obtained from these four senses into a systematic approach for collecting information to complete the picture on the patient's health.

How to prepare a patient for assessment

Introduce yourself to the patient; inform them of the role you will be playing in their care. It is preferable to obtain the health history of current and previous illnesses when the patient is dressed or covered to maintain their dignity and to minimise anxiety. Remember that the patient may be worried and possibly frightened, as they will just have been admitted to hospital. Keep in mind that the patient may consider an assessment an invasion of privacy because you will be observing, touching sensitive, private and perhaps painful body areas.

Examination requires the patient's consent, therefore, give an explanation of what is proposed by briefly explaining what you will be doing, why it is necessary, how long it will take, and why changes to position will be required. Obtain the patient's verbal acceptance before you begin (NMC, 2008).

Begin by using A to F format as your nursing assessment:

Airway
Breathing
Circulation
Disability – central nervous system
Exposure – once the initial assessment is completed and the need for advanced life support is excluded the patient will need to be exposed for a thorough top to toe assessment
Fluid – homeostasis and IV/SC infusions
Family.

Within this process you should include formal examination of each system to prevent you from missing any critical information about the patient's condition.
Your assessment should incorporate a review of the

■   patient's notes
■   charts
■   investigations and results that are available.

(HELP, 2002)

There are four core physical assessment skills:

■   inspection
■   palpation
■   percussion
■   auscultation.

Within the general care area nurses are expected to be competent at inspection and auscultation. Palpation and percussion is viewed as an expanded role. Therefore, nurses should undertake educational programmes (with assessment of competence) before using these skills in practice. Nurses are reminded to be aware of their professional accountability (Chapter 41).

Inspection

All assessments begin with inspection. Inspection starts from the moment you first meet the patient, throughout the health history and physical assessment. Inspection uses visual skills to gather information on a particular system or on the patient as a whole (Rushforth *et al.*, 1998). This incorporates vision, hearing and smell to observe for normal conditions and deviations because of disease. Look for obvious and subtle signs, which will then require further investigation during the assessment.

> **Box 6.1 Observations for each body system**
>
> ■ Colour, e.g. urine with a renal assessment
> ■ Size, e.g. skin redness in patients with sepsis from cellulite
> ■ Location, e.g. of pain in pancreatitis
> ■ Movement, e.g. restricted from breathlessness
> ■ Texture, e.g. surgical emphysema
> ■ Symmetry, e.g. of thorax during breathing (chest trauma)
> ■ Odour, e.g. smell of breath in diabetic keoacidosis
> ■ Sounds, e.g. audible wheezing in patient with severe asthma

Auscultation

Auscultation involves listening for sounds produced by the body, but unless nurses have undergone further training it is restricted to the lungs (see Chapter 15). Some sounds can be heard with the ear alone, e.g. gurgling of patients with airway secretions. However, most are very soft and so need to be channelled through a stethoscope (Jarvis, 2008).

The stethoscope should be placed against the patient's skin and not over clothing as this reduces the validity and accuracy of the sounds (O'Neill, 2003). Auscultation involves pressing the stethoscope firmly against the skin.

When auscultating for breath sounds make comparisons between each lung so listen to right then left apex, middle zones, bases and axillae. Compare each side, comment upon abnormal breath sounds: fine/course crackles, wheeze, bronchial, stridor. If present discuss the location, where is the sound greater.

A few tips for using a stethoscope in clinical practice:

■ provide a quiet environment;
■ ensure the area to be auscultated is exposed;
■ ensure the ear pieces fit snugly into the ears to ensure good passage of sound down the auditory canal (O'Neill, 2003);
■ the tubing should be around 48 centimetres. The shorter length of tubing reduces background noise (3M Healthcare, 2003);
■ warm the stethoscope head in your hand;
■ listen to and try to identify the characteristics of one sound at a time;
■ close your eyes to help focus your attention;
■ stretch the stethoscope tubing to improve sound transmission (McGrath and Cox, 1998).

Palpation

Fingertips are the most sensitive part of the hand and so are used for palpation. Palpation uses touch, consisting of varying degrees of pressure to assess texture, temperature, moisture, organ location and size, swelling, vibration, pulsation, rigidity/spasticity, crepitation, masses and pain (Jarvis, 2008).

To accurately do this you will need short fingernails and warm hands to provide patient comfort. If you are to palpate tender areas ensure you do this last (Epstein *et al.*, 2003).

Percussion

Percussion involves striking one object against another to produce vibrations and sound waves, and requires a skilled touch and trained ear to detect slight sound variations. Therefore, nurses in practice do not perform this skill unless they have undertaken advanced educational training.

To aid your process of assessment the key steps are detailed in Figure 6.1 (produced by two nurses, Fontaine and Munro, within their hospital in 2004).

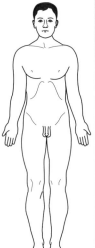

Airway
- **Talk** to patient
- **Look** for chest movement
- **Look** for accessory muscle use
- **Listen** for sounds of breathing/noisy breathing
- **Feel** for expired air
- **Identify** potential risks

NB Noisy breathing is always abnormal

Circulation
- **Look** for distress/agitation
- **Look** for pallor, sweating
- **Feel** radial pulse and volume
- **Count** pulse rate
- **Check** capillary refill time
- **Check** arterial blood pressure
- **Check** core and peripheral temperature
- **Identify** potential risks

Fluid homeostasis
- **Look** at mucous membranes
- **Look** at skin turgor
- **Look** for peripheral oedema
- **Check** input volume
- **Check** urine output
- **Identify** potential risks

Blood glucose regulation
- **Check** capillary blood glucose
- **Identify** potential risks

Breathing
- **Look** for distress
- **Look** for chest expansion
- **Look** at rhythm – regular/irregular
- **Look** at depth
- **Look** for symmetry
- **Look** for accessory muscle use
- **Count** respiratory rate
- **Listen** for noisy breathing
- **Listen** for cough
- **Listen** and look for secretions
- **Identify** potential risks

Disability – level of consciousness
- **Use** AVPU then calculate Glasgow Coma Score (GCS)
- **Identify** potential risks

Disability – motor impairment
- **Use** GCS
- **Identify** potential risks

IV/SC infusions
- **Check** prescription chart
- **Check** fluid to be infused
- **Check** volume infusing correlates with prescription
- **Check** site for phlebitis
- **Assess** pain score
- **Check** urine output
- **Identify** potential risks

Figure 6.1 Nursing assessment *aide-mémoire*

Documentation

It is important to make a note in the patient's documentation each time an observation, care or intervention is given for the following reasons:

1 subtleties of a patient's clinical condition are forgotten quickly;
2 communicating to other healthcare professionals about the patient's condition and responses to interventions – the patient's notes should be up-to-date and contemporaneous;
3 a written record carries the greatest weight with adjudicating parties (Cox and Roper, 2005), e.g. in the event of a complaint.

Begin documentation with

■ general information including age, race, sex, general appearance, communication skills, behaviour, orientation and level of co-operation;
■ follow on with the patient's complaint – using their words;
■ previous medical history;
■ drug history;
■ allergies;
■ family history if relevant;
■ all information obtained using various assessment techniques – complete one body system before proceeding to the next (depending upon your role you would also include investigation results and your overall impressions);
■ plan of care.

Nurses are encouraged to be conversant with local and national protocols on documentation.

Accuracy

Analyse vital signs together because two or more abnormal vital signs provide important clues to your patient's problem. Take observation measurements at regular intervals, as a series of readings provides more valuable information than a single set. If an abnormal value is demonstrated, take that vital sign again to ensure it is accurate. It is important to note that normal readings vary with a patient's age, size and abnormal physiology, which because of chronic conditions is normal for the patient.

Think about interpreting observations and relate them to the patient's condition. Two examples to ensure accuracy in assessments are:

1 Always check capillary refill before using pulse oximetry because if capillary refill is abnormal then pulse oximetry can be inaccurate (poor peripheral perfusion).
2 When using skin turgor to assess for volume depletion remember rapid weight loss and advanced age of patient also lead to decreased turgor.

Prevention of in-hospital cardiac arrest

Rates of survival and complete physiological patient's recovery following an in-hospital cardiac arrest are poor in all age groups, e.g. fewer then 20 per cent of adults having an in-hospital cardiac arrest will survive to go home (Nolan *et al.*, 2005).

Regular monitoring and early, effective treatment of seriously ill patients improves clinical outcomes and prevents some cardiac arrests (Resuscitation Council (UK), 2006). There is now guidance for the emergency admission of acutely ill adults, particularly to the ward care areas in terms of physiological parameters (NCEPOD, 2007). Nurses are encouraged to be conversant with such guidelines. Other guidelines are available to help improve morbidity and mortality and suggest intervention dependent upon assessment, e.g. BTS (2008). The frequency of assessment should correlate to the patient's severity of illness.

When patients deteriorate they display common signs that represent failing respiratory, cardiovascular and neurological systems. This is the basis for monitoring vital sign observations. In recent years the use of early warning scoring systems has been used to aid the identification of at risk patients.

Modified early warning systems to detect deterioration

It has long been recognised that the patients with the highest mortality in critical care units comprise those patients admitted from the hospital wards (Goldhill *et al.*, 1999a), and are more prone to developing a cardiorespiratory arrest due to severe physiological abnormalities. Thus, a pro-active approach to intervention is crucial. But the success is dependent upon the quality (usually) of assessment.

As a result of all these factors the Comprehensive Critical Care (DOH, 2000a) report recommends the use of an early warning tool to identify which patients are critically ill or deteriorating, and to prevent admission or readmission to a critical care unit (ICS, 2002). Hospitals are using various types of early warning systems to help staff to identify which patients are at risk, using physiological parameters monitored during routine ward observations (Ball, 2002). The main advantages of these tools are that the patient's abnormal physiology will be picked up earlier in the development of critical illness, enabling staff to take a pro-active approach to acute care. The key to these early warning systems working is for ward teams to use them on all patients on the ward to ensure the capture of the individuals that may go on to develop critical illness. For some patients this will begin the process of referral to a critical care unit.

For a full discussion on modified early warning systems please read Chapter 38.

Time out 6.2

1 What questions would you ask a patient to elicit information on the descriptive characteristics of their main symptom and the associated problems?

2 Consider how the four physical assessment techniques could assist with the detection of abnormal physiology. Take examples of recent patients you have been involved with.

3 Using the early warning tools available consider the key features that will assist you to identify a deteriorating patient.

In-hospital resuscitation

If the deteriorating patient is either not identified early enough, or if identified, does not respond to the interventions commenced, then they will further deteriorate and can go on to develop a cardiorespiratory arrest.

The guidance on management of cardiac arrests used in hospitals throughout the UK is developed by the Resuscitation Council (UK).

For all in-hospital cardiac arrests, ensure that:

- cardiorespiratory arrest is recognised immediately;
- help is summoned using the standard telephone number, e.g. 2222 – as this is centrally located it is imperative that information regarding the location is given;
- CPR is started immediately using airway adjuncts, e.g. a pocket mask, and if indicated defibrillation is attempted as soon as possible.

Sequence for the collapsed patient in a hospital:

1 Ensure personal safety.
2 Check the patient for a response by gently shaking shoulders and asking loudly, 'Are you all right?' If you do not get a response then call for help and commence using the cardiac arrest algorithm (Resuscitation Council (UK), 2006).

Implications for practice

- Nurses need to have full awareness of the correct method of carrying out a patient assessment.
- All nurses need to continually develop their assessment skills as their role progresses.
- At all times a systematic approach should be adopted when conducting a comprehensive assessment.

Summary

This chapter provides a presentation of the key areas and skills that are required to undertake a patient assessment, including history taking and physical examination of a patient who is acutely ill. Through a comprehensive assessment nurses are able to adopt a pro-active approach in the identification of acute and critical illness.

Chapter 7

Nutrition

Philip Woodrow

Contents

Learning outcomes

After reading this chapter you will be able to:

■ understand the risks of, and effects from, malnutrition during illness;

- assess which types of nutrition are most appropriate for individual patients;
- plan and provide nutritional care for patients, including preventing or minimising complications caused by feeding.

Fundamental knowledge

Anatomy and physiology of the gastrointestinal tract.

Introduction

Nutrition is fundamental to health, providing energy for body function, repair of damaged tissue and healing. Mortality rates reflect malnutrition (Kennedy, 1997). Some patients are malnourished on admission, but many become more, rather than less, malnourished during their hospital stay (McWhirter and Pennington, 1994; Campbell *et al.*, 2002). Malnourishment is especially high among older people – up to half of older people admitted to hospital being undernourished (Cornish and Kennedy, 2000). Up to 40 per cent of hospital patients remain malnourished throughout their stay (Pearce and Duncan, 2002).

Sicker patients may

- be unable to eat;
- be nil by mouth;
- have diets restricted by disease (e.g. renal diets);
- have poor appetites (e.g. from nausea or pain).

so may need nutrition or supplements through an alternative route. Malnourishment frequently remains unidentified until it has progressed (Kinn and Scott, 2001), often to the extent of causing complications.

Nurses seldom see what is given to, or eaten by, their patients. While many patients can report what they have eaten, sicker patients may forget, be confused or have impaired communication.

Nutritional support is often delayed or overlooked (Kinn and Scott, 2001), and prescribed regimes are often not completed (Marshall and West, 2006). Giving only half a prescribed antibiotic regime would be considered unacceptable, yet giving only half of prescribed nutrition appears to be condoned.

Nutrition can be significantly improved through good teamwork and communication between the various professionals involved (Kinn and Scott, 2001); nurses have an important role in identifying patients at risk of malnutrition, assessing nutritional needs and initiating action. Depending on individual patient's needs, that action may be provided through the nursing staff themselves, or through other healthcare professionals, such as dieticians. This chapter focuses on the knowledge nurses in practice need to be able to assess and provide nutritional support, not the more specialised aspects that other healthcare professionals may undertake.

Malnutrition

In a healthy body glycogen stores can compensate for moderate starvation before body protein is metabolised for energy. Once stores are exhausted, the body uses alternative sources of energy, breaking down body fat and protein for energy – catabolism, equivalent to autocannibalism – 1–2 per cent of muscle is broken down each day (Skipworth *et al.*, 2006). This is likely to cause

- skeletal muscle weakness, delaying mobilisation and rehabilitation;
- respiratory muscle weakness, predisposing patients to chest infection;
- immunocompromise, also exposing patients to greater risks from infection;
- reduced metabolism (van den Berghe, 2000), so delaying tissue repair.

Energy

Nutrition should ideally balance energy supply with energy expenditure. Nutritional energy is usually measured in kilocalories (kcal). Energy can also be measured in kilojoules (kJ). 1 kcal = 4.184 kJ.

The two main sources of energy are:

- carbohydrates (including sugars)
- fats.

Diets (oral, enteral or parenteral) usually mix both sources. While nutrition is important to recovery, limiting nutrient load is more likely to improve outcome, especially in sicker patients (NICE, 2006a). Aggressive feeding regimes, advocated a decade ago, are now seldom seen. There are formulae for calculating energy requirements, but patients requiring this level of nutritional support should be referred to dieticians.

Very ill/malnourished people who have not eaten for 5 days are at high risk of 'refeeding syndrome'. Suddenly restoring normal supplies of nutrients to starved people increases insulin release, taking sugar, water and micronutrients (potassium, phosphate) into cells, causing life-threatening fluid, electrolyte and other imbalances (Mehanna *et al.*, 2008). Hypophosphataemia causes hypo-magnesaemia. So patients at risk of this syndrome should have feeds (enteral or parenteral) introduced at half their estimated requirement for 24–48 hours (NICE, 2006a), with electrolyte and micronutrient imbalances restored. Before feeding, vitamin B supplements should be given.

Carbohydrates are starchy foods which are metabolised into sugars. Blood sugar needs insulin to cross cell membranes. Inside cells, mitochondria metabolise sugar into adenosine triphosphate (ATP), the energy used by all cells. Sugar provides much ATP while producing relatively little metabolic waste (carbon dioxide, acids, water). Sugar is, therefore, the best single source of energy in illness.

Intravenous 5% glucose provides 'free water' that crosses cell membranes to provide intracellular hydration. It is not a significant source of energy – 1 litre of 5% glucose contains only 836 kJ; many chocolate bars provide more.

Glycaemic control

Hyperglycaemia induces a systemic inflammatory response, provoking cytokine release and so causing a range of complications (Jeschke *et al.*, 2003). Since van den Berghe *et al.*'s (2001) study in patients following cardiac surgery, studies in other groups of patients have also demonstrated improved survival and outcome from tight glycaemic control (e.g. Essposito *et al.*, 2002; Cely *et al.*, 2004; Langley and Adams, 2007; Scalea *et al.*, 2007).

Fat

Obesity is endemic in Western society, doubling in the UK within two decades (Foxton, 2003). Obesity causes much ill-health, but acute illness is not an appropriate time to begin dieting. Fat is a useful energy source, although fat metabolism produces significantly more waste products (carbon dioxide, metabolic acids, water) than glucose, potentially worsening

- respiratory problems
- acidosis
- oedema.

Nitrogen balance

Protein is a major nutrient, used for muscles and plasma proteins. Nitrogen is a source of amino acids (protein), so nitrogen balance indicates muscle metabolism:

- negative nitrogen balance: loss exceeds supply = catabolism (muscle break-down);
- (neutral) nitrogen balance: existing body tissue is maintained;
- positive nitrogen balance: supply exceeds loss = anabolism (muscle building, although some will also be stored as fat).

Surplus protein cannot be stored. High protein diets have no known benefit, and with renal impairment may be harmful, so excess protein should be avoided (Thomas and Bishop, 2007).

In health, the only significant loss of body nitrogen occurs as urea and other chemicals in urine, so nitrogen balance can be reliably calculated by comparing nitrogen intake in food with nitrogen loss in 24-hour urine collections. Illness may increase nitrogen loss from other sources, such as wound exudate and diarrhoea, so 24-hour urine collections become increasingly unreliable as patients become sicker.

Translocation of gut bacteria

The gut has a rich blood supply to enable absorption. Lack of food causes gut atrophy within hours, impairing gut barrier function and so allowing gut bacteria to translocate into the bloodstream (Guzman and Kruse, 2001; Kudst, 2003). Blood from the gut flows to the liver, where specialised macrophages called *Kupffer cells* destroy pathogens. But ischaemia also compromises liver function (see Chapter 34), exposing the lungs and other organs to infection from gut-derived pathogens.

Enteral nutrition prevents gut atrophy, significantly reduces risks from endogenous infection and reduces the risk of damage to other organs (Zarzaur *et al.*, 2000; Fukatsu *et al.*, 2001), even if nutrition absorbed is insufficient to meet energy demand. So even if nutritional needs are primarily met through parenteral nutrition, small volumes of enteral feeds are often prescribed for gut protection.

Surgery

Traditional practices of prolonged starvation before and after surgery are harmful. Practice has improved, but could improve further. Prolonged pre-operative fasting has largely been eradicated by admitting many patients on the day of elective surgery, but many patients are malnourished on admission. Post-operative mortality is higher among patients with low serum albumin (Palma *et al.*, 2007). When patients are admitted for gut surgery, their gut pathology has often contributed to undernourishment, for example, Crohn's disease.

'Enhanced recovery' protocols promote pre-operative anabolism so that patients can benefit more from post-operative nutrition:

■ solid foods up to 6 hours pre-operatively;
■ 800 ml clear carbohydrate drink before midnight;
■ 400 ml carbohydrate drink 2–3 hours pre-operatively;
■ clear fluids up to 2 hours pre-operatively;
■ commence oral food 4 hours post-operatively.

(Fearon *et al.*, 2005)

Unless advised otherwise, all drugs should be given pre-operatively (RCN, 2005a). Enhanced recovery

■ reduces pre-operative thirst, hunger and anxiety (Fearon *et al.*, 2005);
■ reduces post-operative hyperglycaemia and insulin requirements (Fearon *et al.*, 2005);
■ improves cardiac output and splanchnic perfusion (Revelley *et al.*, 2001).

Early post-operative feeding is both safe and beneficial, even following gut surgery (Skipworth *et al.*, 2006; Hans-Geurts *et al.*, 2007).

Absence of bowel sounds is not a contraindication for feeding. Bowel sounds are largely caused by movement of air or gas. Air is swallowed while eating, so patients who are starved are unlikely to have sufficient air to cause bowel sounds. While patients with paralytic ileus will not have bowel sounds, patients with no bowel sounds may have absence of peristalsis or absence of air. Nurses should, therefore, encourage early nutrition whenever possible.

Oral nutrition

Oral nutrition is the safest, simplest and cheapest form of nutrition, provided the patient is able and willing to eat. However, plated food can bring problems of assessing needs/intake, as plated food is generally distributed and cleared away by support staff (Grieve and Finnie, 2002). Nutritional state should, therefore, be assessed. Strategies that can help improve nutrition include:

- 'red trays' – placing meals of patients at risk on a red tray helps identify priorities for observing and helping with oral intake, and support staff should not clear away red trays until a nurse has seen what has been eaten;
- rotas of voluntary workers for meal-time support;
- protected meal times, giving patients the opportunity to eat food provided (RCN, 2008b).

Oral supplements may be needed. Any patient with additional or complex nutritional needs, or having an 'at risk' score, should be referred to dieticians.

Enteral nutrition

Where oral diets prove impossible or inadequate, tube feeding into the gut is both the safest and cheapest alternative.

At rest, gastric pH is below 4, providing a hostile environment for any invading micro-organisms. Resting feeds allows gastric acidity to return to normal, although optimum rest periods remain unclear. It should be long enough for the stomach to empty. Resting the gut overnight for 6–8 hours seems physiological – patients taking oral diets would not eat overnight. However, if patients have taken little oral diet in the day, overnight nasogastric supplements may allow time for the appetite to develop before the main meals the next day.

Diarrhoea

Diarrhoea is caused when more fluid enters the bowel than can be absorbed during transit time. Excess water entering the gut, or decreased ability to absorb fluid (e.g. increased motility), can result in diarrhoea. Likely causes of diarrhoea include:

- antibiotics
- gut infections – e.g. *C difficile*, *Norovirus*
- excessive gut fluid
- hypoalbuminaemia
- malabsorption.

Passage of faeces through the colon usually takes about 12 hours. This delay is partly caused by the presence of gut commensals (harmless bacteria). However, antibiotics destroy gut bacteria, so increasing the likelihood of diarrhoea.

Diarrhoea occurs in only 3 per cent of enterally fed patients not receiving antibiotics, compared with 41 per cent of enterally fed patients receiving antibiotics (Guenter *et al.*, 1991).

Gut absorption is partly affected by osmotic pressure. Osmotic pressure attracts water. Normally gut osmotic pressure is low, while capillary blood is relatively high. This draws water from the gut into capillary blood. Blood osmotic pressure is created mainly by albumin (the main plasma protein). Low levels of serum albumin, common in acute illness, reduces water absorption from the gut, resulting in more watery stools.

Giving drugs to reduce gut motility (such as codeine phosphate) facilitates absorption of more water, and so reduces diarrhoea. However, diarrhoea removes gut pathogens, so slowing down motility may facilitate translocation of problem pathogens into blood.

Tubes

Fine-bore nasogastric tubes (5–8 French gauge) are recommended (NICE, 2006a), as they cause less oesophageal erosion/ulceration, and are better tolerated (Best, 2007). Tube placement on insertion, and before each feed, should be tested by aspirate, pH being no more than 5.5 (NICE, 2006a). X-ray assessment should not be used routinely to assess placement of gastric tubes, although should be used for post-pyloric (jejunostomy) tubes, and the 'whoosh' test (injecting air into the tube) should never be used (NICE, 2006a). If prolonged tube-feeding is anticipated, a percutaneous gastrostomy (PEG) should be considered.

Total paralytic ileus prevents enteral feeding, but paralysis most often affects the stomach, and least often affects the bowels. As most nutrients are absorbed in the ileum, feeding directly into the small bowel (jejunal tubes) can provide effective nutrition.

Aspirate

Gastric residual volume (aspirate) is the most widely used method to evaluate feed tolerance (Conzalez, 2008). Although fine-bore tubes can be aspirated, it is more difficult, and can damage tubes. So unless patients have wide-bore (Ryle's) tubes, which are not recommended, aspiration should only be performed occasionally, when indicated (e.g. to test tube placement), and not routinely.

Previous practices of tolerating only up to 200 ml are now generally being replaced by the North American guidelines:

- <200 – maintain feed;
- 200–500 – maintain feed, but careful bedside evaluation;
- >500 – withhold feed and reassess patient's tolerance.

(Conzalez, 2008)

Unless excessive, aspirate should be returned, to prevent imbalances from loss of gastric acid, electrolytes and feed (including fluid). If absorption is poor, gut motility can be increased with prokinetic drugs (e.g. metoclopramide, low-dose erythromycin (Booth *et al.*, 2002; Nguyen *et al.*, 2007)).

Blockage

While fine-bore tubes cause less oesophageal irritation than wide-bore ones, they are more likely to block. Risk of blockage can be reduced by

- flushing regularly with water;
- flushing tubes after drug administration;
- giving drugs in syrup/linctus form rather than crushing tablets.

(Thomas and Bishop, 2007)

Parenteral nutrition

Whenever possible, patients should be fed enterally. If the gut cannot be used, parenteral feeding (directly into the bloodstream – sometimes called total parenteral nutrition – TPN) is preferable to starvation. Likely reasons for not using the gut are

- total paralytic ileus (rare);
- following complicated gut surgery it is occasionally necessary to rest the gut to allow healing;
- severe inflammatory bowel/gut conditions.

Disadvantages of parenteral nutrition are

- expense;
- gut atrophy and translocation of gut bacteria from non-use of the gut;
- (usually) hyperglycaemia/hypertriglycidaemia;
- infection risks (from intravenous cannulation and the infusion being feed given for 24 hours).

Parenteral feeds contain concentrated glucose (range 10% to 50%), which may cause thrombophlebitis. Some feeds have to be delivered into central veins, but general practice is that all TPN is given centrally. If a central line is inserted, and only needed for feeding, a peripherally inserted central catheter (PICC) is usually chosen. If a shorter central line (internal jugular, subclavian, femoral) is used, parenteral nutrition should be given through a dedicated lumen – a lumen that has not been used for anything else. Due to the higher infection risk, feeding through a femoral line is not recommended.

Parenteral feeds containing fat, protein and glucose are white; those containing only glucose and protein are clear. Feeds also contain other nutrients, each of which should be individually prescribed for each patient, with prescriptions checked against the bag label before administration. Nutrients may be damaged by exposure to light, so bags should be covered.

Large volumes of intravenous glucose may exceed insulin production, so blood sugar should be monitored regularly (initially hourly). Many patients need insulin infusions with parenteral nutrition.

Assessment

Patients are usually seen first and most often by nursing staff, who are, therefore, best placed to initially assess nutritional needs, and so prevent further muscle wasting. NICE (2006a) defines malnourishment as any of:

- body mass index (BMI) <18.5 kg/m²;
- unintentional weight loss >10% in last 3–6 months;
- BMI <20 kg/m² and unintentional weight loss >5% within last 3–6 months;

recommending nutritional support for any of these, and anyone who

- has eaten little in last 5 days;
- is unlikely to eat little in the next 5 days;
- has poor absorptive capacity;
- has high nutrient loss;
- has increased nutritional needs (e.g. hypercatabolic).

Visual observation may indicate:

- dehydration
- undernourishment
- obesity.

Subcutaneous fat loss (leaving loose skin) often indicates malnutrition. Some muscles, such as biceps, can be felt, indicating muscle wasting. However, muscle and fat wasting may be masked by oedema. Nutritional status should be assessed within 24 hours of admission, to enable early intervention.

Patients and/or relatives should be asked about diet, although problems may be denied. Weight loss may indicate malnutrition, although oedematous patients will gain rather than lose weight. Breathlessness or nausea frequently cause malnourishment in hospitalised patients. Ketonuria indicates catabolism of body tissue. A patient's condition may also suggest dietary problems. For example, breathless patients are often malnourished because eating exacerbates their breathlessness; alcoholics are often malnourished, because while alcohol supplies carbohydrates (energy), it contains few other nutrients. Seeing what patients eat (e.g. from finished plates) and recording their dietary input is a simple, but often neglected, nursing observation.

Many nutritional screening tools have been developed – Fulbrook et al. (2007) found 14 in their pan-European survey, but the British Association for Parenteral and Enteral Nutrition (BAPEN) recommend MUST (Malnutrition Universal Screening Tool – MAG, 2003).

MUST combines scores for body mass index (BMI – kg/m²), weight loss and disease to identify risk of malnutrition:

0 = low risk
1 = medium risk
2 or more = high risk.

Guidance is included for actions with each score. While MUST is relatively simple, most sicker in-hospital patients score 'high risk', necessitating referral to the nutritional support team (dieticians). While this is laudable from patient-safety perspectives, availability of nutritional support teams is often limited (Fulbrook *et al.*, 2007), so any significant delay in the dietician review should be documented, with nurses and other available staff meanwhile optimising nutritional input.

The Subjective Global Assessment (SGA – Detsky *et al.*, 1987) is a simple and easy-to-use assessment tool (Sirodkar and Mohandas, 2005), and can be downloaded from www.hospitalmedicine.org/geriresource/toolbox/subjective_global_assessmen.htm.

Implications for practice

- Many patients admitted to hospital are malnourished.
- Malnourishment often persists and sometimes progresses in hospital.
- Length of stay, morbidity and mortality all increase with malnutrition.
- Nutritional status of all patients should be assessed within 24 hours of admission.
- The MUST screening tool is recommended by NICE (2006a).
- Patients taking oral diets but 'at risk' should be given red trays (or other means to identify they take priority).
- Patients suffering from, at risk of, malnutrition should be referred to dieticians and other appropriate professionals.
- Patients unable to eat an oral diet should be enterally fed whenever possible.
- Before stopping/reducing enteral feeds, consider factors that may reduce gut motility; consider prokinetics.
- Absence of bowel sounds is not a contraindication for enteral/oral diets.
- If the gut is unable to absorb adequate diet, parenteral nutrition should be provided.
- Nursing care includes assessing and monitoring nutrition and potential complications to minimise risks to patients.

Clinical scenario

Robert Jones, 56 years old, is admitted with an acute exacerbation of chronic obstructive pulmonary disease (COPD). He is being treated with oxygen therapy and drugs, including intravenous antibiotics, steroids and 2-hourly nebulisers. He weighs 62 kg and is 1.7 metres tall; his skin appears dry and loose.

1 How would you assess Robert's nutritional needs? List his risk factors for malnutrition. Find the MUST screening tool from your workplace and calculate his MUST score (including body mass index – BMI). From reading this chapter, are there any additional means of assessment could you use?

2 Based on your assessment, what action would you take? Identify the options for nutrition. List the benefits and risks of each.

3 Devise a care plan to minimise risks identified. Include how to monitor Robert's nutrition to meet any changing needs.

Bibliography

Key reading

In recent years, many major reports have focused on nutrition, including RCN (2005a, 2008b) and NICE (2006a). The Joanna Briggs Institute (2008) offers a useful review, while Mehanna *et al.* (2008) review refeeding syndrome.

Further reading

Lochs *et al.* (2006) provide international (ESPEN) guidelines for nutrition in specific gastrointestinal disorders. Holmes (2007) offers a nursing review of malnourishment in hospitals. Thomas and Bishop (2007) is an established key text for dieticians.

Chapter 8

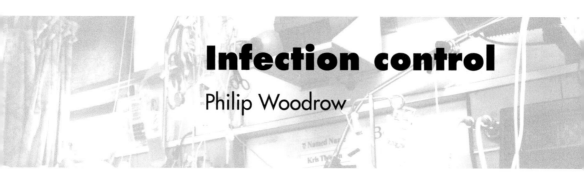

Infection control

Philip Woodrow

Contents

Learning outcomes

After reading this chapter you will be able to:

- understand the significance of infection control;
- understand how the chain of infection can be broken;
- be able to identify high-risk factors for spread of key problem organisms.

Introduction

Media 'scares' have given infection, and infection control, high profiles that, at least as far as public confidence is concerned, has often been counter-productive. Behind media hype, however, there are justified causes for concern. Approximately one in ten people entering UK hospitals acquires infection (Breathnach, 2005), and of those who do, approximately one in ten die from those infections. Hospital-acquired infection rates have remained virtually unchanged for a quarter of a century (Weston, 2008). Remembering Florence Nightingale's premise that 'Hospitals should do the sick no harm', infection is, therefore, a serious concern for all health professionals, and its prevention an important duty. This chapter outlines some ways infection can be reduced, and describes some of the more problematic organisms and related nursing care. Specific treatments are not generally discussed, as these should be guided by local microbiologists, and change rapidly with developments of both new drugs and microbial resistance.

People at risk

Falling standards are frequently blamed for infection, yet health services may be victims of their own success. Immunity declines with age, so countries with ageing populations, like the UK, also have increasingly at-risk populations. Many illnesses further compromise immunity, with sicker people being most at risk. Yet sicker people receive more treatments, many of which are invasive. Each invasive treatment/procedure increases infection risks. Medical advances have enabled people to live to greater ages, further increasing numbers of people at high risk. But increasing microbial resistance to antibiotics ('superbugs') raises the spectre of antibiotic-resistance epidemics (Cars *et al.*, 2008). Preventing all infections is unrealistic, and a blame culture is counter-productive. What can realistically be achieved is reducing infection and mortality rates. Staff who understand implications of infection, especially sepsis, are more likely to reduce risks to their patients. All patients are at risk of hospital-acquired infection, but high-risk factors are summarised in Box 8.1.

Box 8.1 High-risk factors for infection

- Sicker patients
- Immunocompromise (e.g. low white cell count, chemotherapy, steroids)
- Invasive equipment/treatments (especially vascular, and especially central lines)
- Very old/young

Colonisation and infection

Millions of microbes exist on and within human bodies. Some are transient, many are resident. Human bodies are not sterile, and eradicating all body organisms is neither practical nor desirable. As long as bacteria colonise, but do not infect, they are generally harmless (*commensals*), and many are helpful. Infection occurs when organisms cause a pathological response in the host. Typically, most infections are from opportunist pathogens – organisms that are virtually harmless to healthy people, but which infect those made vulnerable by age, disease or treatment.

Infection may be endogenous (when organisms translocate to another part of the body, such as from the gut into the blood, or from colonies on indwelling equipment) or exogenous (from outside the host). The gut normally contains at least 500 species of bacteria (Hall and Horsley, 2007). Approximately one-quarter of hospital-acquired infections occur in lower respiratory tracts, with a further quarter being urinary tract infections (Breathnach, 2005). Harbath *et al.* (2003) suggest that exogenous cross-infection from people and equipment accounts for up to one-third of hospital-acquired infections, making at least 20 per cent of infections preventable.

Micro-organisms

Most hospital infections are bacterial. However, problem viral and fungal infections have increased recently, while development of other organisms, such as the prion which causes Creutzfeld-Jacob Disease, has attracted significant attention.

Bacteria are classified as gram negative or gram positive, according to whether they retain crystal violet-iodine complex stain. Problem gram positives include:

- *Staphylococci* (e.g. MRSA)
- *Clostridium*
- *Enterococci.*

Gram negatives include:

- *Pseudomonas*
- *Acinetobacter*
- *Enterobacter*
- *Escherichia coli*
- *Klebsiellae*
- *Proteus*
- *Serratia*
- *Helicobacter pylori.*

Traditionally, gram positives were viewed as community organisms, while gram negatives were found in hospitals and caused more serious infections. However, gram positive development of widespread antibiotic resistance (Humphreys, 2001), such as MRSA and *Clostridium difficile*, have created notorious epidemics and problems.

MRSA

Probably the most prevalent hospital-acquired infection, and the one the public are most aware of, is methicillin-resistant staphylococcus aureas (MRSA). The UK has the highest rate of MRSA infections in Europe, with mortality rates increasing each year (Crowcroft and Catchpole, 2002).

There are many different strains of *Staphylococcus*, and although not all have developed multiple resistance, many have – Vincent (2000) suggests as many as

81 per cent. Resistance varies, with no antibiotics fully effective against all strains. Highly resistant strains may cause few problems to carriers, but readily infect sicker, immunocompromised patients. The UK has 17 epidemic strains of MRSA (EMRSA), of which EMRSA 15 and 16 are most widespread, difficult to control and cause most MRSA septicaemias (RCN, 2005b; Winter, 2005). Most (70 per cent) cases of MRSA occur in over 65s (Morgan *et al.*, 2000). Cunningham *et al.* (2005) suggest MRSA cross-infection is more likely to occur with overcrowding and rapid turnover.

Up to half of the population are colonised with *Staphylococcus* (Lim and Webb, 2005). People who are not colonised readily become carriers of transient organisms. Although impractical to screen and treat all staff carrying MRSA, identified carriers should be treated to reduce risks to patients. Most hospitals have policies for screening all patients for MRSA. Typically, the nose, throat and groin are swabbed, and samples of urine and sputum (if possible) are sent. Hospitals also have policies for treating MRSA. After patients have washed in antibacterial soap, clean bedding and linen should be provided to prevent recolonisation. Whenever possible, infected patients should be nursed in side rooms (Grundmann, 2006).

Clostridium difficile

Aptly named, this is a difficult organism to treat. Strain 027 is especially virulent, causing many high-profile outbreaks and deaths since 1999 (Kelly and LaMont, 2008). About 3 per cent of adults carry *C. difficile* in their gut, colonisation rates increasing markedly in the over 65s (Pépin *et al.*, 2005; Hall and Horsley, 2007), but infection is usually from ingestion. In-hospital patients treated with broad-spectrum antibiotics are especially at high risk of *C. difficile* infection (Voth and Ballard, 2005; Hall and Horsley, 2007). Pépin *et al.* (2005) found less than one-tenth of patients infected were under 65 years of age, while over half were over 85.

C. difficile is the single main cause of hospital-acquired diarrhoea (Voth and Ballard, 2005), which is often profuse, causing life-threatening dehydration. In the 2002 Quebec epidemic, nearly one-quarter of those infected died within one month (Pépin *et al.*, 2005). Relapses are common (Poxton, 2005). Infection is usually treated with metronidazole or vancomycin. As *C. difficile* is a gut infection, this is usually prescribed orally, although there is no evidence that intravenous administration of metronidazole is less effective. Toilets/commodes should be cleaned with a chlorine-based disinfectant agent after each use (Hall and Horsley, 2007). *C. difficile* is highly resistant, and alcohol handrubs appear to be ineffective, so everyone having contact with infected patients should wash their hands in soap and water (Pratt *et al.*, 2007). With most people (staff and visitors) now used to alcohol handrubs, it is probably wise to remove these from the immediate bed area and display notices to wash hands instead.

Vancomycin-resistant Enterococci (VRE)

Bowels normally carry more *enterococci* than any other gram positive organism (Mascini and Bonten, 2005). *Enterococci*, responsible for one-third of healthcare-associated infection (Gould, 2008), are usually relatively easily treated. But emergent strains resistant to most antibiotics pose a major threat. Although there have been only isolated outbreaks of VRE in the UK, this mutation is endemic in the USA (Ridwan *et al.*, 2002), where it is the third major cause of nosomonial septicaemias (Mascini and Bonten, 2005). It often co-infects with MRSA, to which it can transfer vancomycin resistance (Zirakzadeh and Patel, 2006). Vancomycin is widely used to destroy resistant organisms, so once resistance to this develops, there are few ways to destroy infecting organisms. Soap and water handwashes are ineffective against VRE (Lim and Webb, 2005), and it can survive more than a week in the environment (Zirakzadeh and Patel, 2006). Some recent antibiotics, such as linezolid, have been developed to treat VRE, but with asymptomatic carriage in Europe being fairly common (Mascini and Bonten, 2005), VRE epidemics are probably a crisis waiting to happen.

Pseudomonas

Pseudomonas causes one-tenth of all hospital-acquired infections (Thuong *et al.*, 2003), more than any other gram negative organism. It thrives in temperatures between 5–45°C and many different environments, but is especially found in moist areas, such as baths, washbasins and toilets (Berthelot *et al.*, 2001; Lim and Webb, 2005). One-quarter of hospital staff carry *pseudomonas* (Haddadin *et al.*, 2002).

Acinetobacter

Acinetobacter baumannii (Acb) infections are increasingly being encountered, with up to one-quarter of the population being colonised by it (Allen, 2005). It is also often found in soil, sewage and water (Pitt, 2007). Recent emergence of multi-resistant strains (Munoz-Price and Weinstein, 2008) pose significant risks for healthcare.

Viruses

There are many viruses that can cause infections, although generally viral infections are less serious than bacterial ones.

Norovirus outbreaks frequently occur during winter months. This typically causes vomiting (often projectile) and profuse watery diarrhoea, which can cause life-threatening dehydration. It is highly contagious, so patients infected should be isolated. Incubation is rapid (24–48 hours) (Hairon, 2008), so by the time it is detected, most people (staff and patients) will have been exposed to the virus. Preventing spread to other wards is, therefore, the priority (Hairon, 2008).

Media coverage of Asian Bird Flu (H5N1) outbreaks in the Far East, and isolated bird infections in the UK and elsewhere, generated widespread concern about this virus. To date, H5N1 has not mutated into a human virus; all human infections have been through direct contact with infected birds. The virus has, however, diversified, causing death in more than half its human victims (Pareek and Stephenson, 2007). Human infection in the UK is currently unlikely, although any suspected case should be reported to medical staff and investigated. Incubation often occurs in two to five days (Writing Committee..., 2008).

Fungi

The most widespread fungal infection in hospital remains *Candida* (Soni and Wagstaff, 2005), an opportunistic organism that typically infects the mouth and external female genitalia in susceptible patients. In the USA it causes up to one-tenth of nosocomial septicaemias, usually through cannulae (Almirante *et al.*, 2005). Although still the most prevalent strain, incidence of *Candida albicans* is declining while infections from other azole-resistant *Candida* species is increasing, probably due to increased use of Fluconazole in the 1990s to treat people with HIV (Hajjeh *et al.*, 2004). Although fairly easily treated, infection is too often missed by failing to assess vulnerable patients. Fungal infections typically cause white coating on tongues and rashes in skin folds.

Controlling infection

All staff should try to prevent infection. Infection occurs only if there is:

- a source
- means of transmission *and*
- means of entry.

Removing one link breaks this chain of infection. There are many sources of infection in hospital, the main source often being within patients themselves (endogenous infection). Although known problem sources should be treated, such as with 'deep cleaning', transmission of micro-organisms from one patient to another is a greater problem. Family and friends rarely move between patients, so although they should be encouraged to use alcohol rubs when entering and leaving wards, they present relatively minor risks. Greater risk of transmission occurs with staff and equipment moving between patients. Hand hygiene (see below) and cleaning down equipment, before and after patient contact remains the best way to prevent cross-infection (WHO, 2005). Readers should ensure they are familiar with local policies on hygiene and decontamination. Generally, staff should use alcohol rubs before and after patient contact, and equipment should be cleaned with a moist wipe after patient use.

Even if contact transmission were eradicated, airborne microbes can be transmitted through

■ dust
■ airborne skin scales
■ droplets (such as from coughs).

Close proximity of beds significantly increases risks of airborne infection (Eggimann and Pittet, 2001). Unfortunately, recent financial pressures have encouraged some hospitals to seek misguided short-term financial savings by closing wards and crowding patients into those wards remaining open. Invasive procedures, especially dressing changes, should whenever possible be planned to avoid bed-making, when airborne skin scales are likely to increase. Dirty linen should be carefully folded, and linen skips brought to the bedside. Low staffing levels and high workloads correlate with increased cross-infection (Allen, 2005; Coia *et al.*, 2006), largely because busy staff attempt to cut corners, such as basic hygiene.

Skin generally forms a protective barrier against microbes entering the body. But any break in the skin (wounds, cannulae or other indwelling equipment, such as urinary catheters) provide bacteria with possible means of entry. Intravenous cannulae cause at least one-third of bloodstream infections (Eggimann and Pittet, 1998). Wearing non-sterile gloves when handling any invasive equipment significantly reduces numbers of bacteria that can enter the body (Pratt *et al.*, 2007). Peripheral cannulae should be replaced every 48–72 hours (Pratt *et al.*, 2007) and any unnecessary cannulae removed. Charting insertion dates of cannulae, and other invasive devices, can facilitate prompt changes. Drugs should be given through whichever least-invasive route will be effective, so prescriptions for intravenous drugs should be reviewed at least daily to assess whether oral, or other, administration is feasible.

Hand hygiene

Since Semmelweis' work, starting in 1843 and published in 1861, studies have consistently shown hand hygiene to be the single most important way of reducing cross-infection, yet nearly two centuries later compliance with hand hygiene remains poor. Widespread introduction of alcohol handrubs, which are quicker and more accessible than hand-washing, has improved compliance (Tvedt and Bukholm, 2005). Decontamination is largely caused by drying of the alcohol, so it is important to allow sufficient time for drying to occur before touching patients. Efficacy of rubs vary, so readers should check with local guidelines how much rub to use. Hands should be decontaminated before each patient-care episode (Pratt *et al.*, 2007).

Most hospitals have policies against wearing jewellery and wrist-watches, which can facilitate microbial colonisation (RCN, 2005c).

Uniforms

Uniforms frequently harbour microbes (RCN, 2005c). Wearing plastic aprons during patient-care activities can reduce transfer from resident or transient organisms onto or from clothing (RCN, 2005c), although in the busyness of most wards aprons are not always put on at appropriate times, and some staff move between patients without discarding aprons.

Implications for practice

- Invasive techniques and dressings should, when possible, avoid times of dust disturbance.
- Strict asepsis must be observed when breaking any intravenous circuit or treating any open wound.
- Adequate laundry facilities should be provided for staff to change uniforms daily.
- Hand hygiene should be observed before and after each aspect of care, and before approaching and after leaving each bed area.
- Alcohol handrubs should be available by each bed.
- Peripheral cannulae should be changed every 48–72 hours.
- Invasive devices which are not necessary should be removed as soon as possible.

Summary

Infection remains, and is likely to remain, a problem in search of solutions. Intense public and media concern about hospital-acquired infections, especially 'superbugs', is generally accompanied by at best limited insight into realities of illness and healthcare. The World Health Organisation (WHO, 2005) places hand hygiene as central to its global safety challenges.

Financial pressures of recent years have resulted in some actions that seem to place targets and short-term financial savings above costs in mortality and morbidity. Paradoxically, financial cost of treating infections have probably exceeded initial savings. Eradicating all infections is impractical, but many patients admitted to hospital die unnecessarily from hospital-acquired infections. Minimising infection risks is fundamental to safety for everyone. Local infection control teams are a valuable resource for advice, and should be involved whenever infection, or potential sources of infection, cause concern.

Clinical scenario

Joyce Cantrell is admitted from a residential home, unwell. On examination in A&E she is found to have abdominal cramps, has a dry, coated tongue, and seems to have eaten little since yesterday morning. Vital signs are:

- temperature 38.4°C
- heart rate 108 bpm
- blood pressure 103/54 mmHg.

No respiratory rate is recorded. She suffers from mild dementia, and cannot remember whether she took her lisinopril this morning. Her nearest family live many miles away, and seldom visit her. In A&E she is incontinent of urine, and subsequently catheterised. An IVI of normal saline 250 ml/hour is commenced.

Following admission to an acute medical ward, where you are looking after her, she develops profuse green diarrhoea, and C. *diff.* is suspected.

1   List your main concerns from the above history.

2   How can infection risks to Joyce, or others, be minimised?

3   Following local protocols, devise a plan of care for Joyce.

Bibliography

Key reading

National guidelines have been published by Pratt *et al.* (2007). Readers should be familiar with relevant local policies. The RCN (2005b) provides a thorough nursing review of MRSA.

Further reading

Detailed information about specific organisms can be found in almost any microbiology text. Articles frequently appear in most journals, the *Journal of Hospital Infection* specialises in the topic. Recent nursing reviews include Storr *et al.* (2005), Chalmers and Straub (2006) and Wiseman (2006).

Part 2

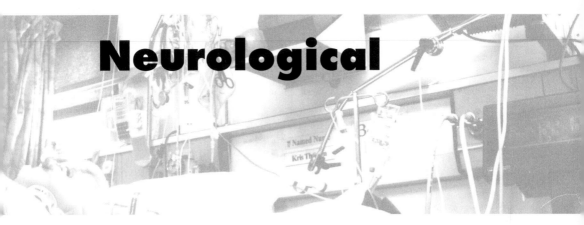

Neurological

Chapter 9

Neurological assessment

Philip Woodrow

Contents

Learning outcomes

After reading this chapter you will be able to:

- understand the importance of detecting neurological changes;
- explain how to undertake neurological assessments in general wards.

Fundamental knowledge

Neurological anatomy and physiology.

Introduction

Patients may be admitted with acute neurological problems, or suffer neurological complications from disease to other parts of the body. While patients with identified neurological problems will usually be transferred to specialist wards/units, nurses working on general wards should be able to assess significant acute neurological changes to enable early intervention. Nurses can assess their patients' neurological function through

- changes in mood or behaviour;
- AVPU assessment;
- Glasgow Coma Scale assessment;
- pupil size and reaction to light.

This chapter does not discuss neurological assessments that may be available in other departments of the hospital (e.g. CT scans) or in specialist hospitals (e.g. intracranial pressure monitoring).

Behaviour

Often, the first detected sign of neurological deterioration may be a change in behaviour. This may be detected by nurses, other staff in the area, or relatives/friends. Nurses should, therefore, not only use their own observations, but note any changes reported by others – this may be as subtle as, 'He seems rather tired today.' A possible, but not the only, reason for a change in behaviour is a neurological pathology. There are many possible changes in behaviour, but common examples are

- tiredness/lethargy;
- aggressiveness;
- confusion or altered cognition;
- motor impairment (e.g. dribbling, dysphagia, dysphasia, weakness);
- hallucinations.

With any change in behviour, the patient's neurological status should be assessed further, although the possibility of the patient just having an 'off day' should be considered.

Clinical information

Basic neurological assessment is included in the Modified Early Warning Score (MEWS – see Chapter 38).

Alert	MEWS score 0
V – responds to verbal stimuli	MEWS score 1
P – responds to painful stimuli	MEWS score 2
Unresponsive	MEWS score 3

Most UK hospitals use MEWS, or an adaptation of it.

'Alert' is normal, so if any patient is not alert, their response to voice should be assessed. This can be as simple as saying 'Hello', or 'Are you alright?' If the person responds in some way (verbally, or looking at the speaker), they are responsive to voice. If there is no response, the speaker should attempt a few more phrases, in case the person has some hearing impairment. If the person has dysphagia, they may respond by looking but be unable to speak. Responding to voice does not exclude neurological problems, so as with any of the other causes for concern identified below, further neurological assessment should be made (e.g. Glasgow Coma Scale *and* medical assessment). Being unresponsive to voice, but responding to pain, indicates a lower level of consciousness, and being unresponsive is generally a very poor sign. Assessing response to pain should only be undertaken if the person is not alert and does not respond to voice. Response to pain is discussed more fully in the section on Glasgow Coma Scale (see below).

AVPU enables quick initial assessment, and corresponds with the Glasgow Coma Scale (Kelly *et al.*, 2004). As observations are usually recorded by healthcare assistants, it is important that they report any abnormal vital signs, such as deterioration in AVPU score. AVPU should be assessed on admission, to enable detection of any subsequent changes.

While AVPU is useful, it does not distinguish between new and pre-existing impairment. As early warning scores are intended to alert staff to acute changes, some hospitals have adapted AVPU to include a trigger for new changes. For example, East Kent Hospitals University Trust has added 'new agitation' (with a score of 1) to its adaptation of MEWS.

Grossly abnormal blood sugar (high or low) almost invariably causes acute confusion, so if blood sugar has not recently been measured, this should be checked with any new confusion.

Nurses may be alerted to neurological changes from abnormal blood results. For example, severe hyponatraemia (typically <120 mmol/litre) often causes cerebral oedema. Results indicating impaired kidney function (see Chapter 30) may also show the presence of neurotoxins.

Glasgow Coma Scale

GCS indicates level of consciousness, using three different assessments:

- eye opening
- best motor response
- best verbal response.

No response in each category scores 1, so the minimum possible score is 3. Each step above no response scores 1 above the step below. So:

- eye opening: spontaneously = 4
- best verbal response: orientated = 5
- best motor response: obeys command = 6

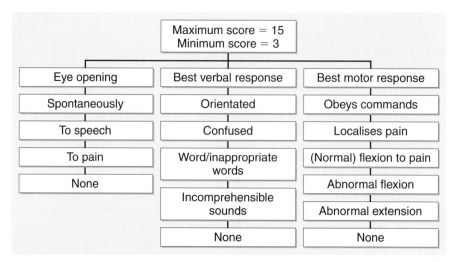

Figure 9.1 **Glasgow Coma Scale**

scores the maximum 15. A score of 14 should not cause concern, but:

- 13 = mild impairment
- 9–12 = moderate impairment
- 3–8 = severe impairment (coma), usually needing intubation to protect the airway.

GCS is a widely used and useful assessment. However, it indicates level of consciousness, not neurological deficit. So if the patient has one-sided weakness, the stronger limb(s) should be assessed.

Impaired motor and verbal responses usually indicate more significant problems than impaired eye responses (Teoh *et al.*, 2000), so as well as obtaining an aggregate score, each assessment should be separately charted – many hospitals include a section for each of the three aspects assessed, with the assessment being noted as a graph, so that trends can be easily followed.

Responses to pain

Assessing response to pain should only be undertaken if the patient shows no higher level of consciousness. For initial AVPU assessment, vigorously shaking the patient's shoulder may be sufficient. A normal response to pain is for the peripheral nervous system to initiate a spinal reflex withdrawal to pain, or guarding. Such responses, therefore, only confirm the peripheral nervous system is intact; they provide no information about the central nervous system. Conversely, if patients have a peripheral nervous system deficit (e.g. hemiparesis from a stroke), stimulating the peripheral nervous system may not elicit a response even though the central nervous system may be intact. So for any more advanced assessment, including Glasgow Coma Scale, pain assessment should seek to directly stimulate the central nervous system.

Russell (2008) identifies three central stimuli:

- trapezium squeeze – pinching and twisting the trapezius muscle, between the head and shoulders;
- supraorbital pressure – running a finger along the bony ridge at the top of the eye;
- sternal rub – grinding the sternum with knuckles; Lower (2003) suggests this should leave imprint of knuckles on patient's skin and an imprint of your nails on your fingers.

Lower (2003) and Waterhouse (2005) identify a fourth central stimulus:

- mandibular pressure (using the index and middle fingers, push upwards and inwards on the angle of the patient's jaw for a maximum of 30 seconds).

For an initial assessment, where decisions about treatment or withdrawal may be based on responses, each of these may be useful. But the sternal rub and mandibular pressure probably are inappropriate for repeated assessments, and all repeated stimuli should be used cautiously. Where tissue damage is suspected, painful stimuli should not be inflicted on that area – for example, supraorbital pressure should not be used if facial bones are unstable or fractured (Russell, 2008).

Frequency

Informal assessment, such as behaviour, should be assessed by all staff whenever they are near patients. But in general wards, there are currently other means of continuous neurological assessment. Charted observations, such as AVPU and GCS, are necessarily intermittent. Frequency of performing these observations must be a clinical decision based on risk assessment: what is the maximum time that can be left between observations that is likely to provide sufficient early warning of significant changes? Where there is no identified neurological concern, AVPU is usually scored with routine observations (e.g. every 4–12 hours). If there is a new concern about neurological deterioration, the time interval will probably be 10–15 minutes, with intervals being relaxed if the condition stabilises or improves. NICE (2003a) have offered guidelines for GCS scores in A&E triage:

- half hourly for 2 hours or until GCS reaches 15;
- then hourly for 4 hours;
- return to half hourly if there is any deterioration;

but even in an A&E department the advisability of these times is questionable. As with other nursing observations, each nurse is individually professionally accountable: observations that are either too frequent or too infrequent may reasonably be questioned.

Pupil reaction

Pupil size and response are controlled through the third cranial nerve (occulomotor), so any abnormality indicates a problem with this nerve, or the brainstem. To assess pupil response, a bright light is needed. For patient safety, as the bulb is held near the eye it should not protrude beyond the rim of the torch (MHRA, 2008). Assessors should check the bulb is sufficiently bright beforehand – infrequent use means torch-lights are often too dim to stimulate a reliable response.

Normally, pupils dilate rapidly in darkness and constrict rapidly in light, with both pupils remaining equal in size. So, pupils should be inspected first:

■   Are the pupils equal in size?
■   Are pupils a reasonable size for the amount of light?
■   What is the pupil size (measured in millimetres)?

Small pupils in a normal level of daylight (or artificial light) are often caused by opioids. If the patient's consciousness seems newly impaired, and opioids have recently been given, the patient probably needs opioid-reversal (naloxone – e.g. Narcan®). Excessively dilated pupils may indicate either nerve or brainstem damage, but can also be caused by eyedrops, especially those containing atropine. Unequal pupils may indicate nerve compression – for example, fluid (oedema, intracranial bleeding) may cause a shift in the brain mid-line, so pressing on one side of the nerve. However, some people have slight inequalities in pupil size (Waterhouse, 2005) – Patil and Dowd (2000) suggest these occur in one-fifth of people. Inequality may also be caused by false eyes or pupil damage.

The next stage assesses pupil response. Any bright overhead lighting should be turned off, and if sunlight is bright, curtains/blinds may need to be closed. The patient's eyes should then be covered, to allow pupils to dilate. This can often be achieved by asking patients to close their eyes, and then open them, but sometimes nurses may need to shade the patient's eyes with their hand. Once pupils have had time to dilate, the light should then be shone from the side to the centre of the open eye:

■   Do the pupils react to light?
■   Is reaction normal (brisk) or slow?
■   Is reaction equal in both pupils?

Pyrexia

Raised body temperature is usually caused by increased metabolism and/or infection, but a far less common possible cause of pyrexia is hypothalamic damage. The hypothalamus, in the brainstem, regulates body temperature, so if this is damaged, thermoregulation fails, typically causing pyrexia. Damage may be permanent (e.g. stroke) or transient (e.g. oedema), and may or may not be treatable.

Implications for practice

- Changed behaviour may indicate neurological deterioration, so all staff should be encouraged to observe and report worrying changes.
- AVPU assessment should be part of regular 'routine' observations, and recorded on admission.
- Where AVPU scores below 'alert', or where there is any concern about changes in behaviour, Glasgow Coma Scale and/or pupil assessment should be made.
- Glasgow Coma Scale indicates level of consciousness; it does not assess the peripheral nervous system (e.g. weakness from stroke).
- Pupil reaction assesses function of cranial nerve III, but can be affected by drugs (e.g. opioids).

Summary

Acute neurological events can occur to anyone in hospital. Fortunately MEWS, and most early warning scores include AVPU assessment. Concerns may also be raised by noticeable changes in behaviour. Whenever a patient is not alert, or there is any cause for concern, further neurological assessments, such as Glasgow Coma Scale and/or pupil size and reaction to light, should be made.

Clinical scenario

Two weeks after surgery for a fractured neck of the femur, Charlotte Norrington becomes acutely confused. Pre-operatively, Charlotte was a fit and active 76-year-old, who lived independently in her own home. On admission her vital signs and blood results were all within normal limits. The surgery has been successful, but post-operatively her recovery was slow, and she was transferred to a rehabilitation ward. The HCA now reports that she seems to be talking nonsense, and that she is dribbling (bilaterally) when eating her food. AVPU is the only trigger that scores on MEWS, but her biochemistry shows progressive hyperkalaemia (now 6.8) and hyponatraemia (now 114) since admission. On examination, the doctor wonders whether she might have had a small stroke, although Charlotte appears to have equal strength on both sides of her body.

1   List the possible factors that could cause, or contribute to, acute neurological deterioration. What significance could hyperkalaemia and hyponatraemia have for her neurological and other aspects of physiological function?

2   What further investigations might you, or the medical team, make to identify possible causes for Charlotte's confusion?

3   From your answers above, list likely interventions that might be beneficial. Discuss your answers with senior colleagues on your ward.

Bibliography

Key reading

As with many other nursing procedures, the Marsden Manual (Dougherty and Lister, 2008) provides authoritative guidance. Articles on neurological assessment, and the Glasgow Coma Scale in particular, occasionally appear in nursing journals; Waterhouse (2005) and Dawes *et al.* (2007) are currently the most recent and reliable from UK nursing journals.

Further reading

Despite being A&E focused, and some questionable recommendations, NICE (2003a) is worth reading. Hickey (2003a) remains an important text on neurological nursing.

Chapter 10

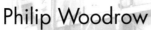

Acute pain management

Philip Woodrow

Contents

Learning outcomes

After reading this chapter you will be able to:

- understand physical and psychological effects of unrelieved pain;
- effectively assess acute pain;
- understand benefits, limitations and problems of widely used analgesics.

Fundamental knowledge

Nerve conduction (including A and C fibres); Gate Control
Theory (Melzack and Wall, 1988).

Introduction

Pain is unpleasant, so preventing pain is desirable for humanitarian reasons: the
purpose of nursing is to minimise distress and suffering (RCN, 2003a). But pain
management is often poor (Carr, 2000; Ng *et al.*, 2000; Schafheutle *et al.*, 2001;
Manias *et al.*, 2002). Pain is not just a psychological phenomenon; it also has
physiological consequences that can delay recovery from illness, and increase
morbidity, mortality and financial costs. Likely physiological effects of pain
include:

- stress
- poor sleep
- shallow breathing (atelectasis; chest infection)
- delayed healing.

Preventing pain, therefore, improves physical and physiological outcomes, enabling earlier discharge.

Pain is frequently a problem for patients in acute hospitals, yet knowledge of
pain, and, therefore, its management, is often limited (Carr, 2000; Twycross,
2002; Coulling, 2005). This chapter outlines the main causes of pain in acute
illness and how to relieve it. Neuropathic pain is briefly discussed. Analgesics and
common side effects are described, but readers wanting further information about
pharmacokinetics should consult pharmacology texts. Pain is individual to each
patient, so needs individual assessment, and individualised treatment (McCaffery
and Pasero, 1999). Acute pain is usually a symptom of a problem. So although
pain relief should be provided, causes for the pain should also be investigated.

Types of pain

Nociceptive pain occurs when signals travel from tissues through afferent pain-
conducting nerves (nociceptors) to the brain. Such pain is generally a warning
sign of tissue damage (Sternbach, 1968; International Association for the Study of
Pain, 1979).

Somatic pain from skin, muscles and joints often causes especially sharp pain,
these tissues being rich in the A delta (A) nerve fibres, sending rapid signals to the
brain. These nerve fibres usually localise the pain clearly, enabling patients to
identify where pain originates. Somatic pain causes sharp responses, such as
crying, screaming or cringing.

Pain from deeper tissues (*visceral pain*) is usually transmitted more slowly, and
less specifically, through C fibres. Visceral pain usually persists longer, often
causing guarding or defensive responses.

Poor localising of pain may cause it to be *referred* to nearby nerve pathways leftover from embryo development. Common, but not inevitable, examples of referred pain are

- liver → thoracic cavity;
- gall bladder → shoulder;
- bladder → back of legs;
- cardiac → left side of jaw/left arm.

Phantom pain has long been recognised, but is sometimes too easily dismissed. More than half of amputees suffer pain 'in' the amputated limb (Watt, 2001). Causes of phantom pain are debated; there may be psychological aspects, but nerve fibres to the amputated limb remain intact above the stump. Unfortunately, phantom limb pain seldom responds to treatment (Richardson, 2008).

A psychological phenomenon

Pain signals travel to the cerebral cortex of the brain, which interprets them in contexts of previous experiences. Pain is the interpretation of these signals, not the signals themselves. So if signals can be interrupted before reaching the cerebral cortex, pain will not exist. Equally, if the cerebral cortex interprets other signals as painful, then pain exists. Melzack and Wall's (1988) Gate Control Theory suggests that low-grade stimulation of A signals in the dorsal horn of the spinal cord can relieve pain by blocking the 'gate' to C fibre signals. It is probable that scratching an itch, or using Transcutaneous Electrical Nerve Stimulation (TENS), both of which cause low-grade tissue damage, relieve pain through this mechanism.

Neuropathic pain

Types of pain discussed above have clear physiological causes (tissue damage) and reasons (protection). Neuropathic pain is caused by damage to central or peripheral nerves, but has little protective/warning function. Neuropathic pain is relatively common, can occur quickly (within hours), may remain undiagnosed, and so inadequately treated. It occurs in up to 3 per cent of patients seen by acute pain service (Hayes *et al.*, 2002), and nearly one-fifth of trauma patients (Crombie *et al.*, 1998). When traditional approaches to acute pain management prove ineffective, pain is likely to be at least partly neuropathic.

Detailed discussion of neuropathic pain is beyond the scope of this chapter, but

- gabapentane
- pregabalin
- amitryptaline
- tramadol

are often effective. Doses often need to be incrementally increased. Ketamine may also be useful (Visser and Schug, 2006).

Assessing pain

Pain assessment is often poor, resulting in post-operative pain often being under-treated (Rakel and Herr, 2004). Because pain is individual to each patient, each patient should be asked about their pain:

■ Do they have pain? If so, where?
■ Ask them to describe it (use open phrases, such as 'What is it like?' 'When does it occur?').

Patients may not report pain because they

■ do not want to appear 'weak';
■ think busy staff have higher priorities;
■ expect to suffer pain;
■ have not been fully informed about ways to relieve pain.

(McCaffery and Pasero, 1999)

Many assessment tools are available, and are reviewed by McLafferty and Farley (2008), but most acute wards use tools based on numerical scales (such as 0–3; see Figure 10.1), where the lowest figure represents no pain, and the highest figure represents the worst pain imaginable. An advantage of the 0–3 scale is that it follows the WHO 'analgesic ladder' (see Figure 10.2).

The 0–3 pain score
0 = None at rest or on movement
1 = None at rest, slight on movement
2 = Intermittent on rest, moderate on movement
3 = Continuous at rest, severe on movement
Movement: ask patient to cough, observe facial expression and/or ask patient to try to touch the opposite side of the bed.

Figure 10.1 **0–3 pain score**

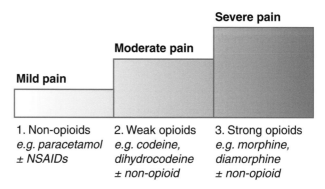

Figure 10.2 **WHO analgesic ladder**

This 'ladder' provides a simple step-by-step guide to increase, or decrease, analgesics.

Alternative assessments for patients who cannot use verbal or visual rating scales include the Behaviour Pain Scale Tool (Young *et al.*, 2006), which uses such visual signs as facial expression and position. Although not ideal assessments, other non-verbal signs may indicate pain:

- sudden hypertension and/or tachycardia;
- position and other body language;
- interaction with, or information from, visitors.

(Hawthorne and Redmond, 1998; Murdoch and Larsen, 2004)

Assessing cognitively impaired adults is reviewed by Murdoch and Larsen (2004).

Analgesics

Drugs are the main, although not the only, means of relieving acute pain. Nurses in acute care should, therefore, have reasonable knowledge about options available, so they can request prescriptions of specific drugs (including drugs to alleviate side effects), and choose the most appropriate analgesic prescribed. Patients should be informed about benefits and side effects of drugs.

Opioids

Opioids act on specific receptors, mainly in the brain and spinal cord, which cause side effects such as

- nausea (the most common)
- constipation
- respiratory depression
- hypotension
- sedation
- urinary retention
- pruritis
- anxiety/restlessness.

(Macintyre and Ready, 1996)

Not all side effects occur in all patients, and mixing analgesics optimises pain relief while minimising problem side effects (Kehlet, 2001). When opioids are prescribed

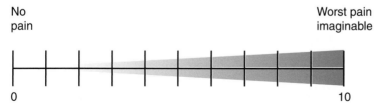

No pain

Worst pain imaginable

0

10

Figure 10.3 **Visual analogue scale**

- reversal agents (e.g. naloxone)
- anti-emetics
- laxatives

should be routinely prescribed 'PRN'.

Naloxone (flumazenil) reverses opioids such as morphine, diamorphine, fentanyl and pethidine. While naloxone reverses serious side effects such as respiratory depression, it also reverses analgesia, so it should be given incrementally, and pain reassessed. Naloxone has a shorter half-life than opioids, so further doses may be needed to prevent the return of serious side effects.

As well as being unpleasant, nausea and vomiting can cause

- stress responses (see Chapter 13)
- dehydration
- electrolyte imbalance.

Although opioids reduce gut motility, opioid-induced nausea is mainly caused by stimulation of the vomiting centre in the brain (Golembiewski and O'Brien, 2002). So anti-emetics which primarily increase gut motility (e.g. metochlopramide) are unlikely to provide relief (Wigfull and Welchew, 2001). Anti-emetics which target the vomiting centre (e.g. ondansteron/zofran, prochlorperazine, cyclizine) are more effective, and may be given in combination with each other (Strunin *et al.*, 1999).

While opioids are potentially addictive, likelihood of developing addiction from short-term use for acute pain is remote. Generally, patients should be given the analgesia they need, without doses being withheld for fear of addiction.

Morphine remains the 'gold standard' opioid. Long-acting preparations (e.g. Zomorph®, OxyContin®) provide good background analgesia, while short-acting ones (e.g. Oramorph®, OxyNorm®) are useful for breakthrough pain.

Diamorphine (*heroin*), chemically engineered morphine that crosses the blood–brain barrier more easily and so is more powerful, is rarely used in acute care in the UK.

Fentanyl is widely used for epidurals, and for transcutaneous patches. Viscusi *et al.* (2007) suggest that fentanyl patches are as effective as intravenous morphine, although can take up to 24 hours to become fully effective. Patches should remain in place for 72 hours. Intravenous fentanyl is largely limited to patients being invasively ventilated, although Hewitt and Jordan (2004) suggest it is safer than most opioids with asthma. Compared with morphine, other benefits include:

- reduced histamine release, so less pruritis (itching);
- less likely to cause hypotension;
- less sedative.

Fentanyl derivatives, including alfentanil, sufentanil and remifentanil, are most commonly used in day case surgery or as continuous infusions in critical care units.

Pethidine is generally less useful than other opioids as it

- is shorter acting (effect 2–3 hours);
- produces a long-lasting neurotoxic metabolite (norpethidine);
- is highly addictive;
- provides no more pain relief than morphine.

(McQuay and Moore, 1998)

However, when other opioids prove problematic or ineffective, it may be worth considering.

Codeine

Oral codeine phosphate (30 mg, 60 mg) is useful for moderate pain. It is also used to treat diarrhoea. Tylex contains 30 mg of codeine; co-dydramol contains 8 mg of codeine.

Non-opioids

Although weaker than opioids, non-opioids have important roles in acute pain management. The WHO (1996) recommends paracetamol for mild pain, and paracetamol combined with other non-steroidal anti-inflammatory drugs (NSAIDs) and/or an opioid for moderate to severe pain.

Paracetamol

Paracetamol has an 'opioid sparing' effect – reducing opioid doses reduces side effects. Although a mild analgesic, regular paracetamol (1 g, 6 hourly) should generally be prescribed whenever opioids are given. Some compound moderate analgesics (e.g. co-codamol and co-proxamol) contain paracetamol, so additional paracetamol should not be given with these.

NSAIDs

Conventional NSAIDs (e.g. ibuprofen) may cause

- bronchoconstriction (wheezing) in up to one-fifth of aspirin-sensitive asthmatics;
- oliguria/renal failure;
- prolonged clotting (bruising/bleeding);
- gastric ulceration/bleeding;

so should only be used for a short time (Macintyre and Ready, 1996). Selective cox 2 NSAIDs (e.g. celecoxib, etoricoxib, lumiracoxib) claim to cause less gastrointestinal irritation, with less platelet aggregation, so causing less disruption to clotting (Sikes *et al.*, 2002; Arboleya *et al.*, 2003); however, their use should still be avoided with renal impairment or hypotension (Fitzgerald and Patrono, 2001).

Patient-controlled analgesia (PCA)

Intravenous, or subcutaneous, analgesics can be administered by patients themselves through a PCA pump. Giving patients control within maximum (dose, preset lock-out) limits, usually achieves better analgesia, and is preferred by patients (Snell *et al.*, 1997). Morphine is the most widely used PCA opioid, although Michelet *et al.* (2007) found that adding small doses of ketamine reduced morphine consumption and so reduced side effects such as respiratory depression. Typical regimes are 1 mg doses with 5 minutes' lock-out.

PCA analgesia does not suit everybody. About 12 per cent of patients find them difficult to use (Mackintosh, 2007). Some patients are frightened to use PCA analgesia; often, encouragement is needed, with reassurance that overdose is almost impossible, as drowsiness from morphine would prevent them activating further doses. Neither staff nor relatives should ever activate delivery.

Patients receiving PCA analgesia should be closely monitored for

- vital signs (respirations, oxygen saturation, pulse, blood pressure)
- level of consciousness
- nausea
- pain
- dose used.

Usually, observations should be made hourly. Many hospitals have specific charts and protocols for PCA analgesia. If possible, it is best not to nurse patients using PCAs in side rooms.

PCA analgesia may be needed for a few days. Infusions should be changed according to local protocols. When discontinued, suitable step-down analgesics should be prescribed – usually medium-strength analgesics, with PRN opioid. Ng *et al.* (2000) found that more than one-fifth of PCAs were discontinued prematurely.

Epidurals

Epidural analgesia usually effectively relieves severe pain (McLeod *et al.*, 2001; Marret *et al.*, 2007), and is often used following abdominal or vascular surgery (Mackintosh, 2007). Epidurals usually mix opioids (morphine or fentanyl) with local anaesthetics (usually bupivacaine). Bupivacaine can be used on its own, usually for bolus doses. Unfortunately, one-quarter of epidural catheters are misplaced (Ballantyne *et al.*, 2003), giving either insufficient block, or necessitating increased doses with increased risk of side effects. Epidurals can be patient-controlled, but usually run continuously, so overdose can occur. Patients receiving epidural analgesia should, therefore, be closely observed by staff familiar with epidural care.

As with PCAs, most hospitals provide courses and protocols for managing epidurals. Observations (usually hourly) should include:

- vital signs (respirations, oxygen saturation, pulse, blood pressure)
- level of consciousness

- nausea
- pain
- dose delivered
- level of block (usually tested by cold spray)
- checking the dressing is intact, not leaking (no wet sheets) and no signs of haematoma.

Epidurals often cause hypotension (Weetman and Allison, 2006), which may need additional intravenous fluids (colloids). Hypotension and possible weakness/numbness make it advisable to use hoists the first time patients transfer from bed post-operatively. Initial mobilisation will usually be by physiotherapists.

Epidural use is usually limited to a maximum of 4 days, as infection risks rise significantly after this time.

Insertion site haematoma is rare, but may cause fatal sepsis or meningitis (Darouiche, 2006). Prophylactic heparin should, therefore, not be given before and after removal of catheters; most hospitals have protocols for when to omit heparin. Catheters usually have distinctly coloured tips (e.g. blue) – when removing the catheter check the tip is intact, and if in any doubt, inform the anaesthetist.

Non-pharmacological approaches

Analgesics, especially opioids, are the mainstay of acute pain management. But some pain may be relieved or reduced by simple comfort measures, such as

- smoothing creases in sheets;
- relieving prolonged pressure;
- turning pillows over;
- placing limbs in a comfortable, well-supported position;
- reducing noise and light;
- touch, explanations, reassurance and empowerment strategies.

With chronic pain, patients may have developed strategies to ease it. TENS, other complementary therapies (e.g. hot/cold pads, aromatherapy, therapeutic massage) and relieving anxieties (reassurance, relaxation, distraction) may help reduce discomfort.

Implications for practice

- Pain is a complex phenomenon involving both physiological transmission of pain signals and cognitive interpretation.
- Pain is individual to each person, so should be assessed individually.
- Promoting comfort and alleviating/minimising pain is fundamental to nursing care.
- Acute pain management often necessitates opioid drugs.
- Regular paracetamol should be prescribed with regular opioids.

- Consider also non-opioid and non-pharmacological ways to relieve pain.
- Evaluate effectiveness of pain relief, and observe for side effects.
- Causes of pain should be investigated.

Summary

Pain is unpleasant, but also complicates and delays healing, so should be relieved for both humanitarian and physiological reasons. Acute pain is frequently experienced by acutely ill patients, yet is often poorly managed. Nurses should assess each patient's pain frequently, and have sufficient working knowledge of commonly used analgesics to select the most appropriate way to alleviate pain and side effects of analgesics. Most acute hospitals employ acute pain specialists, who should be actively involved in management of more complex pain, including (usually) epidural management.

Acute pain often needs opioids, although non-opioid drugs can provide useful synergy with opioids, and non-pharmacological approaches should be considered. Evaluating and documenting effectiveness of pain relief helps optimise its effect and minimise its complications.

Clinical scenario

Michael Newberg, aged 73, had an elective Hartmann's procedure (major bowel surgery) two days ago. Due to insufficient staffing levels, his fentanyl and bupivacaine epidural infusion was discontinued and the catheter removed overnight; he was prescribed regular codeine 60 mg with paracetamol 1 g at 6-hourly intervals with as required intramuscular morphine 10 mg. On the morning ward round he admitted feeling pain, and was given a morphine injection. He also identified shoulder pain, for which he has since been given a heat pad. Now, two hours following the morphine injection, his respiration rate is only ten breaths per minute.

1 How would you assess Michael's pain? Identify the strengths and limitations of your preferred methods of assessment.

2 Evaluate the likely benefits and adverse effects of the various post-operative analgesics provided so far for Michael.

3 Identify changes for managing Michael's pain, together with the reasons for your recommendations and how you would evaluate their effectiveness.

Bibliography

Key reading

Classic texts include McCaffery and Pasero (1999) and McMahon and Koltzenburg (2005).

Further reading

Useful handbooks for pain management include Bennett (2006) and Mann and Carr (2006). Weetman and Allison (2006) review epidurals.

Chapter 11

Psychological disturbances

Tina Moore

Contents

Learning outcomes

After reading this chapter you will be able to:

- identify causative factors of psychological disturbances;
- discuss the normal sensory process;
- analyse present practices and suggest/implement strategies to minimise manifestation of clinical features;
- be involved in effective transfer strategies.

Fundamental knowledge

Physiology of stress (Chapter 13); transferring patients (Chapter 37).

Introduction

The goal of acute/critical care is to support the patient during their illness and conserve life as far as possible. Sometimes, these actions contribute to the patient's discomfort, pain and anxiety (Pattison, 2005). Hospital admission within itself can be a highly stressful experience for both patient and their family. Combined with the effects of acute/critical illness detrimental consequences on physiological and psychological well-being occur. Such psychological disturbances can have a long-term effect and been linked to post-traumatic stress disorder (PTSD) (Cuthbertson *et al.*, 2004; Jones *et al.*, 2005).

Much of the literature pertaining to the psychological needs of patients originate from the intensive care environment. However, the characteristics of acute/critical illness will be the same wherever the patient is located (DOH, 2000a). A great deal can be learnt from the experiences of intensive care nurses.

This chapter identifies the types of psychological disturbances that patients can develop and discusses appropriate preventative measures.

Delirium

A variety of labels are used to describe these psychological disturbances, potentially leading to confusion among staff. Common terminology includes:

- psychosis
- post-traumatic stress disorder
- delirium
- ICU syndrome
- sensoristrain.

Despite these multiple labels, there is congruency between the contributing factors. Psychological symptoms correlate to the diagnosis of delirium as identified by *The Diagnostic and Statistical Manual of Mental Disorders* (DSM: American Psychiatric Association, 2000) and include:

- disturbance of consciousness
- disorientation
- confusion
- hallucinations
- delusions.

Symptoms develop over a short period of time (usually hours). Although the DSM is American in origin, it is widely adopted within the Mental Health setting in the United Kingdom. The description used for delirium is pertinent to the psychological disturbances experienced by the acutely/critically ill patient.

Delirium has been referred to as '*every man's* psychosis' (Clark, 1993), an appropriate expression as everyone is susceptible in developing this disorder; there is no discrimination. Delirium within ICU is indeed a real issue, as estimations indicate that the prevalence of delirium (in ICU) can range from 20 per cent to a staggering 80 per cent (Ely *et al.*, 2004; Thomason *et al.*, 2005) indicating that it is an unrecognised problem. This will have implications when patients are transferred to general wards. These figures could escalate due to increases in the number of older people and more severely ill patients being admitted. There is also the recognition that delirium occurs post-operatively and with long-term hospitalisation (particularly with the older person). There is an urgent need to take action to reduce these figures. Lessons should be learnt from the failures of the past and strategies adopted in order to heighten an awareness of this problem.

Delirium has been defined as an acute, reversible organic mental syndrome with disorders of attention and cognitive function, increased or decreased psychomotor activity and a disordered sleep–wake cycle (Borthwick *et al.*, 2006). It can fall into one of three categories:

- hyperactive (hyperalert)
- hypoactive (hypoalert)
- mixed.

(Meagher, 2001)

Contributing factors

The cause of psychological disturbance is multifactoral, but these can be bracketed under three main headings.

Pathophysiological

Cerebral illness associated with advancing in age, e.g. dementia and Alzheimer's disease, or a history of alcohol or substance abuse (Borthwick *et al.*, 2006) can lead to delirium. Other contributing factors include:

- metabolic and haemodynamic instability (particularly those aggravating an underlying chronic systemic illness)
- hypoxaemia
- acidosis
- electrolyte imbalances
- severe infections
- intracerebral abnormalities.

Pharmacological/medical condition

Overuse of sedation and analgesia (Borthwick *et al.*, 2006) and the sudden withdrawal of narcotics can cause an acute delirious episode. Other drugs that have an influence include:

- corticosteroids
- inotropes

- antibiotics
- antiarrythmic drugs.

Environmental (sensory imbalances)

This is the largest influence. Nurses can and do have a great deal of control over environmental stressors that patients are exposed to. The situation contributes to the patient becoming dependent and so feels helpless. Some patients may also feel isolated, both socially and environmentally. When confronted by an intensive barrage of stressors or stimuli, they are probably less emotionally resilient and less able to adapt to them.

Sensory deprivation and sensory overload indicate that external environmental stimuli are having an adverse effect upon people's ability to make sense of their surroundings. Sensory deprivation is defined as an absolute reduction in variety and intensity of sensory input, with or without a change in pattern. Homeostatic mechanisms create a situation where the individual strives to maintain an internal balance, a variation in stimuli to the cerebral cortex as mediated by the reticular activating system (RAS).

Time out 11.1

1 Find out how the brain processes information received from the five senses.
2 What are the normal processes that occur to enable us to control the stimulation of the environment?
3 How do you think these processes alter for a patient who is exposed to environmental stressors?

The reticular activating system

The RAS acts as a filter that removes most (99 per cent) of the information received via the senses, which prevents the cerebral cortex from being overloaded with irrelevant information and, therefore, helps to maintain sanity.

It has an adaptation level that is stimulated through our five senses. This initiates cortical activity, necessary for normal perception, learning and emotion. When this regulating system is upset, disturbances in sensory input occur, triggering compensatory adjustments. When these adjustments fail, behaviour becomes disorganised.

There are three main causes of upset to RAS balance:

1 reduced sensory input – poorly functioning receptors block adequate stimuli and result in sensory underload;
2 relevance deprivation – a reduction of the patterning or meaningfulness of the stimulation;
3 alteration of the RAS – changes the mechanisms for general arousal and alerting.

Due to additional stressors acutely/critically ill patients' responses to isolation are markedly intensified. This may lead to sleep deprivation. These experiences may not allow the patient to derive meaning from the environment. The intensity of the environment and the supportive devices create feelings of fear. Fear reduces the patient's ability both to hear what is happening around him and make appropriate interpretations of sound. When the deprivation barrier cannot be overcome, the unfulfilled need for sensory input leads to behaviour characterised by regression, disorganisation of sensory co-ordination and difficulty in thinking coherently.

Clinical features

Personal experience suggests that within a few days of acute/critical illness, symptoms associated with delirium can begin to manifest. Delirium is often a frightening experience both for patients and their relatives. Disorientation is probably the most common clinical sign and other symptoms are variable depending on the severity of the illness. Mild delirium includes an inability to concentrate or remember complete thoughts. Patients can appear to be alert and wakeful, but the next moment absent and drowsy.

Patients are usually quiet, sleepy and slow in responding and may have vivid hallucinations with hypoactive delirium. Some may become withdrawn and passive (Borthwick *et al.*, 2006). Some patients may refuse contact with others, often showing no expression in their faces and sometimes looking very frightened and tense (American Psychiatric Association, 2000). This range in symptoms may account for the diversity in figures offered by Ely *et al.* (2004) and Thomason *et al.* (2005). Patients are often misdiagnosed as depressed (Borthwick *et al.*, 2006).

The hyperactive form may be more easily recognised due to agitation and severe aggression. Some patients risk unintentional self-harm, through dislodging critical life support and monitoring equipment, and may even harm others. Other clinical features include:

- fidgeting
- pulling clothes
- disorientation
- complex commands not being followed
- inappropriate verbal responses
- abnormal vital signs (Borthwick *et al.*, 2006)
- patients may shout or call out.

Disorientation and confusion regarding the identity of people such as relatives, and even themselves occur in the more serious form. Hallucinations are a result of the cortex attempting to arrange available stimuli and to find meaning in the environment, thus maintaining arousal. To patients these hallucinations represent their real world, often making it difficult to determine reality from fiction. An alert state is the result of highly co-ordinated interplay between the cortex and the reticular formation. Hallucinations are often visual (some may see writing on walls) and sometimes manifest as paranoid delusions. Bizarre bodily sensations are quite usual (patients attempting to pick off objects from bedclothes/themselves) (American Psychiatric Association, 2000).

Physiological symptoms include:

- Tachycardia – adrenocorticotrophic hormone (ACTH) stimulates the secretion of catecholamines (adrenaline and noradrenaline) enabling the 'flight or fight' response.
- Hypertension – vasodilatation occurs, increasing blood supply to the organs, enabling coping with emergencies.
- Tachypnoea (increased oxygen consumption). The bronchus is dilated allowing an increased intake of oxygen/inspired air, which increases respiratory rate allowing more oxygen supply to the muscles.
- Increased serum glucose, caused by glycogenesis.

If prolonged, haemodynamic and respiratory deterioration will occur. Agitation leading to hypermetabolism at muscular level will contribute to metabolic acidosis, possibly resulting in worsening organ dysfunction. Physiological arousal will then be sufficient to cause exhaustive coping mechanisms which result in a fatal outcome.

Management

Preventative measures are more effective than treatment. All activities should be invested in identifying those patients at risk and having a preventative strategy implemented (removing the underlying causes, and treating the signs and symptoms) before diagnosis.

Although staff caring for the acutely/critically ill patients are aware of psychological issues, acute physical symptoms are often given higher concern and priority than psychological ones because of the life-threatening situation. Uncertainty and unfamiliarity with the patient's initial clinical signs of delirium (Granberg-Axèll et al., 2001) could also account for the low priority. Care of the patient goes beyond physical intervention. In his writings in relation to intensive care, Dyer (1995) suggests that although the presenting illness did play a role, the key factor in the development of the psychological impairment was the environment. Indeed, Dyer (1995) identifies linkages between unwitting exposures to experiences in intensive care that are akin to those employed as a means of torture.

Assessing the patient

Nurses consistently underestimate or fail to notice psychological complications later reported by patients. When faced with a confused, agitated patient, consider possible physiological causes. When these have been eradicated, consideration should be given to the environment or treatment as the possible cause.

Where possible the same nurse should be involved in the care, this will aid consistency and credibility of patient monitoring. The assessment should include the patient's behaviour, emotions and perceptions of the environment. The patient's ability to communicate, hear, see, move and understand should be noted, in addition to any medication that could modify the patient's perception and interpretation of information. There are various assessment tools now available for monitoring agitation and sedation, e.g. the Delirium Detection Score (Otter *et al.*, 2005). However, anecdotal evidence suggests that these tools need to be utilised more effectively in clinical practice and possibly adapted to suit local needs.

Reality orientation

Nurses should understand the importance of reality orientation and the need for structuring sensory input, explaining any treatment or procedure. Reality orientation can also be detrimental to some patients, so this should be treated with caution. The amount and intensity of information should be given on an individual basis and only after constant assessment and evaluation. This process should start as early as possible.

When sensory disturbances are likely, patients need to be warned and reassured that it is common and temporary (if this is the case). Discussing symptoms relating to psychological disturbances should reassure the patients that they are not going mad. Patients have a need to order the stimuli in their own environment into a meaningful pattern. Without explanation of the objects and machines in the patient's environment, s/he is left alone with meaningless machinery, thus heightening anxiety. Prior reassurance to the patient that their experiences are part of their illness process may help to avoid/minimise feelings of disorientation, isolation and fright (Hewitt, 2002).

Orientating the patient to day–night cycles, through the use of digital clocks (patients forget how to read normal clocks) and calendars should help. Patients need to keep in touch with the outside world and the use of radios, televisions and newspapers, and visits from their friends/family should be encouraged. Wherever possible, visual stimulation should be increased by appropriate positioning of the patient or supplying a mirror to enlarge his visual field.

Alterations in sensory experiences could manifest as perceptions of altered body image. This may cause the patients to view their body as less perfect and so withdraw from others. Nurses should provide patients with correct information about themselves in reference to the environment.

There is a possibility that nurses' communication with acutely/critically ill patients may still be task-focused, relatively uninformative, nurse controlled and associated mainly with physical procedures (Ashworth, 1980). However, effective communication is a key strategy in preventing delirium. Explanation of patients' condition and progress is essential. Information provided must be on the level of their (the patient) comprehension. Communication between nurses and patients is likely to be as vital as it is difficult.

Other strategies include: minimising unfamiliar noises; explaining a new noise; creating a familiar environment; having the patient's pictures near them; explaining and removing supportive devices as soon as possible; encouraging family contact.

Therapeutic use of touch

Patients should be allowed time to communicate feelings. If unable to do so verbally, tactile communication should be encouraged. This helps the patient respond in whatever way he can and should make him feel an active participant in the conversation and activities about him. For an unconscious patient unable to open his eyes, verbal communication or touch may be an important part of their limited stimulation. Touch may help reduce the physiological effects of stress. Worrell (1977) found evidence that nurses intentionally minimise tactile contact as a sequence of their own coping mechanisms. There is widespread concern among staff and visitors that touching the critically ill person may paradoxically produce harmful physiological effects on the patient. Some studies have found that touch has a negative/positive effect on physiological response.

Transfer (to different locations of care)

Discharge to the ward has the potential to cause relocation stress. Well-documented major characteristics include apprehension, anxiety, depression, increased confusion and loneliness. Discharge planning processes need to be in place to reduce this to prepare the patient for their transfer to different areas of care. Discharge planning processes need to be in place in an attempt to reduce the stress involved in relocating (Chapter 13). After being transferred to the ward, some patients may still have nightmares from their experiences. Reducing non-essential monitoring and nursing care prior to discharge will help to reduce dependence. The aim is to empower patients to take more control in the decision-making processes and participating more in their own care.

Pharmacological treatment

This intervention should be viewed as a last resort if preventative measures do not work; or if the patient is displaying unsafe behaviour to self and others including insomnia, agitation and delusions.

Once physiological influences have been ruled out, Haloperidol is recommended for hyperactive delirium (Hales and Yudofsky, 2004). Cardiac monitoring is required if used in high doses due to the risk of QT prolongation. If the patient's mental status does not improve then referral to a psychiatrist may be indicated.

Implications for practice

- Acutely/critically ill patients are considered to be at high risk of developing psychological disturbances.
- Nurses should conduct a comprehensive assessment in an attempt to identify those patients at risk.
- Patients should be isolated (side room) only when necessary.
- Patients should be warned of symptoms or the potential symptoms caused by

psychological disturbances, explaining the normal processes that may be affected.

■ Family members should be encouraged to be involved in the patient's care.

Summary

The manifestation of psychological disturbances is a real issue because it has detrimental effects on both psychological (humanitarian) care and physiological responses (e.g. stress response). It is also an experience which may be increasing among patients. In minimising the occurrence of psychological disturbances, nurses should aim to identify those at risk through a comprehensive assessment. They should promote a normal sensory environment for patients and assist them with perceptual or thought disturbances.

Borthwick *et al.* (2006) rightly indicate that nothing has improved since the 1950s, when these problems were identified to date. Too little time is assigned to preventative measures (Dyer, 1995). There is an urgent need for nurses to develop appropriate strategies to minimise/prevent the risk of psychological disturbances occurring. This may help to reduce the morbidity associated with this particular disorder.

Clinical scenario

Kathleen Winsor, a 64-year-old retired school teacher, is admitted to the acute ward after presenting in A&E with severe headaches and photophobia. She is pyrexial, B/P 160/110, heart rate 98 irregular.

A provisional diagnosis of meningococcal meningitis has been made. Kathleen is nursed in isolation and requires hourly monitoring.

1 Describe your assessment of Kathleen in relation to her psychological needs.

2 What criteria would you use to determine whether Kathleen is at risk of developing symptoms in relation to psychological disturbances?

3 Discuss the strategies that need to be adopted in order to minimise the risk of developing psychological disturbance for Kathleen.

Bibliography

Further reading

Dyer (1995), although written some time ago, makes interesting reading and is still applicable today.

Chapter 12

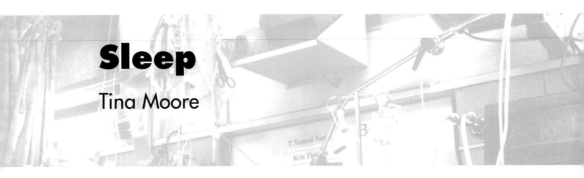

Sleep

Tina Moore

Contents

Learning outcomes

After reading this chapter you will be able to:

- identify the stages of sleep;
- identify the factors affecting sleep;
- understand the affects of sleep deprivation on acutely/ critically ill patients;
- suggest strategies required to prevent/reduce the effects of sleep deprivation.

Fundamental knowledge

Circadian rhythms, stress response (Chapter 13).

Introduction

Sleep deprivation continues to be a major problem for patients in hospital. This problem has been compounded by a historical lack of interest in the topic both in terms of literature and nursing intervention. Often, sleep is an overlooked and neglected aspect of the plan of care (Honkus, 2003). The facilitation of sleep is one of the main duties of the nurse at night-time.

Sleep deprivation may be viewed as an inevitable part of acute/critical illness. Despite this, nurses have an influence over the patient's environment and hold a responsibility to promote as much sleep as possible. Adequate sleep is essential for these patients as the effects of sleep deprivation can have detrimental consequences on their already compromised well-being.

This chapter will discuss the normal physiology of sleep, pathophysiology of sleep deprivation and strategies to promote sleep. Little new material appears to be available and, therefore, older research remains relevant and so used in this chapter.

Purpose of sleep

Sleep has been defined as a state of unconsciousness from which individuals can be aroused by sensory or other stimuli (Horne, 1998) and is considered a basic need for survival. This is a natural and beneficial state, essential for the physiological and psychological well-being of humans. There remains little conclusive evidence available relating to the purpose of sleep. Most literature discusses the relationships between the quantity/quality of sleep and the effects of sleep deprivation on the individual. It is believed that sleep has restorative function and provides protection from fatigue in addition to compensating for energy deficit acquired during daily activities.

The amount of sleep required is variable. On average adults who are allowed to sleep without restriction sleep about 8 hours per night (Merritt, 2000). The ageing process is associated with changes in normal sleep patterns, increased nocturnal awakenings, sleep deficiency and early-morning awakening. In addition to this the number of naps and the length of naptime may be increased for those over 75 years of age, increasing total sleep time.

Sleep cycle

Sleep is a complex, active process (Honkus, 2003) that involves both the reticular activating system (RAS) (Chapter 11) and circadian rhythm. The RAS is associated with the level of arousal and wakefulness, and thus, a contributing factor with the sleep/wake cycle. Circadian rhythm of sleep and wakefulness represents a relationship between activity and inactivity (Mahowald and Schenck, 2005).

The mean time for one normal sleep cycle is 70–120 minutes (Morton and Fontaine, 2009) but can be variable, with an average of six cycles in 24 hours. The hypothalamus is responsible for the timing of these cycles.

Some patients have problems sleeping before entering hospital, and coupled with acute illness and interventions compound the lack of sleep. Critically ill patients spend more time in the lighter sleep stages, therefore, noise from monitors and normal hospital night-time activities can easily disrupt their sleep. Noise in general (from staff forgetting that it is the patients' night-time) and noisy patients, although challenging, should be kept to a minimum. Often, acutely/critically ill patients require hourly invasive and non-invasive monitoring. Non-invasive monitoring can still disturb the patient (e.g. automated blood pressure monitors).

Normal sleep is divided into five stages. The first four stages relate to non-rapid eye movement (NREM), also known as slow wave sleep (SWS) and the fifth stage is rapid eye movement (REM). NREM sleep is believed to be restorative sleep for the body, while REM sleep is believed to be restorative sleep for the brain's mental processes (Shapiro, 1993). Sleep is, therefore, a time of energy conservation and renewal.

NREM

- Stage 1 (sleep latency) equates to a transitional state of the lightest level of sleep, lasting no more than 7 minutes (Carskadon, 2004). Characteristics include aimless thoughts, drifting sensation, frequent myoclonic (brief rhythmic jerks) of the face, hands and feet. Individuals can easily be awakened.
- Stage 2 (light sleep) lasts 5–15 minutes. Individuals are more relaxed but can still easily be awakened.
- Stages 3 and 4 (deep, slow wave sleep) are the deepest levels of sleep and random stimuli does not arouse the individual. Sleep time is variable in these stages (15–30 minutes).

In the average young adult NREM constitutes 50 to 60 per cent of the total sleep time for stages 1 and 2 (Urden *et al.*, 2006), implying that younger patients can tolerate sleep disturbances better than the older person.

REM

- Stage 5 is sometimes referred to as paradoxical sleep and usually counts for 20–25 per cent of the total night's sleep (Guyton and Hall, 2005). Here, some parts of the brain are active, while other parts are suppressed. During REM the individual is more difficult to awaken than in any of the other stages. Sleep is longer and more intense; as a result sleep deprivation is probably more significant when it occurs during this stage.

Within the sleep cycle there is normal progression through repetitive cycles starting with NREM stages 1, 2, 3 and 4, followed by stages 3 and 2 and then the REM stage (see Figure 12.1).

Sleep changes accompany normal ageing and include increased fragmentation of night-time sleep due to periods of wakefulness and less time spent in the deeper stages of sleep.

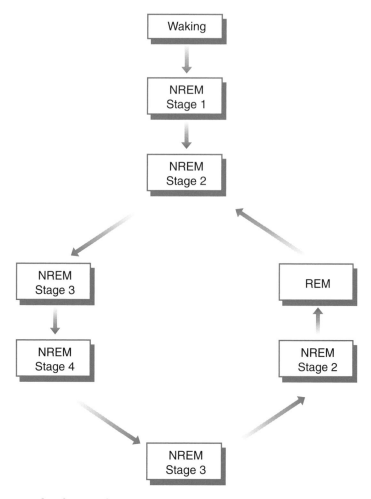

Figure 12.1 **The sleep cycle**

Physiology of sleep

There is a deficit of research evidence in this area.

Time out 12.1

1 Reflect upon your experiences during night duty; consider the factors that can cause sleep disturbance with acutely ill patients.
2 Have you personally suffered from sleep deprivation? What were the causes? How did you feel?

Table 12.1 The physiology of sleep

Stage of sleep	Physiological affects
NREM – parasympathetic nervous system predominates	• Protein synthesis and tissue repair (e.g. the repair of epithelial and specialised cells of the brain, skin, bone marrow and gastric mucosa) (Guyton and Hall, 2005). • In addition growth hormones are secreted by the anterior pituitary gland and functions to promote protein synthesis while sparing catabolic breakdown. • During sleep the brain's cortical activity is depressed, causing reduced brain stem activity and lowering of the metabolic rate (reduces respiratory rate, heart rate and blood pressure), which can sometimes be erratic (Guyton and Hall, 2005). • Core body temperature is reduced. • Muscle tone and reflex activities are depressed and deep tendon responses are practically absent (Fox, 1999).
REM – sympathetic nervous system predominates	• Sudden dilation of the pupils (Guyton and Hall, 2005); caution should be adopted when monitoring pupil reaction. Premature ventricular contractions and tachydysrhythmias associated with respiratory pauses may occur during REM (Urden et al., 2006).
In preparation for the physical activity, the release of catecholamine peaks around 6 a.m. (Todd, 1997) and may be responsible for episodes of ischaemia and early-morning cardiac death and strokes.	• Secretory rates of adrenocorticotropic hormone and cortisol are higher in the early hours of the morning (between 4 a.m.– 6 a.m.) thus putting the body in a 'stressed like' state. So avoid early-morning stimulation.

Sleep deprivation

A sleep disorder exists when the inability to sleep well produces impaired daytime functioning or excessive sleepiness (Fox, 1999). An integrated review on sleep in acute care settings by Redeker (2000) concluded that few studies have shown the outcome of sleep disturbance in those environments.

As discussed, sleep is of great biological and psychological importance. Factors affecting sleep are many. Discussed below are a few significant reasons for sleep pattern disturbances in hospital. However, conflicting evidence exists which highlights the complexity and subjectivity of sleep and possible environmental influences:

■ Environmental disturbances, such as noise (staff, machinery, other patients); lighting; store room positioning.
■ The design of ward areas (lack of privacy). An obvious conclusion of higher noise levels were recorded in areas with more patients (Southwell and Winstow, 1995; Meyer *et al.*, 1994).
■ The delivery of patient care often requires frequent disruption to the patient throughout the day and night (Honkus, 2003).
■ Subjective factors such as limited amount of personal space; limited privacy; restricted capacities (e.g. caused by intravenous tubes); pain; discomfort; anxiety and worry are significant contributory factors.
■ Age (Southwell and Winstow, 1995). However, no age difference was found by Simpson *et al.* (1996).
■ Psychological stress (Honkus, 2003), although this could be a cyclical problem. This would be dependent upon the variety, magnitude and frequency of stressors.
■ Medications – beta blockers may cause nightmares.

The relationship between hospitalisation and sleep disturbance is well documented (Redeker and Whykpis, 1999; Southwell and Winstow, 1995; Redeker, 2000). Patients who are acutely/critically ill may spend 40 to 50 per cent of their sleep time awake and of the remaining sleep time only 3 to 4 per cent in REM sleep (Lee, 1997).

The combination of the physiological problems and the experiences that patients have during their period of acute/critical illness (environment, treatment, illness itself) contribute to the patient feeling fatigued or tired. Symptoms vary between individuals but influencing factors include: age, premorbid personality, motivation and the environment. A night's disturbance of sleep can compromise the patient's immune system (Dinges *et al.*, 1994), thus making them more susceptible to hospital-acquired infections.

Approximately 70 per cent of growth hormone secretion takes place during deep sleep and decreased thyroid-stimulating hormone and adrenocorticotropic hormone also occurs (Kubitz, 1999), thus having an affect on wound healing.

Sleep also has a psychological restorative function. Decreased REM sleep leads to impaired memory for cognitive functioning (Stevens, 2008) and lack of sleep leads to memory lapses and difficulty in remembering what they have experienced.

NREM sleep deprivation symptoms include fatigue, anxiety and increased severity of illness. REM deprivation is more detrimental, often occurring within 72 hours of REM deprivation (Urden *et al.*, 2006). Symptoms include irritability, apathy, decreased alertness and increased confusion. Continued loss may lead to perceptual distortion and significant disturbance in mental/emotional function, ranging from disorientation and restlessness to auditory and visual hallucinations with personality changes (including paranoia).

Promoting sleep

Human beings possess a 24-hour biological clock that is resistant to change and long-term disruption can be fatal. The provision of adequate sleep is an important but often overlooked component of care. The goal is to foster as much uninterrupted sleep as is possible, while continuing with the safe monitoring and intervention of care.

Each patient has a 'right' to undisturbed sleep. However, this 'right' is often impossible for the acutely/critically ill patient due to the fact that all patients have a fundamental 'right' to be looked after safely. Those patients who require nursing intervention at night should be nursed efficiently and quietly, with the minimum of disturbance to themselves and other patients.

Nurses should treat disturbance to the patient's sleep seriously and take appropriate action to prevent it. Continual assessment of the patient's normal sleep pattern should be undertaken, together with the patient's current sleep pattern. However, in reality this may be seen as an impractical task as many wards only have one qualified nurse on duty. Nonetheless, healthcare assistants could be trained and involved in this assessment. This should be undertaken by communication, documentation, discussion and individual care-planning to determine whether the patient's individual's needs are being met. Potential threats to disturbed sleep should be identified, involving consideration of all environmental factors and subjective perceptions of the patient involving sleep.

Wherever possible a minimum of at least four hours of uninterrupted sleep each 24 hours should be achieved in order to maintain minimal performance. Frequent naps (20 or 90 minutes in length) should be encouraged. Accurate knowledge of the sleep cycle and the functions of sleep will assist nurses in monitoring patients safely, while ensuring that they achieve optimal quality of sleep. At night only essential monitoring should be carried out. There should be a policy in place providing advice and guidance on how nurses can arrange care at night to ensure that optimum sleep is enhanced (Honkus, 2003). For the safety of the patient, however, machine alarms should *not* be turned off.

Clustering patient care activities is vital in order to maintain normal sleep cycles. This requires careful planning and sometimes means that the nurse must act as an advocate to the patient in relation to other members of the team.

During REM sleep the patient's vital signs may change, resulting in concern that the patient's condition is worsening. Consequently, nurses may increase the frequency of monitoring the patient, adjust intravenous fluids and measure vital signs in response. Hence, patients may not get the sleep they require. Nurses must be aware of these factors and observational data must be analysed with this in mind, as unsubstantiated actions may have detrimental effects.

At night low lighting should be used (but bright enough to enable close monitoring of patient, particularly of skin colour). Artificial light can replicate differences between day and night (with higher levels during day and lower levels at night); this may help patients determine day and night differences and thus aid maintenance of circadian rhythm. Therapeutic use of light has been demonstrated as an effective treatment for circadian sleep disorders and depression (Terman *et al.*, 1995).

A study by Southwell and Wistow (1995) highlighted the differences in nurses' and patients' perceptions, with nurses reporting less frequently on noise. Therefore, consideration of the patient's perspective and experiences needs to be adopted (Hofhuis and Bakker, 1998). Noise levels should be reduced to a minimum by staff wearing soft-soled shoes, speaking quietly and avoiding unnecessary conversation during the night. Unnecessary and noisy phone calls should be avoided (some wards have a silent flashing bulb/light to alert a telephone call) and plan supplies and equipment in advance. The room temperature and ventilation should be regulated.

Other strategies include the use of curtains or screens for privacy and dignity, but this should be done with discretion as screens cannot compromise the monitoring of the patient.

Visitors should be made aware of the importance of sleep, not only for the patient but also for themselves. Indeed most clinical areas now adopt a restful period of two hours in the afternoon, where only essential care is carried out. This allows the patient to rest during the day thus increasing total sleep time for 24 hours. This is not an ideal situation as patients should benefit from continuous sleep, but it is better than losing their sleep entirely.

The transferring of patients from critical care areas back to a general ward should be avoided during the periods of 22.00 hours and 07.00 hours (NICE, 2007a); should this occur it should be recorded as an adverse incident.

Implications for practice

- Nurses should include sleep in the assessment and planning of care.
- Older patients are more susceptible to sleep deprivation.
- Sleep deprivation can have detrimental physiological and psychological effects on the acutely ill patient.
- At night only essential care and monitoring is performed to maintain a safe level of care. Obviously if the patient's condition dictates the level of monitoring and intervention is increased accordingly.
- Ensure that the benefits of intervention outweigh those of undisturbed sleep.
- Clustering of care should be performed to allow maximum time for undisturbed sleep.
- If patients are disturbed in their sleep during the night, consider restful periods during the day.

Summary

Adequate sleep is an essential component of acute care. Disturbances to sleep affect a significant amount of patients. Sleep has physiological and psychological restorative functions, and the promotion of sleep should be viewed as a natural part of care.

Clinical scenario

Yamin, 56 years old, has been admitted from the ward to the HDU with uncontrolled type-two respiratory failure. He requires CPAP therapy, with hourly monitoring of vital signs and arterial blood gas via an arterial line.

1   State why Yamin is at risk of developing sleep deprivation.

2   What symptoms would you expect this patient to have? Provide a rationale for your answer.

3   At night his temperature is significantly lowered, his blood pressure decreases, his heart rate is labile with the occasional premature ventricular contraction (PVC) and his respiratory rate increases and is irregular. There is also a reduction in his oxygen saturation levels. State a reason for these physiological changes.

4   What strategies can be adopted to promote sleep?

Chapter 13

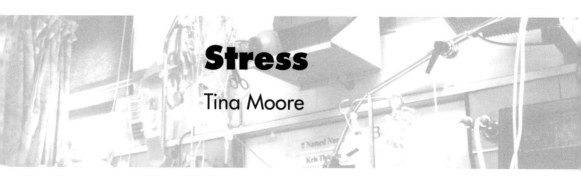

Stress

Tina Moore

Contents

Learning outcomes

After reading this chapter you will be able to:

- identify the major causes of stress within the acute care setting for both the patient and nurse;
- discuss the physiological changes that occur in response to stress;
- understand and implement the management of stress.

Fundamental knowledge

Acute pain management (Chapter 10); psychological disturbances (Chapter 11); patient-centred care (Chapter 2); nutrition (Chapter 7); family care (Chapter 4); transferring patients (Chapter 37).

Introduction

It is debatable as to whether caring for the acutely/critical patient is more stressful than other areas of nursing. Equally, it is not clear if acute care nurses experience a larger amount of stress in total. Stress is a subjective phenomenon, dependent upon multiple variables, e.g. the nurse's level of competence and experience; severity of patient's illness; past experiences; perceptions of the situation and complexity of decision-making. Taking into consideration these variables, any clinical environment has the potential to be stressful.

This chapter aims to identify some of the sources of stress confronting both the patient and nurse. It is divided into two sections: the patient's perspective and the nurse's perspective. While it is identified that transfer has a large impact (stress) on the patient and their family, readers are directed to read Chapter 4 for discussions in this area.

There are various definitions of stress available. Each contains many meanings, making them confusing and ill defined. Nevertheless, common attributes are seen within all of them, in that they all state the relationship between environmental influences and the individual.

Stress is a response, by the body, to a stimulus that disturbs or interferes with normal equilibrium. So, stress can be viewed as a response to perceived demand. Therefore, it is a situation that is created when an individual is faced with any stimulus that causes disequilibria between normal homeostatic functioning (Morton and Fontaine, 2009). This function is dependent upon the individual's ability to perceive and appraise the situation. Consequently, any situation can activate stress, and so has become a natural component of our lives.

There is a tendency to concentrate on the negative components of stress and where possible attempt to avoid stress-provoking situations. Stress can and does act as a motivator, as seen in some individuals who work and thrive in 'highly stressful' environments. A certain amount of stress is considered to be desirable for adaptation to occur. However, problems arise when coping mechanisms fail and stress becomes counter-productive. Signs include lack of concentration, anxiety and insomnia.

Stressors

The inability to cope with excess demand will possibly lead to prolonged stress and abnormal responses (either physical and/or psychological), eventually affecting quality of life and performance. Stressors originate from multiple sources, e.g. biological (injury or illness); psychosocial (interpersonal conflicts, poor communication); environmental (unfamiliarity with the surroundings, technology).

Stressors can be harmful, threatening or indeed challenging. An individual's ability to cope will be different, depending upon the perception, appraisal and supportive mechanisms in place, as well as their health status. Individuals will differ in the extent to which they perceive an event as controllable, predictable and a challenge to their capabilities and self-concept. The more uncontrollable an event seems, the more likely it is to be perceived as stressful.

Strategies of coping are thoughts and acts that the individual uses to handle the demands of stressful interactions. They are considered to be the mediator between the stressful event and its outcomes. Coping strategies can be problem-focused and/or emotion-focused (Tuncay *et al.*, 2008). Problem-focused strategies are directed towards alerting the stressor. Cognitive (interpersonal) forms involve the identification of the problem and generating solutions to manifestations of stress.

Emotion-focused strategies involve developing/regulating accompanying distressful emotions. This involves distancing, escape-avoidance, self-control, positive appraisal and acceptance of responsibility (Tuncay *et al.*, 2008). Nurses can assist patients in dealing with their subjective interpretation of the traumatic event because modes of coping arise from the individual's cognitive appraisal of the stressor. Different patients may view similar situations in different ways, resulting in different consequences for long-term adjustment. Early intervention should emphasise realistic perceptions of hesitation.

Models of stress

There are various models of stress in existence. Stimulus-based models relate to the relationship between the external causes of stress and the individuals who are exposed to it. These models may be useful in identifying external stressors, such as noise, poor air quality, etc. However, they fail to identify the individual's responses to the stressor(s).

Probably the most well-known model is Selye's (1956) General Adaptation Syndrome (GAS), an example of a response-based model involving physiological responses to stress. It recognises the individual's ability to respond and adapt to their environment. This is demonstrated by all organisms in three progressive phases:

1 Alarm state – the body mobilises to confront the threat 'fight' and 'flight'.
2 Resistance, or adaptation – here a lot of physical and nervous energy is used up. Coping mechanisms vary. However, if the stressor continues it will withdraw physical and emotional energy.
3 Exhaustion and death – response to stress initially is appropriate and useful in aiding the patient to cope, responses in the long term are likely to be detrimental to recovery.

The transactional model described by Lazarus (1966), who was influenced by the work of Selye, expressed the belief that fundamentally the concept of stress referred to the relationship between the organism and the environment rather than the organism or environment alone. Hence stress is viewed as a dynamic, interactional process. Within the acute care environment, an amalgamation of the transactional and response-based models seems to be the most useful in enabling the identification of, and coping with, stress.

1 Think of a situation when you felt stressed – what were the causes? In your opinion do you think that stress could be preventable?
2 Describe the feelings you had.
3 Now consider the patients that you have cared for. What have been the causes of their anxiety?
4 Can you identify common themes of stress?

The patient's experience

Causes of stress in the patient presents in different ways:

- physical or psychological discomfort
- staff interaction
- family
- fear of dying
- difficulty in communicating fears, pain
- sense of isolation
- vulnerability, loss of control, powerlessness
- environment and unsettled pattern of activity
- effects of drug therapy.

Clinical features

The patient's physiological response to stress can cause considerable added strain on failing organs and incorporates the stress response as previously discussed (Chapter 11).

Psychological responses to stress include anxiety, worry and apprehension. Major symptoms include feeling of estrangement from others, tendency to relive the trauma repeatedly in memories and dreams. Sleep disturbance (Topf and Thompson, 2001) and difficulty in concentration may also be apparent.

Stressful situations can precipitate physiological and psychological reactions. The stress response (physiological) relates to a cascade of metabolic and neurohormonal changes that create a defensive mechanism in order for coping to take place.

Stress-induced hyperglycaemia is attributed to hypersecretion of the counter regulatory hormones: catecholamines-adrenaline (epinephrine) and noradrenaline (norepinephrine); glucagons; cortisol and growth hormone. Release of adrenaline and noradrenaline results in decreased insulin and increased glucagons secretion by the pancreas. The effect is a surge in circulating glucose derived from glycogenolysis, gluconeogenesis and impaired peripheral utilisation of glucose. Hyperglycaemia itself impairs peripheral glucose utilisation and residual insulin secretion. Patients who have reduced insulin production or those with borderline insulin secretory reserve are unable to increase insulin production. Secretion is, therefore, inadequate to counteract these intense catabolic effects.

The sympathetic branch of the autonomic nervous system plays a key role in the stress-mediated glycaemic response. Catecholamines exert an overall inhibitory effect on insulin by activation of adrenergic receptors in the pancreatic beta cells that produce insulin (Ganong, 2005). Ketoacidosis may develop in patients with the most severe insulin deficiency. This activity results in increased heart rate, respiratory rate and blood pressure.

Responses to stressors are useful as a coping strategy in the short term but could have detrimental affects to recovery in the long term. The continued breakdown of protein stores will lead to muscle wasting and fatigue; suppression of the inflammatory response will initiate infection and the increased extracellular fluid volume will produce oedema and altered fluid balance (Adam and Osborne, 2005).

Management

Acute illness involving admission to a critical care unit, equally, patients being transferred back to the ward from critical care, creates predictable stressors. Being able to predict the occurrence of a stressful event (even if the individual cannot control it), can usually reduce the severity of the stress. Where possible, preventative strategies should be adopted, particularly when the stressor is environmentally orchestrated and foreseen. In the event of booked admission to critical care, nurses should take advantage of planned visits to enable the patient and family (where appropriate) to psychologically prepare for admission. This should be optional for the patient as some patients' stress levels may increase when confronted with a critical care environment and hence be counterproductive.

The acutely ill patient's condition can deteriorate very quickly with a rapid reversal of their coping strategies. This is something that nurses often cannot control or indeed predict. By including the patient (where possible) in the decision-making process can foster a sense of control. A holistic approach to the delivery of care should be adopted.

Nurses should develop a caring, non-judgemental relationship and try and understand the patient's perspective, allowing them to express themselves freely. Coping can be judged only in terms of the consequences. Attend to the patient's psychological and emotional needs by talking to them rather than letting care be physiologically led. Nurses should introduce themselves at the start of the shift and reinforce this information throughout the course of the period of time. Visits should be encouraged from the family and friends, who can bring in familiar objects to help orientate the patient.

Severe hyperglycaemia is best treated by intravenous infusion of insulin via a sliding scale regime (see Chapter 33). Opiates can be used as a form of pain control as well as a sedative but there are contraindications and side effects to consider. Benzodiazepines and haloperidol can be administered as supplements to the opiate regimen. Benzodiazepines, e.g. diazepam, have active metabolites including oxazepam that can accumulate in acutely/critically ill patients.

To minimise the effects of stress, effective and efficient discharge planning is required, which includes: high levels of liaison and communication between ward and unit staff to smooth the transition.

Stress in the nurse

Caring for the acutely ill patient may be stressful. If stress remains unrecognised or unalleviated, burnout is likely to occur. The quality of care may deteriorate (clinical errors) and staff may avoid or distance themselves from all but the absolutely necessary interaction with the patient. Staff dissatisfaction at work may become evident in the form of sickness and absenteeism.

Causes

Causal factors of stress tend to be interpersonal (conflicts within a multi-disciplinary team, bureaucracy, inadequacies of nursing care by others) and extra-personal (environmental).

Stress can interfere with individuals' appraisal of their situation – 'can't see the wood for the trees' syndrome. Clinical features of stress may be:

- emotional – increasing irritability;
- behavioural – indecisiveness;
- physical – increasing suspiciousness and distrust;
- cognitive – inability to concentrate or listen;
- physiological – stress response (as discussed earlier).

(Roberts 1986)

Long-term stress can lead to ill-health, e.g. gastric ulcers, coronary heart disease and a compromised immune system.

Management

Management comprises of prevention and coping strategies, taking ownership in working towards reducing stress to a controllable level, but in order to do this, stress needs to be of a manageable level. Stress challenges us to take a mental helicopter to a point above the situation so that we can get a different view on it (Davidson, 1999) and be prepared to entertain new thoughts and ideas and develop a new focus and perspective.

Coping with stress needs a supportive working environment through preceptorship and effective teamwork. Keeping a diary/journal as a way of expressing oneself may be useful. The use of reflection through clinical supervision may help nurses critically examine their practice and learn through this process. In doing so, they should develop critical analytical skills, identifying areas for future development. Debriefing can be offered by a supervisor, but requires great skill. Emotions brought to the surface in a debriefing need to be examined in private and not at the bedside.

Nurses need to be able to prioritise the management and delivery of care. By adopting this approach could enable nurses to manage their time and efforts more effectively and efficiently. Prioritising involves nurses thinking ahead and making some predictions about possible intervention/patient outcomes. This also involves breaking work down into a series of tasks and placing these tasks in a logical order. Implications for these tasks should be examined.

Implications for practice

- Stress can and does have detrimental effects upon the nurse and patient.
- Patients are at risk of developing internal and external stressors that may compromise their health and recovery from illness.
- Nurses are responsible for identifying potential patient stressors and adopting strategies to prevent or minimise their effects.
- Appropriate strategies need to be utilised to help individuals cope with stress.
- Involvement in reflection and clinical supervision may help to support nurses and possibly reduce stress.

Summary

Stress is an individual concept that manifests itself in different ways. Our perceptions of the situation or experience will determine how we react to stress. Ideally, predicting and avoiding stressful situations is the best strategy to adopt. If this is unavoidable, as in many situations, then a variety of strategies may be adopted.

Clinical scenario

Susan Butcher (D grade, qualified for six months) has been working on the acute care ward for two weeks. It is a busy 28-bedded unit, constantly full to its bed capacity. At interview she was informed that she would have a preceptor and be well supported. This in her opinion has failed to happen.

Colleagues have noticed that she is becoming increasingly irritable, has made errors of judgement, is constantly late for work and looks tired. She has been heard to say that she cannot cope with the demands of the job and wants to leave.

1 Identify the stressors for Susan.

2 Discuss the detrimental affects that could occur.

3 Devise a plan of action to help support Susan and increase her coping strategies.

Chapter 14

Acute neurological pathologies

Philip Woodrow

Contents

Learning outcomes

After reading this chapter you will be able to:

- describe to patients causes of acute neurological problems discussed here;
- plan effective nursing care for patients with these conditions;
- care safely for patients with acute neurological complications.

Fundamental knowledge

Neurological anatomy (including brain stem, hypothalamus, pituitary gland, formation of cerebro-spinal fluid; myelin; sympathetic and parasympathetic nervous system control; autonomic nervous system).

Introduction

Some patients may be admitted to hospital with neurological problems, but others develop complications after admission for other pathologies. More so than many pathophysiologies discussed elsewhere, nursing care significantly contributes to recovery from acute neurological disease; problems, and so nursing care, are often similar, so this chapter begins by identifying key problems caused by brain damage, then describes acute neurological conditions:

- traumatic brain injury (TBI)
- epilepsy
- Guillain–Barré Syndrome (GBS)
- spinal cord injury.

Neurological disease may impair consciousness and/or movement, so all patients are vulnerable, and rely on staff to maintain their safety. For example, impaired gag reflexes may expose patients to risks from aspiration, so a clear airway should be maintained by nursing patients in the recovery position. Conditions affecting peripheral nerves, such as Guillain–Barré Syndrome, limit mobility, exposing people to risks of tissue damage.

Stroke, a major cause of morbidity and mortality, is not discussed, partly because it is a huge and currently rapidly changing topic, and partly because new admissions should be fast-tracked to specialist stroke units. Subarachnoid haemorrhage, often devastating with poor prognosis, is also not discussed as it usually necessitates ICU admission, but is discussed in Woodrow (2006).

Many central nervous system pathologies (including cerebral oedema) share similar symptoms, so this chapter begins by describing common symptoms and nursing care.

Psychological

The less patients can do for themselves, the more they rely on nurses to meet fundamental activities of living. Intimate aspects of care may be psychologically threatening to patients, especially as many patients with neurological pathologies are young. Neurological problems often cause anxiety and frustration, especially as recovery may be protracted. Personality changes may include:

- reduced inhibition
- inflexible thinking

- memory deficits
- greater irritability.

(O'Neill and Carter, 1998)

Frontal lobe brain damage is especially likely to cause aggressiveness and loss of inhibition. Neurological problems, especially epilepsy, often bring social stigmas (Lanfear, 2002), and sometimes legal restrictions, such as suspension of driving licence – the DVLA website details current restrictions. Physical limitations or acute confusion/aggression can make these patients labour-intensive and stressful for nurses. Relatives exposed to aggression or confusion may experience similar distress.

Thermoregulation

In health, the hypothalamus regulates body temperature. Cerebral damage may affect hypothalamic function, causing pyrexia (Rossi *et al.*, 2001). Pyrexia increases metabolism, consuming more oxygen and nutrients. Peripheral nervous system dysfunction may impair thermoregulation by loss of vasodilatation, shivering and sweating reflexes. Temperature should, therefore, initially be assessed frequently. Pyrexia may necessitate antipyretic drugs, such as para-cetamol, to provide cerebral protection. Inducing mild hypothermia helps prevent cardiac arrest from ventricular fibrillation (Fukuda and Warner, 2007), although hypothermia can cause other complications, such as

- reducing oxyhaemoglobin dissociation which reduces oxygen delivery to tissues;
- coagulopathies.

Inducing hypothermia, therefore, remains a debated aspect of management.

Blood sugar

Severe brain injury usually causes hyperglycaemia (Hunningher and Smith, 2006) from catecholamine (adrenaline) release, although blood sugar may be labile, swinging rapidly from hyperglycaemia to hypoglycaemia. Blood sugar should initially be monitored hourly, with frequency reduced if it remains stable. Glucose infusions, such as 5% glucose, should be avoided (Eynon and Menon, 2002), as these may increase cerebral oedema.

Nutrition

Cells need energy to survive. Cell energy (adenosine triphosphate – ATP) is produced by mitochondria (in cells), normally from glycolysis (breakdown of glucose in the presence of oxygen). Unlike most body cells, brain cells store little ATP, so rely on almost continuous perfusion. Oxygen is vital – cerebral hypoxia is a major cause of secondary death from traumatic brain injury (TBI). TBI increases metabolism, so high-energy intake is needed to match hypermetabolism (Hunningher and Smith, 2006). Inadequate nutrition causes muscle wasting (see Chapter 7), which in trauma patients may delay recovery and discharge.

Peripheral nervous system diseases, such as Guillain–Barré Syndrome, may reduce gut motility. Dieticians should be actively involved in multidisciplinary care. Large-volume feeds may necessitate increasing gut motility with drugs such as metoclopramide.

Diabetes insipidus

Diabetes (fountain-like) describes the classic symptoms of polydipsia and polyuria. It usually refers to diabetes mellitus, where lack of insulin causes hyperglycaemia, which causes osmotic diuresis (polyuria) resulting in hypo-volaemia and polydipsia. In diabetes insipidus, pituitary gland damage may reduce antidiuretic hormone production, resulting in reduced renal reabsorption of water (polyuria), and so hypovolaemia and thirst. Urine is dilute but, unlike diabetes mellitus, glycosuria is absent. If caused by cerebral oedema or other transitory damage, diabetes insipidus resolves once the cause is removed.

Traumatic brain injury (TBI)

Traumatic brain injury is the largest single cause of morbidity and mortality in young (<45) people (Werner and Engelhard, 2007). Each year nearly 1.5 million people in the UK suffer TBI (Menon, 1999), especially from road traffic accidents (Allen and Ward, 1998) and, to a lesser extent, contact sports such as rugby and boxing (Collin and Daly, 1998). Patients with severe TBI (= Glasgow Coma Scale 3–8) are usually comatose, so need urgent anaesthetic review for probable intubation, ventilation and transfer to intensive care (NICE, 2007b). Patients with less severe injury may be transferred to other wards, and patients who recover from severe TBI may progress to specialist neurological rehabilitation units or whichever wards have available beds. Recovery from severe injuries may take years, and may remain incomplete: one-third of people recovering from severe traumatic brain injury have long-term disabilities (Bader and Arbour, 2005).

Time out 14.1

Reflect on patients you have nursed who had head injuries. What problems and needs were caused by their traumatic brain injury? List the care and treatments these patients were offered.

Damage at the time of injury is essentially irreversible, but early and effective treatment of secondary damage (inflammation, oedema) significantly reduces morbidity and mortality (Werner and Engelhard, 2007). Secondary damage is usually caused by

- hypotension (90 per cent have ischaemic damage at autopsy)
- hypoxia
- hyperglycaemia
- hypercapnia.

(Moppett, 2007)

Reversing all these improves outcome. Oxygen therapy (15 litres via non-rebreathing mask) is usually the first priority.

The National Collaborating Centre for Acute Care (2007) recommend life-saving decompressive surgery within four hours of traumatic brain injury. However, neurosurgery is usually only possible at regional centres. Key aims of early treatment are

- reversing hypoxia
- reversing hypotension
- optimising cerebral perfusion pressure.

Patients with TBI are often admitted to intensive care for elective sedation and ventilation. Until transfer, treatment targets are likely to be similar to those listed in Box 14.1.

Box 14.1 Likely targets for early treatment of traumatic brain injury

- PaO_2 >13 kPa
- $PaCO_2$ 4.5–5.0 kPa
- Systolic BP >120 mmHg
- MAP >90 mmHg
- Blood sugar 4–9 mmol/litre
- ICP <20–25 mmHg
- CPP 60 mmHg
- Control seizures

Trauma often causes multiple injuries, necessitating other support and care. For example, trauma may cause lung contusion, necessitating respiratory support. Because injuries may be extensive, some may have been missed during, or developed since, initial assessment. Nurses should actively assess all needs and potential problems of patients with TBI and trauma. With trauma, the possibility of spinal fractures should be considered. Hard collars are used until spinal fractures have been excluded. Support collars may also be useful if soft tissue injury is suspected.

Base of skull fractures, which may remain unidentified until x-rayed, could result in nasal tubes penetrating the brain, so nasal tubes should be avoided until base of skull fractures have been excluded. Base of skull fractures may leak cerebro-spinal fluid (CSF), which may drain from the nose (*rhinorrhoea*) or ear (*otorrhoea*), often forming a yellow ring, or 'halo sign', around bloodstains on linen (Hickey, 2003b).

Immobility predisposes patients with traumatic brain injury to deep vein thromboses (DVT), so prophylaxis is usually commenced. DVT prophylaxis should not be withheld for fears of it causing intracranial bleeding, as risks of this are slight (Hunningher and Smith, 2006).

Although anti-epileptic drugs are not usually given routinely, up to one-quarter of people with traumatic brain injury develop seizures (Moppett, 2007), so nurses should observe for signs of fitting. Steroids are not beneficial (Hunningher and Smith, 2006).

Spinal injury

Higher spinal injuries, especially cervical, cause greater functional loss. Injury may be complete or incomplete. Incomplete injury is caused by initial inflammation; once this subsides patients may recover some function during the early weeks.

Early deaths from spinal injury are usually caused by respiratory failure. Injuries above C3 often cause respiratory paralysis, while injuries lower than C3 often cause respiratory compromise (March, 2005). Spinal shock is the other main life-threatening complication (Harvey, 2008).

Spinal cord injury can also cause

- acute (volume-responsive) kidney injury
- paralytic ileus
- deep vein thrombosis from venous stasis
- double incontinence

and problems with most other systems and functions. Many patients develop severe pain and spasticity (Harvey, 2008). Patients with cervical spine injury ideally should be admitted to ICU (Hadley, 2002), for later transfer either to specialist units or to wards within the hospital. Early immobilisation is generally beneficial.

Lower spinal injuries cause fewer problems, as most thoracic and abdominal functions remain intact. Thoracic and lumbar injuries affect legs (DVTs, immobility), so until stabilised patients should be log-rolled to prevent further injury. Of people with paralytic injury, 38 per cent develop DVTs within three months (Anderson and Spencer, 2003). Lower abdominal organs (bladder and bowels) may be affected.

Life-threatening complications have usually resolved once patients transfer to general wards, but other complications may persist. Nursing care should include:

- pain assessment, analgesia
- bowel care
- DVT prophylaxis
- mobilisation and rehabilitation, active (or passive) exercises.

Many need specialist input, such as chronic pain specialists and physiotherapists, but nurses should be actively involved in all care. A bowel management plan is valuable; Coggrave (2008) reviews bowel care strategies. Abdominal massage is recommended by Ash (2005). Manual evacuation of faeces may be necessary (RCN, 2008a); this is reviewed by Kyle *et al.* (2004).

Patients and families are likely to be anxious about their future; most (85 per cent) people surviving the first 24 hours are alive ten years later (Winter and Knight, 2005).

Autonomic dysreflexia

This common complication of spinal injuries above T6 (Cherian *et al.*, 2005), and sometimes as low as T10 (Keely, 1998), often occurs six months following injury, but can occur at any time.

At rest, these patients have excessive parasympathetic stimulation, causing underlying bradycardia and hypotension. On stimulation, absence of inhibitory neurotransmitters causes excessive sympathetic reflex responses (Harvey, 2008) – life-threatening hypertension and tachycardia. Other symptoms include:

■ headache
■ sweating
■ flushed face and neck
■ pale below the lesion
■ nausea
■ blurred vision.

(Harvey, 2008)

Distended bladders (sometimes as little as 200 ml) (Cherian *et al.*, 2005) and bowels (NPSA, 2004; Furlan *et al.*, 2007) are the main causes. Other significant causes include fractures, pressure ulcers and ingrowing toenails (Harvey, 2008). Causes should be quickly removed if possible, hypertension monitored and treated. Once the stimulus is removed, antihypertensives may cause profound hypotension. Prophylactic prevention includes monitoring bladder and bowel function, intervening early to prevent distension in patients who have suffered upper spinal injuries.

Epilepsy

Epilepsy is the most common serious neurological disease in the UK, occurring in one in every 200 people (Sisodiya and Duncan, 2004). Fits may also be caused by acute neurological problems, injury or cerebral hypoxia. Two-fifths of seizures are caused by brain damage from disease or trauma (Lanfear, 2002), such as

■ traumatic brain injury
■ raised intracranial pressure (e.g. secondary to liver failure)
■ hypoxia
■ meningitis.

Epilepsy is unpredictable. Patients with history of fitting may develop seizures in response to many other factors.

When fitting commences its duration and consequences are unpredictable. So immediate actions should be to

- summon help;
- assess;
- maintain a clear airway (if compromised, place in recovery position; insert a guedel airway if possible, but without forcing the mouth open);
- deliver high-concentration oxygen if apnoeic;
- maintain safety (remove likely hazards, supporting the person with pillows);
- maintain privacy and dignity (screen them from other people).

Nurses should note

- when the fit began and ended;
- which parts of the body were affected.

During seizures, especially the tonic phase, patients can still hear and understand their surroundings, so staff should calmly reassure them about what is happening. Seizures can be very distressing to family, friends and other patients, so offering them reassurance is also valuable.

Seizures may be partial (starting in one hemisphere of the brain) or generalised (starting in both hemispheres). Tonic-clonic seizures (formerly called *grand mal* or *convulsions*) cause generalised alternation of muscular spasms, often with loss of breathing, clenching of teeth and single or double incontinence. Seizures may be preceded by an 'aura', which may warn people who have previously experienced fitting. Often their eyes roll upwards. Fitting causes excessive muscle activity, producing heat and so pyrexia (Thomas and Hirsch, 2003). Seizures usually only last a few minutes, but often leave a headache, confusion or tiredness (NICE, 2004a).

Benzodiazepines (lorazepam, diazepam) are first-line drugs for treating fits (Marik and Varon, 2004; Stokes *et al.*, 2004; Walker, 2005); if fitting continues, propofol or thiopental are recommended for adults (Stokes *et al.*, 2004). If fitting stops quickly, outcome is usually good; if fitting persists for 30 minutes, one-quarter of patients die (Thomas and Hirsch, 2003).

Status epilepticus is often, although not universally, defined as seizures lasting more than 30 minutes (Thomas and Hirsch, 2003), although Marik and Varon (2004) suggest that 5 minutes would be a better definition. Prolonged fitting usually necessitates transfer to intensive care (Walker, 2005).

Half of people who have fits may experience further seizures within five years (Sisodiya and Duncan, 2004), so they should be advised about risks. People may choose to wear medi-alert bracelets, although the stigma sometimes attached to epilepsy may discourage others from doing this. UK law prohibits epileptics from driving until they have been free of fits for one year.

Guillain–Barré Syndrome (GBS)

This syndrome occurs where peripheral neuropathy causes acute neuromuscular failure (Winer, 2008). Once considered a single disease, it comprises similar but separate peripheral nervous system pathologies, including

- acute inflammatory demyelinating polyneuropathy (AIDP)
- acute motor axonal neuropathy (AMAN)
- acute motor and sensory axonal neuropathy (AMSAN)

and a few rarer pathologies. AMAN is more commonly found in China and Japan, whereas AIDP is more common in North America and Europe (Kuwabara *et al.*, 2002). This chapter focuses on AIDP.

Guillain–Barré affects 1–2 per 100,000 of the UK population (Pritchard, 2008), making it one of the most common neurological pathologies. Two-thirds of cases are preceded by infections a few weeks beforehand (Pritchard, 2008). The syndrome causes ascending demyelination of peripheral nerves, especially motor nerves, resulting in progressive muscle weakness. Sensory nerves usually remain unaffected.

Problems experienced often include (see Box 14.2):

- *Pain*, usually severe, exacerbated by touch and anxiety. Opioid analgesia is often needed, although neuropathic analgesics such as carbamazepine, gabapentin or amitryptyline are also useful (Hughes *et al.*, 2005; Pritchard, 2008). Muscle weakness often prevents patients from making themselves comfortable, so patients should be positioned comfortably.
- *Respiratory failure* can be caused by muscle weakness, and may need intensive physiotherapy and sometimes non-invasive ventilation.
- *Hypersalivation* and loss of gag reflex from autonomic dysfunction can create risks of aspiration, requiring oral suction. Facial muscle weakness may cause dribbling.
- *Hypotension* from widespread peripheral vasodilatation (poor sympathetic tone).
- *Hypertensive episodes* from failure of normal negative feedback opposition to sympathetic stimuli.
- *Dysrhythmias*, including tachycardia and bradycardia from dysfunction of nervous control.
- *Sweating* from autonomic dysfunction, so nurses should provide frequent washes and changes of clothing for comfort.
- *Thrombosis* from venous stasis (immobility) and poor perfusion, so patients should have prophylactic subcutaneous anticoagulants and thromboembolytic stockings.
- *Limb weakness*, necessitating passive exercises to prevent contractures and promote venous return; analgesia cover is often needed for this.
- *Incontinence* from bladder muscle weakness.

Box 14.2 Main problems caused by Guillain–Barré Syndrome

- Pain
- Respiratory failure
- Hypersalivation
- Hypotension
- Hypertensive episodes
- Dysrhythmias
- Sweating
- Thrombosis
- Limb weakness
- Incontinence

(BSRM/RCP, 2003)

Recovery is unpredictable, relying on regrowth of damaged nerves. Intravenous immunoglobulin (IVIg) usually reverses the condition (El-Ghariani and Unsworth, 2006), although recovery usually takes some weeks. Otherwise, treatments are mainly supportive, preventing the above complications. Rehabilitation should include active exercise (Hughes *et al.*, 2005), so physiotherapists should be involved at an early stage. A significant minority can suffer long-term pain and depression (Kogos *et al.*, 2005).

Implications for practice

- Central nervous system pathologies/problems can cause hyper/hypoglycaemia, pyrexia and various neuro-endocrine complications.
- Primary damage from traumatic brain injury is largely irreversible, but most deaths and many disabilities are caused by secondary complications; preventing complications improves survival and reduces morbidity.
- Spinal injury can cause extensive disability, necessitating nursing interventions for many activities of living.
- Autonomic dysreflexia commonly occurs after spinal cord injury, and can cause sudden life-threatening hypertension.
- Lorazepam is usually the drug of choice for stopping fitting.
- Tonic-clonic seizures can be life-threatening – assess using ABCDE.
- Peripheral neuropathies are less immediately life-threatening, but can cause prolonged dependence on others, and severe cases may cause respiratory failure.
- Neurological diseases can be particularly frustrating for patients and families; many bring social stigma and legal restrictions. Psychological and social care and support are, therefore, especially important.
- Skilled nursing care makes a significant contribution to survival and recovery following traumatic brain injury.

Summary

Patients with neurological conditions may be referred to specialist centres, but many are admitted to and remain in general hospitals. This creates challenges for nurses working in those hospitals. The frustrating nature of many of these conditions, and sometimes their effects on cognition, can make caring for these patients and their families especially stressful. Yet the quality of nursing care is especially important to outcome for these patients. This chapter has discussed some of the more commonly encountered neurological conditions, and nursing interventions, seen in general hospitals.

Clinical scenario

You are making the admission assessment for Tom Walker, 26, who has Guillain–Barré Syndrome.

1 List, in order of priority, your main potential concerns and baseline observations you would undertake.

2 Tom has not previously suffered from this disease, but heard that an acquaintance of his died from it. This makes him very anxious. He and his wife want to know what is likely to happen to him. Write down how you would explain the disease to him.

3 Devise a plan of nursing care for Tom's first few days on your ward.

Bibliography

Key reading

Harvey's (2008) book about spinal cord injury is written primarily for physiotherapists, but chapters on background and pain management are especially useful for nurses. Moppett (2007) reviews traumatic brain injury, while NICE (2007b) provide updated guidelines. Stokes *et al.* (2004) provide UK guidelines for epilepsy, albeit targeting primary/secondary care, while Walker (2005) reviews status epilepticus.

Further reading

Ash (2005) and Cherian *et al.* (2005) review autonomic dysreflexia. Sheerin (2005) provides a nursing review of spinal cord injury. Werner and Engelhard (2007) review traumatic brain injury. Pritchard (2008) and Winer (2008) review Guillain–Barré Syndrome. DVLA website: www.dvla.gov/uk/drivers.htm.

Part 3

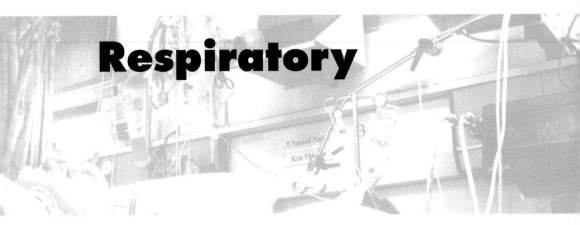

Respiratory

Chapter 15

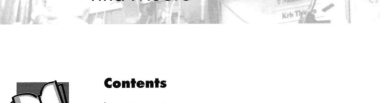

Respiratory assessment

Tina Moore

Contents

Learning outcomes

After reading this chapter you will be able to:

- assess and interpret the patient's respiratory status;
- identify signs of hypoxaemia and hypercapnia (carbon dioxide retention);
- demonstrate knowledge and understanding of Type 1 and Type 2 respiratory failure.

Fundamental knowledge

Respiratory physiology; gaseous exchange; carriage of gases; the transfer of oxygen (O_2).

Introduction

Deterioration to the patient's respiratory function is one of the first indicators of acute illness (BTS, 2008; Resuscitation Council, 2006). Respiratory disorders are a major cause of critical illness (DOH, 2000a) and accounts for one of the main reasons for admission to the critical care unit.

The primary purpose of respiratory assessment is to determine the adequacy of gas exchange, oxygenation of the tissues and excretion of carbon dioxide (CO_2) (Moore, 2007). By undertaking a full and systematic respiratory assessment the nurse is in a firm position to act upon findings (from the data collected) and ensure that prompt and appropriate medical/nursing interventions are initiated.

This chapter examines the process of respiratory assessment and its implications in recognising the two types of respiratory failure. It is beyond the scope of this chapter to discuss hypoxaemia (this is addressed in Chapter 19).

Time out 15.1

1 List the information you require when assessing a patient's respiratory status.
2 On your next shift, observe how many patients have an identified respiratory problem. Write down the causes.
3 Now look at their observation charts, medical/nursing notes – how many of these patients have had a comprehensive respiratory assessment performed? Think of reasons for your answer.

Respiratory assessment

Wherever possible the same nurse should be involved in the assessment/ monitoring of the patient's respiratory status for the duration of a shift. This should enable the identification of subtle as well as overt changes. Depending on the severity of respiratory impairment history-taking may be limited and so observational skills will need to be relied upon (Moore, 2007). During assessment significant factors that influence the patient's respiratory function should always be taken into consideration, for example:

- Obesity – patients with large or distended abdomens may not be able to sit upright and could suffer impediment of the diaphragm, affecting lung expansion.
- Circulatory problems – pulmonary oedema, anaemia – impede gas exchange.
- Environmental influences, e.g. exposure to the cold, may cause shivering, distorting assessment findings.
- Trauma – particularly of the chest.
- Known allergies may cause anaphylaxis.
- Pathophysiological problems which can cause abdominal distension, e.g. bowel obstruction, ascites, pancreatitis.

- Smoking history (including passive smoking).
- Employment, e.g. painter, farm worker.
- Medication, e.g. bronchodilators, steroids.
- Social factors/home factors, e.g. damp housing, living with relative with tuberculosis (TB)
- Pregnancy – fluid retention is caused by increasing oestrogen levels resulting in oedema. Progesterone levels rise six-fold through pregnancy (Lumb, 2005) and have a significant effect on the control of respiratory and arterial blood gases. In addition, an enlargement on the uterus in the third trimester causes the diaphragm to be misplaced, thus affecting lung expansion.

When performing a respiratory assessment, the patient should be positioned upright (wherever possible). This position not only facilitates lung expansion, but also enables access to the anterior and posterior thorax, enabling assessment of accessory muscles. Alternative positions may distort findings and will need to be acknowledged (in the documentation) and when interpreting data. If appropriate, remove the patient's clothing, as this may act as a barrier to visible and possible audible (auscultation) assessment, possibly distorting findings. Some patients may be aware that their respiratory function is being assessed and this may lead to a subconscious response that influences their breathing rate.

Closed questions should be used as much as possible to minimise any distress in the acutely breathless patient. Questions should be prioritised and the patient should be allowed to rest adequately during questioning.

Generally, respiratory assessment can be broken down into four areas – inspection, palpation, percussion and auscultation. Nurses do not perform percussion as a mode of respiratory assessment unless additional training has been undertaken.

Inspection

Rate

The respiratory rate should be counted for one full minute and will be categorised into one of the following:

- *Eupnoea* ('normal' rate) – parameters between 10–17 breaths per minute have been suggested. However, MEWS sets a trigger of 15 and above.
- *Tachypnoea* (greater than 18 breaths per minute) is usually the first indication of respiratory distress. Possible causes include: anxiety, pain, cardiac (e.g. left ventricular) failure, circulatory problems (e.g. anaemia), infection/sepsis.
- *Bradypnoea* (less than ten breaths per minute) could indicate increased intracranial pressure, depression of the respiratory centre (e.g. narcotic overdose), and severe deterioration in the patient's condition.
- *Hypopnoea* (abnormally shallow respirations) may vary with age. Shallow breathing is considered part of the normal ageing process.

Rhythm

The normal respiratory rhythm has regular cycles, with the expiratory phase slightly longer than the inspiratory phase. A short pause is normal between expiration and the next inspiration. Chest movement should be equal, bilateral and symmetrical. Rhythm usually varies between men and women. Men tend to breathe predominantly from their abdomen or diaphragm, women have a tendency to breathe via their thorax or costal muscle. Patients who are sleeping are also inclined to utilise their abdominal muscles. Nurses need to be aware of this difference, as there is an assumption that an increase in respiratory effort relates to the use of abdominal muscles (Moore, 2007).

Altered rhythms indicate an underlying disorder, e.g. Kussmaul breathing (rapid deep respirations due to the stimulation of the respiratory centre in the brain caused by metabolic acidosis) as in diabetic ketoacidosis. Cheyne Stokes respirations (periods of apnoea, alternating with periods of hypoxia) could indicate left ventricular failure or cerebral injury and are sometimes seen in the end stage of life.

Oxygen saturation

All breathless and acutely ill patients should have their oxygen saturation levels checked via pulse oximetry, now considered the fifth vital sign (BTS, 2008; Chapter 16).

Symmetry of breathing

Normally, there is symmetry in chest movement. Failure of the chest wall to rise adequately may indicate fibrosis, collapse of upper lobes or bronchial obstruction. It could also indicate severe pleural thickening that may cause flattening of the anterior chest wall and diminished respiratory effort. The legacy of previous thoracic surgery may be highlighted by the presence of old scars. In the instance of a pneumothorax chest movement may be unequal.

Degree of effort

The use of accessory muscles – sternocleidomastoid, scalenus, trapezius – may suggest difficulty in breathing. The patient may suffer from orthopnoea or even platypnoea (shortness of breath when sitting upright). Patients who have difficulty in expiration may indicate abnormalities of lung recoil and/or airway resistance, e.g. emphysema, pulmonary oedema, asthma. Increased inspiratory effort can imply upper airway obstruction, e.g. anaphylaxis, epiglottis. Tracheal deviation may suggest pneumothorax (possibly induced through treatment), e.g. CVP insertion.

Expiration may be prolonged as seen in asthma or emphysema. The influence of the severity of breathlessness on the restricted activity should be noted. Some patients may breathe through 'pursed lips' on expiration as they try to force the air out of the overdistended alveoli. In addition, nasal flaring can be an indication of respiratory distress in adults, although this is more common in children.

In the presence of a pneumothorax sudden sharp chest pain is made worse by taking a deep breath or cough.

Skin colour

Cyanosis (bluish colour of the skin and mucous membranes) occurs when large amounts of unsaturated haemoglobin are present and may be detectable when oxygen saturation of arterial blood drops below 85 per cent (Moyle, 2002). Therefore, cyanosis is usually considered a late sign of respiratory dysfunction. However, this is subject to considerable variability. Cyanosis is often difficult to appreciate in artificial lighting, unless quite defined, so can easily be missed. Diligence in observation is crucial.

Particular caution needs to be taken when assessing for cyanosis on patients with dark pigmented skin, as skin becomes dusky in colour (Driscoll, 2006), making the detection of cyanosis challenging. In anaemic patients there may be insufficient haemoglobin to produce a blue colour to the mucous membrane.

Peripheral cyanosis (usually seen in poor circulation (Casey, 2001)) is observed in the skin and nail beds and is most noticeable around the lips, ear lobes and fingertips. Central cyanosis suggests circulatory or ventilatory problems and is seen on the lips and under the tongue.

Deformities

Clubbing of the finger digits occurs as a result of a chronic condition forming over a long period of time. This may be indicative of hypoxaemia from chronic pulmonary or cardiovascular disease. Deformities of the posterior thorax can affect the quality of breathing. The diameter of the chest (anterior/posterior) should be compared with the side to side diameter; if the anterior/posterior diameter is approximately double, this indicates a 'barrel chest' (caused by emphysema). Spinal deformities such as kyphosis also influence lung expansion.

Mental status

A reduction in the patient's level of consciousness/altered mental status may indicate hypoxaemia. Symptoms include inappropriate behaviour, drowsiness and confusion and should be reported immediately. If appropriate and immediate action is not undertaken the patient could deteriorate into a state of unconsciousness, possibly developing irreversible brain damage. Assessment of patient's mental status needs to be conducted with care as some patients feel a sense of suffocation and become very frightened and anxious but are not hypoxic. Equally, language barriers/cultural influences must be considered within the assessment process as the patient may simply not understand instructions/questions.

Cough

The assessment of a patient's cough includes observation of the following characteristics:

■   regularity
■   length of time taken to cough
■   presence or absence of pain
■   distinctive sounds (e.g. whoop or bark)
■   strength of cough
■   secretions.

Sputum is a useful indicator of lung pathology:

■   frothy white (sometimes blood-stained) – pulmonary oedema;
■   bloody (frank blood – haemoptysis) – pulmonary embolism or active TB;
■   blood stained (streaks of blood) – pneumonia, abscess, aspiration (of stomach contents);
■   green and purulent – lung infection, pneumonia;
■   yellow/green and copious – advanced chronic bronchitis;
■   black – smoker (tar);
■   old blood – TB, lung cancer.

Palpation

Palpation is used to assess bilateral movements of the chest/diaphragm. It is also used to assess surgical emphysema. See Chapter 6 for further details.

Auscultation

Assessment of breath sounds (with and without a stethoscope) should form part of the nursing assessment. However, current practices indicate that this is variable. Nurses listening to the patient's breath sounds through a stethoscope should have undergone appropriate training. Knowledge of the different types of breath sounds is important to aid description and diagnosis. Without a stethoscope, normal breathing should be quiet. Normal breath sounds are known as vesicular, bronchovesicular and bronchial.

■   Normally, vesicular sounds (low pitched, low intensity – described as 'soft and breezy') can be heard over most of the lung fields.
■   Bronchovesicular sounds should be heard in the anterior region, near the mainstem bronchi and posterior only between the scapulae; sounds are more moderate in pitch and intensity.
■   Bronchial sounds are high pitched, loud and hollow sounding. These sounds are normally heard over the larger airways, and the trachea. If bronchial sounds are heard in other areas this could indicate consolidation of lung

tissue, e.g. in pneumonia (consolidated lung tissue transmits sounds better than air, making it louder).

■ Abnormal breath sounds (known as adventitious sounds) include crackles (as heard in pulmonary oedema); wheezing (normally, an obstruction of the airways by bronchospasm or swelling causes wheezing, e.g. asthma) and rubbing (pleural friction) should be listened for. Stridor (high-pitched sound) usually occurs on inspiration and is caused by laryngeal or tracheal obstruction, requiring immediate attention as this can be potentially life threatening for the patient.

Crackles are discontinuous, non-musical, brief sounds heard more commonly on inspiration. Here, small airways open during inspiration and collapse during expiration causing the crackling sounds. They can be classified as fine, medium or coarse. Attention to their loudness, pitch, duration, number, timing in the respiratory cycle, location, pattern from breath to breath, change after a cough or shift in position is required.

■ Fine crackles – high pitched, soft, very brief and are heard at the base of the lungs near the end of inspiration. Normally represent the opening of the alveoli.
■ Medium crackles – lower in pitch and are heard during the middle/latter part of inspiration.
■ Course crackles – louder, low-pitched, bubbling sounds heard on both inspiration and expiration and are usually associated with mucous which may clear after the coughing.
■ Wheezes include both inspiratory and expiratory.

Respiratory failure

Respiratory failure is a syndrome in which the respiratory system fails in one or both of its gas exchange functions (oxygenation (O_2) and carbon dioxide (CO_2) elimination at rest or during exercise) (Sharma, 2006). This can be acute or chronic. Chronic respiratory failure develops over several days or longer, allowing time for metabolic compensation and an increase in bicarbonate concentration (pH is usually only slightly decreased). While acute respiratory failure is characterised by life-threatening derangements in arterial blood gases and acid base status, the manifestations of chronic respiratory failure are less dramatic and may not be as readily apparent.

Blood gas disturbances occur as a result of alveolar hypoventilation (when either the respiratory rate or tidal volume (normally 500 ml in each breath) is reduced leading to insufficient gas exchange; ventilation:perfusion (V:Q) inequality (Huether and McCance, 2004); physiological shunting, said to occur when pulmonary perfusion exceeds alveolar ventilation; diffusion impairment caused by fluid accumulation; mucous or inflammation. Unventilated alveoli result in vasoconstriction, which then diverts the perfusion to ventilated alveoli, resulting in atelectasis.

There are two types of respiratory failure, dependent upon the cause:

- oxygenation (Type 1)
- ventilatory (Type 2).

The older person is at increased risk in developing respiratory failure due to underlying pulmonary disease, loss of muscle mass and other co-morbid conditions (Sevransky and Haponik, 2003).

Type 1 respiratory failure (oxygenation)

This type of respiratory failure occurs when there is hypoxia without CO_2 retention (hypercapnia) and is typically caused by reduction in inspired O_2; a ventilation/perfusion mismatch and alveolar ventilation (Priestley, 2006). This is the most common form of respiratory failure, and can be associated with virtually all acute disorders of the lung which generally involve fluid filling or collapse of alveoli. Some examples of Type 1 respiratory failure are shock, pulmonary oedema and pneumonia (Sharma, 2006). These are in addition to diseases that affect the lung tissue usually causing a steadily progressive type of breathlessness with a restrictive pattern of lung function, e.g. alveolitis, alveolar cell and metastic carcinoma.

Type 1 respiratory failure is defined as: $PaO_2 < 8\,kPa$; $PaCO_2 < 6\,kPa$ (BTS, 2002).

Clinical features

Respiratory failure may be associated with a variety of non-specific clinical manifestations, making it present without dramatic signs or symptoms. This emphasises the importance of measuring arterial blood gases in all patients for whom respiratory failure is suspected.

EARLY INDICATORS

- Irritability, clouding of consciousness, confusion.
- Restlessness, anxiety, fatigue.
- Cool and dry skin.
- Increased cardiac output/tachycardia/headache (resulting from stimulation of ventilation via the carotid chemo receptors).

IMMEDIATE INDICATORS

- Confusion/aggression.
- Lethargy.
- Tachypnoea.
- Dyspnoea – arising from respiratory diseases, particularly acute, can also be associated with anxiety and panic, exacerbating the symptoms. Airway disease usually causes a pattern of airflow obstruction, e.g. in asthma and emphysema (Seaton et al., 2000).

- Hypotension.
- Tachycardia, bradycardia and a variety of arrhythmias may result from hypoxaemia and acidosis.

- Cyanosis.
- O_2 saturations – less than 75%.
- Diaphoresis (sweating).
- Coma, convulsions.
- Cardiac arrhythmias.
- Respiratory arrest.

Pulmonary arteries respond to hypoxia by vasoconstriction, producing vascular resistance and pulmonary hypertension. Right ventricular enlargement or right-sided heart failure develops later. Nursing care should be directed at preventing the patient from developing late clinical features, through vigilant monitoring and early, appropriate intervention.

Type 2 respiratory failure (ventilatory)

This type of respiratory failure can be caused by increased airway resistance and reduced lung compliance, e.g. severe asthma, chronic obstructive pulmonary disease (Sharma, 2006). Both O_2 and CO_2 blood levels are affected. As the alveoli are microscopic and prone to collapse, under normal conditions, the secretion of surfactant via the alveolar cells facilitates its expansion during inspiration. However, surfactant production is inhibited by hypoxia, acidosis, poor perfusion, smoking and dry gas such as unhumidified oxygen causing atelectasis.

As a result of alveolar hypoventilation the $PaCO_2$ rises resulting in a fall of PaO_2. Respiratory failure that develops slowly allows renal compensation with retention of bicarbonate, often resulting in a near normal pH. Stretch receptors are located in the bronchial smooth muscle and are stimulated by lung hyperinflation. Impulses are sent to the respiratory centre to limit further inflation (avoiding overdistension of the lung) and increase expiratory time. Therefore, when the patient hypoventilates (taking inadequate volumes of air into their lungs) they should be encouraged to take deep breaths to initiate this process.

Type 2 respiratory failure is defined as: $PaO_2 < 8\,kPa$; $PaCO_2 > 6\,kPa$ (BTS, 2002).

Clinical features

In addition to the signs of hypoxaemia the patient may show clinical signs of hypercapnia:

- irritability, aggression, confusion and coma;
- headaches and papilloedema (CO_2 acts as a vasodilator, increasing cerebral flow);

- warm flushed skin and a bounding pulse (CO_2 can cause vasoconstriction by sympathetic stimulation).

> ## Time out 15.2
>
> 1 Revisit your answers from Time out 15.1 activities.
> 2 Based on the information, write draft guidelines for respiratory assessment.
> 3 Discuss your ideas with your colleagues.

Management

Within hospital, a patient with acute respiratory failure should be admitted to an intensive care unit (DOH, 2000a) or a respiratory care unit, but in reality patients may be cared for in general ward areas. In the community, most patients with chronic respiratory failure can be treated at home with O_2 supplementation and/ or ventilatory-assisting devices along with therapy for their underlying disease.

Identifying the type of respiratory failure will determine the form of intervention. Underlying causes of respiratory failure should be treated (e.g. a chest infection or trauma). The goal of management is to enable adequate oxygen delivery to the tissues, so hypoxaemia must be treated as the first priority. Administration of oxygen (Chapter 19) is the fastest and most effective method of treatment, but will do nothing to improve the $PaCO_2$ and may make it worse (Lumb, 2005). It is, therefore, essential to ensure that palliative relief of hypoxia does not result in hypercapnia and arterial $PaCO_2$ should be monitored.

Acute hypoxaemia requires the use of a reservoir bag at 10–15 litres if initial SpO_2 is below 90%, otherwise simple face masks (BTS, 2008). However, some local policies advocate non-invasive ventilation (NIV) therapy.

Type 2 respiratory failure will require additional support, e.g. bi-level non-invasive ventilation; CPAP (continuous positive airway pressure) or full ventilation. Hypercapnia unaccompanied by hypoxaemia, generally, is well tolerated and probably is not a threat to organ function unless accompanied by severe acidosis (Sharma, 2006). Appropriate management of the underlying disease obviously is an important component in the management of respiratory failure.

Implications for practice

- A comprehensive assessment of the patient's respiratory status should be performed on all patients (by a competent nurse) who have an identified respiratory disorder and those who are classified as acutely/critically ill.
- Assessment should include auscultation.
- Assessment should also be used to identify potential respiratory problems.
- Early intervention is essential in order to improve the prognosis of the patients that have identified respiratory problems.
- Hypoxaemia must be treated as the first priority.

Summary

Respiratory disorders are among the most common reasons for admission to critical care units (DOH, 2000a). Yet, anecdotal evidence suggests that the nursing assessment of respiratory function is not performed very well. Often, it is only when the patient has an identified respiratory problem that this form of assessment may be carried out. It is essential for nurses to be aware of the implications of respiratory problems (from whatever cause) and only through a comprehensive assessment can pro-active interventions be undertaken.

Clinical scenario

John Ross, 55 years old, underwent extensive abdominal surgery three days ago. He looks unwell, and is complaining of severe abdominal pain. He is a known smoker. Documentation suggests that John's abdominal pain has never been under control, making movement/mobility difficult.

John is breathing spontaneously but is dyspnoeic. His respiratory rate is 30 per minute, regular but shallow, and he is using his accessory muscles. He has a cough, which is unproductive. He looks pale, and no central cyanosis is present. Auscultation of the lungs indicate reduced entry at both bases with some coarse crackles in the right mid-zone and widespread expiratory wheeze (also heard without a stethoscope).

John's heart rate is variable (artrial fibrillation), with an approximate rate of 120 bpm. He looks pale and clammy. His blood pressure is 160/110 mmHg, and oxygen saturation levels are 87% on 40% oxygen. Blood gas analysis gives: pH 7.38; PaO_2 7.2 kPa; $PaCO_2$ 4.9 kPa, bicarbonate 23 mEq/litre.

John responds to verbal instructions but appears drowsy. He feels cold and slightly clammy.

1 Identify the type of respiratory failure.

2 What type of nursing/medical intervention will John require?

3 What criteria would you use in order to assess the success of treatment?

Chapter 16

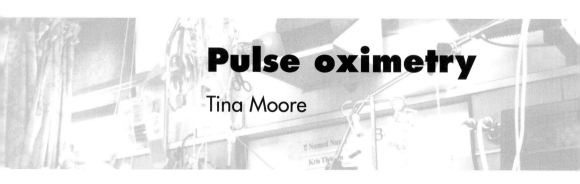

Pulse oximetry

Tina Moore

Contents

Learning outcomes

After reading this chapter you will be able to:

- understand the reasons for using pulse oximetry monitoring;
- demonstrate appropriate use of the pulse oximeter within clinical practice;
- interpret the readings within the context of patient care;
- acknowledge limitations and take appropriate action to minimise these.

Fundamental knowledge

Gaseous exchange; oxygen therapy (Chapter 19).

Introduction

Today, there is more emphasis placed upon the value of pulse oximetry monitoring and is now considered the 'fifth' vital sign (BTS, 2008). Oximeters are now being used in a variety of healthcare settings. The pulse oximeter measures oxygen saturation by differentiating the light absorbance of reduced and oxygenated haemoglobin during arterial pulsations. Some pulse oximeters provide a visual digital waveform and sometimes audible display of arterial pulsation and heart rate. Some have a variety of sensors to accommodate individuals regardless of age, size or weight (Shutz, 2001). Most oximeters found on wards are part of the automated blood pressure monitor.

The uses of pulse oximetry monitoring within the context of acute care will be discussed in this chapter, together with common limitations and strategies suggested to overcome these.

Time out 16.1

1 In any book on physiology, read the respiratory section – particularly the mechanism of breathing and the process of gaseous exchange.
2 Consider why pulse oximeters are used within your area of practice.
3 Discuss the reasons why patients are monitored via this device.

Uses for pulse oximetry

The main function of pulse oximetry is to detect hypoxaemia before it can be detected by sight or before obvious symptoms are displayed. The pulse oximeter provides continuous, non-invasive monitoring of the oxygen saturation from haemoglobin in arterial blood, although, in most areas it is used only for intermittent readings. Where indicated by the patient's condition, continuous monitoring should not be an option but a necessity. It is relatively simple to use and provides immediate results with changes being detected almost straight away.

This monitoring device can be useful in a variety of situations, for example:

- conditions affecting/potentially affecting respiratory status (e.g. acute cardiac failure with pulmonary oedema, acute asthma);
- during diagnostic testing for patients with acute problems (e.g. cardiac or respiratory);
- immediate titration of oxygen therapy (in the absence of arterial blood gas (ABG) (BTS, 2008));
- monitoring for potential hypoxaemia caused by invasive procedures (e.g. suctioning, exercise testing, cardiac catheterisation, bronchoscopy);
- evaluating the effectiveness of oxygen therapy and non-intermittent positive pressure ventilation;
- weaning respiratory support in the absence of arterial blood gases;
- research studies for sleep apnoea.

As pulse oximeters measure the saturation of arterial oxygen and not ventilation or lung performance (e.g. carbon dioxide levels) they will not provide all the answers required when evaluating the patient's ventilatory status. Still they can calculate the SpO_2 status and detect hypoxaemia. When indicated, ABG analysis will be required, to provide additional information such as carbon dioxide, acid base.

How pulse oximetry works

Pulse oximeters measure peripheral arterial blood oxygen saturation (the percentage of haemoglobin filled with oxygen). This is achieved by measuring the absorption of specific wavelengths of light in oxygenated haemoglobin. A probe/sensor (clip-on or adhesive, reusable or disposable) is placed on a site with an adequate pulsating vascular bed, usually the finger (Figure 16.1). One side of the probe has two light-emitting diodes (LED) that transmit red and infrared light wavelengths through pulsating arterial blood to a photo detector on the other side of the probe. The amplitude of light transmitted is measured by the monitor (Figure 16.2) and depends on:

- the volume of the arterial pulse;
- the wavelength of light used;
- oxygen saturation of haemoglobin (Miyasaka, 2003).

The probe needs to be attached to well-perfused (where possible) body parts. In some areas of practice the waveform is used to provide information about the arterial pulsation, so a flattened waveform could indicate a weak pulse.

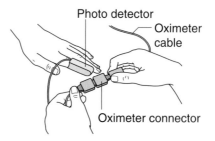

Figure 16.1 **Pulse oximeter probe**

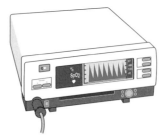

Figure 16.2 **Pulse oximeter monitor**

Oxygen saturation

SaO_2 (abbreviation for saturation of arterial oxygen) is seen on arterial blood gas results, SpO_2 (abbreviation for saturation of peripheral oxygen) and is the value of haemoglobin oxygen saturation as recorded on a pulse oximeter. A saturation of 95% means that 95 per cent of the total amount of haemoglobin in the blood contains oxygen molecules. However, not all patients with the same SpO_2 levels actually have the same amount of oxygen in their blood. Consider two patients, both of whose saturations are 90%. One has an Hb of 6 g/dl and the other of 12 g/dl. The second patient has nearly double the amount of haemoglobin and hence the potential for more oxygen molecules. Therefore, interpretation of the SpO_2 should be carried out within the context of the whole patient profile.

A SpO_2 between 94% and 98% is generally considered to be the normal range for patients below 70 years; 92% and 98% for patients above 70 years and 88% and 92% for those at risk of hypercapnic respiratory failure (BTS, 2008). For some patients above 70 years, a SpO_2 of 94% may be normal and, therefore, they do not require oxygen therapy when clinically stable (BTS, 2008). A result below 90% needs to be taken note of as this could indicate life-threatening conditions, e.g. respiratory failure. However, it is important to interpret results based on as much information about the patient as is possible because normal values vary. When monitoring a patient with pulse oximetry there is a need to establish a baseline and confirm the accuracy of readings by using ABG analysis.

If the patient demonstrates a decrease in SpO_2, assess the patient to determine if intervention is necessary (it could be that the problem is mechanical, i.e. the machine and not the patient). Some treatments result in a decrease in SpO_2 levels, e.g. after suctioning. If the cause of the decreasing SpO_2 cannot be found, the patient's lungs should be auscultated for signs that can indicate fluid or consolidation (Chapter 15). The aim is to rule out any conditions that could decrease arterial oxygenation. ABG analysis may be indicated to determine the underlying cause of the change in SpO_2 levels. Current BTS guidelines provide direction when this may be necessary (BTS, 2008). Increasing SpO_2 levels generally indicate improvement in oxygenation.

Where to place the probe

Manufacturers' guidelines on where to place the probe need to be followed (different devices are designed for different parts of the body). The probe should ideally be placed on an area that is well perfused. This may be difficult,

Time out 16.2

Reflect on situations when you have used pulse oximetry monitoring.

1 What was the rationale for its use?
2 What limitations did you identify in this method of monitoring?
3 How were these limitations overcome?

particularly with the critically ill patient whose saturations need to be monitored. A finger probe is usually the best to use with an adult patient. Alternative routes include the toe and ear lobe. The probe should be moved at least every four hours, to prevent pressure sores or thermal damage (MDA, 2001).

Limitations of use

Despite the many uses of pulse oximetry, there are a number of limitations/factors that influence the accuracy of both technological and physiological readings.

It is well documented that pulse oximeters become unreliable with low SpO_2 (when needed the most). If clinical signs do not give cause for concern there may be problems with connection power sources that need to be checked. Again it is important for the nurse to follow the manufacturer guidelines on using the pulse oximeter.

Table 16.1 offers a quick guide to how to deal with problems in the use of oximetry.

Other factors that may influence the reading include:

- Intravenous dyes used in cardiac output studies which tint the blood and give a lower level reading. Clarification should be sought from the appropriate department in relation to:
  - the type of dye affecting pulse oximetry readings;
  - how long the dye is likely to affect the readings;
  - in what way the readings are affected.
- High levels of carboxyhaemoglobin in patients who smoke (falsely elevated readings).
- High serum bilirubin level (falsely low reading).
- Dark-skinned pigmentation introduces a positive bias of low oxygen saturation (Feiner *et al.*, 2007).

Implications for practice

- Pulse oximetry offers a simple, reliable way to continuously monitor the patients.
- The limitations of pulse oximetry must be acknowledged and appropriate strategies used to reduce/eradicate them.
- Nurses should not rely on pulse oximeter monitoring alone and should analyse data obtained from respiratory assessment (e.g. hypercapnia which may occur in patients with COPD).
- This approach to monitoring should not replace the need for arterial blood gas analysis when indicated.
- Pulse oximetry is inappropriate to use on patients with carbon monoxide poisoning.
- Positioning the probe on the finger will usually provide the best recordings.
- Caution needs to be exercised when monitoring patients with abnormal haemoglobins (e.g. anaemia).
- Pulse oximetry readings must be analysed in the context of the whole person.

Table 16.1 Problems associated with pulse oximetry use

Interference with reading	Appropriate intervention
There is still considerable debate as to whether nail varnish actually affects accuracy of reading. Current evidence suggests that the darker colours, e.g. blue, black, green influence recordings (Hinkelbein et al., 2007). Either way nail polish should be removed as it interferes with patient assessment of hypoxaemia.	Remove all nail polish with nail polish remover. This should be standard practice to enable monitoring of the patient's colour and capillary refill time.
Dark skin reduces the accuracy of pulse oximeters and low oxygen saturation (Fiener et al., 2007).	
Poor perfusion/vasoconstriction, caused by weak pulses, hypotension and hypothermia will cause low, intermittent or unavailable readings.	Warm patient's extremities with a blanket or a warmer pack (leave for a short time to avoid heat injury).
Sudden movements and restlessness may cause the sensor to become partially dislodged, or cause motion artefact (Patterson et al., 2007). This will cause the ability of the light to travel from the LED to the photo detector. Rhythmic movement (e.g. seizures, shivering) may also cause problems.	Explain the importance of keeping still; if the patient is unable to, consider moving the probe to the ear lobe as this may be the most suitable place, as movement least affects the probe.
Interference with the transmission of light – may be caused by dirt (e.g. dried blood).	Keep the patient's skin and the equipment clean.
Pressure sore/thermal damage.	Change the probe position at least every four hours (MDA, 2001) and observe skin.
Research on the effects of bright light (including direct sunlight, fluorescent lights, surgical lamps) shining directly on the sensor probe interfering with the readings remain inconclusive.	Remove the source of light to correct the problem.
Optical shunting occurs when the probe is positioned badly and the light goes directly from the LED to the photo detector missing the vascular bed.	Check position and reposition if indicated.

continued

Table 16.1 continued

Interference with reading	Appropriate intervention
Abnormal haemoglobins can occur in patients with carbon monoxide poisoning due to smoke inhalation. The sensor cannot differentiate between oxyhaemoglobin and carboxyhaemoglobin and will, therefore, provide a falsely evaluated SpO_2 reading.	Do not monitor such patients; ABG analysis should be undertaken instead.
Severe anaemia greater when haemoglobin levels fall to 3 g/dl (Lumb, 2005).	
Equipment malfunction/ Damaged/Poorly positioned probe.	Check the signal strength indicator. A dampened waveform could indicate a reduction in arterial flow, a misaligned sensor could also cause it. In this case the probe will need to be repositioned.
Dysrhythmias.	Test the equipment on yourself or another healthy person. Correlate the pulse reading with the patient's heart rate (if there is a variance it could indicate that not all pulsations are being picked up). Send blood for ABG analysis. A replacement monitor may be indicated.
Intermittent blood flow.	Check pulse rate and capillary refill time.
Possible skin damage from probe sheath.	Check the position and security of the probe. Rotate/transfer the probe to different sites at least four hourly (MDA, 2001).
Alterations to recordings occur when Dynamap® (blood pressure cuff) is used on the same limb.	The pulse oximeter sensor needs to be placed on a finger of the opposite side, as blood flow to the finger will be cut off whenever the cuff inflates. Readings will be inaccurate.

Summary

The benefits of pulse oximetry monitoring are greater than its limitations, as many of these limitations can be overcome through appropriate usage/application. However, it must be remembered that there are certain conditions where it is inappropriate/inadvisable to rely on pulse oximetry readings alone. In this instance ABG monitoring is desirable.

Clinical scenario

Michael Cormer, 34 years old, is admitted to the acute care unit following a three-week history of acute weight loss, shortness of breath and persistent coughing. On admission he is dysponeic, skin colour is pale. He is receiving 35% of oxygen via a facemask.

Assessment data

Blood pressure	130/72 mmHg
Heart rate	130 – sinus tachycardia
Temperature	37.9°C
Respiratory rate	28/minute, very shallow
Oxygen saturations	93%
Haemoglobin	10.7 g/dl

Following a chest x-ray a diagnosis of bilateral pneumothorax had been made. In view of the history and clinical picture the medical staff suspects that Michael has pneumocystis carinii pnuemonia (PCP).

1   Identify the reasons for using pulse oximetry monitoring.

2   Devise a plan of care that is required to ensure safe use of this monitoring device.

3   During the shift Michael's condition deteriorates. He becomes severely dyspnoeic, respiratory rate is 52 per minute, using accessory muscles. Oxygen saturation drops to 80%, heart rate 160 sinus tachycardia. His skin colour is pale and he feels cold and clammy when touched. Evaluate the appropriateness of relying on pulse oximetry readings in Michael's situation.

Chapter 17

Arterial blood gas analysis

Tina Moore

Contents

Learning outcomes

After reading this chapter you will be able to:

- apply knowledge of blood gas analysis safely in the clinical area;
- recognise common acid base disorders;
- understand the treatment for these disorders.

Fundamental knowledge

Respiratory anatomy and physiology (including gas exchange).

Introduction

Arterial blood gas (ABG) analysis is an established method of assessing respiratory and metabolic status. Accurate interpretation of ABG is vital. Nurses providing acute and critical care need to know normal values, causes and associated treatment of abnormal results. This chapter discusses the disorders in acid base balance most commonly presenting in the acutely/critically ill patient.

Respiratory physiology

The control of ventilation occurs through voluntary and involuntary mechanisms. Voluntary control of the muscles of respiration is regulated through the central nervous system (CNS). Here, a person is able to have conscious control over their own breathing rate. Involuntary ventilation depends on the respiratory centre (medulla oblongata and pons). The respiratory centre transmits impulses to the respiratory muscles, causing contraction and relaxation. Normally, carbon dioxide (CO_2) is the main respiratory stimulant. When $PaCO_2$ levels rise the respiratory centre is stimulated to increase the rate and depth of breathing, resulting in increased excretion of CO_2. Low $PaCO_2$ levels eventually inhibit stimulation of the respiratory centre, resulting in an initial increase in the respiratory rate, but eventually becoming slower and shallower. This aids retention of CO_2 to achieve homeostasis. PaO_2 and $PaCO_2$ are guides used to measure O_2 and CO_2 within the blood.

Patients with chronic obstructive pulmonary disease (COPD), through eventual lung damage have alterations in gas exchange. Here, central chemoreceptors become tolerant of high levels of CO_2, relying on hypoxia to stimulate the respiratory drive (hypoxic drive). If these patients are given too much oxygen (O_2) this drive will be inhibited causing respiratory failure and possibly respiratory arrest.

Arterial stab

Indications for ABG analysis are to:

- establish the diagnosis and severity of respiratory failure (limitations of pulse oximetry);
- evaluate interventions;
- manage critically ill patients;
- assess condition immediately following CPR;
- establish a baseline for surgery.

ABGs are only valuable if obtained properly and measured carefully. Some practices indicate that patients should have a stable flow of oxygen for at least 20 minutes before sampling to allow the PaO_2 to equilibrate. Note patient's position, respiratory rate and pattern as the PaO_2 may change significantly with varying body positioning (usually worse in supine position).

For this procedure, blood is usually taken via the radial artery. It is a superficial artery with easy access (making it easier to palpate, stabilise and puncture). The radial artery also has a collateral blood flow (i.e. if damage or obstruction occurs, the ulnar artery will then supply blood to the tissues). Collateral blood flow is confirmed by the Allen test (performed by elevating the hand, occluding both ulnar and radial arteries and releasing compression of the ulnar artery). If adequate collateral circulation is present the hand should flush pink within 5–7 seconds. However, this is difficult to determine in dark-skinned patients.

The pain from an arterial stab must never be underestimated. Informed consent should be obtained (if able). Local anaesthesia can be administered but in practice this seldom occurs. For more frequent measurements an arterial line should be inserted, although these are still rare on general ward areas.

Pre-prepared syringes should be used to obtain the sample (0.5–1 ml of aspirated blood). There should be no air bubbles in the sample syringe. When large air bubbles are mixed with arterial blood, the PaO_2 rises and the $PaCO_2$ usually falls (Marini and Wheeler, 2006).

This procedure involves a high risk of bleeding; therefore, extreme caution should be taken with patients who have bleeding/clotting disorders. At least 5 minutes' pressure should be applied once the needle as been withdrawn, allowing for collapse of the artery and the clotting process to occur. Vigorous shaking of the sample bottle should be avoided as it causes haemolysis. A gentle rolling motion is adequate. The sample should be analysed within 15 minutes (in room temperature), otherwise changes will occur with a rise in $PaCO_2$ and fall in PaO_2 as cells within the syringe continue to metabolise and use O_2.

Patient's sample site and associated limb should be monitored for signs of ischaemic changes (as a result of arterial thrombosis). This can be avoided by varying the sample sites; using the smallest needle possible and confirming good collateral blood flow before cannulation. Nerve trauma and compressive haematoma may occur.

Acid base physiology

pH: normal 7.35–7.45

In chemical terms, pH ranges from a scale of 0 (absolute acid) to 14 (absolute alkaline). The pH concentration of ions measures the acidity or alkalinity in the blood. Human blood is slightly alkaline. A person's well-being depends upon their ability to maintain a normal pH, any deviation can be potentially life threatening. Blood pH below 7.35 is considered acidotic, above 7.45 is considered alkalotic.

The two major organs that regulate acid base balance are the lungs (respiratory) and kidneys (metabolic). The normal by-product of cellular metabolism is CO_2. CO_2 is carried in the blood to the lungs, excess CO_2 combines with the water (H_2O) to form carbonic acid (H_2CO_3), which is a weak acid. The pH will change according to levels of carbonic acid present. This triggers the lung to increase or decrease the rate and depth of ventilation until an appropriate level of CO_2 is established.

Acids are chemicals that can release hydrogen ions (H^+). pH is inversely proportional to the number of hydrogen ions in the blood. So, as H^+ accumulates the pH decreases. H^+ is considered the fuel of life and combines with O_2 to make water. H^+ concentration is critical to the activity of cellular enzymes. Free hydrogen ions are present in the body fluids in extremely low concentrations.

Despite this they are small and highly reactive. Alkalis are chemicals that absorb hydrogen ions. A decrease in H^+ elevates the pH level.

In an effort to maintain the pH within its normal range the kidneys excrete or retain bicarbonate (HCO_3). Reduced levels in blood pH result in retention in HCO_3; increased levels cause excretion of HCO_3.

Anything that interferes with normal functioning of the body (e.g. shock) can disturb acid base balance, therefore, the critically ill patients are at risk of developing problems with acid base imbalances.

It must be noted that the pH does not tell us if the problem is respiratory or metabolic.

ABG analysis

There are four main groups that are analysed:

1   pH
2   respiratory function (oxygen, carbon dioxide, saturation)
3   metabolic measures (bicarbonate, base excess)
4   electrolytes and metabolites (not discussed within this chapter).

In the UK gases are almost always measured in kilopascals (kPa).

Respiratory acidosis (pH < 7.35; $PaCO_2$ > 6.0 kPa)

Respiratory acidosis occurs when alveolar ventilation is insufficient to excrete the metabolic production of CO_2. Therefore, an accumulation of CO_2 takes place. Any condition that causes ventilatory failure can cause respiratory acidosis. These include: CNS depression (e.g. head injury); excessive use of sedatives; impaired respiratory muscle function; atelectasis; pneumonia; massive pulmonary embolism; pain; abdominal distension.

Symptoms include:

- dyspnoea/respiratory distress/hypoventilation
- headache (due to vasodilatation of cerebral vessels)
- restlessness/confusion
- possibly drowsiness/unconsciousness
- tachycardia and dysrhythmias.

Time out 17.1

A 23-year-old male has been admitted, diagnosed with pneumonia. He shows signs of central cyanosis and is dyspnoeic. Arterial gas shows hypoxaemia together with pH 7.29, $PaCO_2$ > 6.0 kPa, HCO_3 26 mmol/litre. Consider what intervention is required.

Intervention is primarily to treat the underlying cause and to increase ventilation. Oxygen therapy will probably be indicated. The patient should be taught how to take deep breaths.

Respiratory alkalosis (pH > 7.45; PaCO₂ < 4.9 kPa)

This occurs when there is alveolar hyperventilation and an excessive loss of CO_2. Any condition that causes hyperventilation can result in respiratory alkalosis. Common causes include: anxiety, fear, fever, sepsis, respiratory stimulants.

Symptoms include:

- light-headedness
- numbness, tingling, confusion, inability to concentrate
- dysrhythmias/palpations
- dry mouth/diaphoreses.

Time out 17.2

A 46-year-old female admitted with a thyroid crisis developed a severe panic attack in the water, while snorkelling with her family. She is hyperventilating (respiratory rate is 44 per minute) and is complaining of dizziness. Blood profile indicates pH 7.54, $PaCO_2$ > 3.8 kPa, HCO_3 27 mmol/litre. What intervention is required?

The aim of treatment is to control the increase in respiratory rate. Patients should be monitored closely for signs of exhaustion respiratory muscle fatigue as reparatory failure can follow.

Metabolic acidosis (HCO₃ < 22 mmol/litre; pH < 7.35)

Metabolic acidosis is the failure to remove/buffer sufficient H^+. This is usually caused by excessive production/accumulation of acids: renal, lactic and ketones. Causes include: diabetic ketoacidosis (production of ketoacids); renal failure (impaired excretion of acids from the kidney); gastrointestinal tract problems (especially associated with the colon's inability to secrete bicarbonate into the gut); loss of base (associated with diarrhoea, intestinal fistulas). It may also be caused by an inadequate buffer system (liver failure).

Metabolic acidosis should be considered a sign of an underlying disease process (Hipp and Sinert, 2008)

Symptoms include:

- headache/confusion/restlessness/increasing lethargy;
- stupor/coma;
- cardiac dysrhythmias;
- Kussmaul respirations (caused by a low pH that causes hyperventilation (as

bodies attempt to 'blow off' carbon dioxide and compensate for acidosis), respiratory rate and depth are increased;

■ warm flushed skin/nausea/vomiting;
■ respiratory depression.

Time out 17.3

A patient has been admitted, diagnosed with DKA. She is drowsy but responsive to pain. Pulse – 136 beats/minute; BP 94/67 mmHg, temperature 39.2°C, respirations – 35/minute. Blood values indicate metabolic acidosis: pH 7.12; HCO_3 8.9 mmol/litre; $PaCO_2$ 2.6 kPa and glucose 34 mmol/litre. Consider the intervention.

The aim of treatment is again to control/treat the underlying cause. The initial goal is to increase the pH above 7.1. Severe acidaemia, i.e. pH <7.10 is potentially fatal, causing ventricular arrhythmias and reduced cardiac contractility. Bicarbonate is not normally given unless in severe acidaemia.

Metabolic alkalosis ($HCO_3 > 26$ mmol/litre; pH > 7.45)

Metabolic alkalosis happens when plasma bicarbonate is increased, often caused by an excessive loss of metabolic acids. Causes include lactate administration in dialysis; excessive ingestion of antacids; loss of acids: vomiting, excessive nasogastric suctioning, hypokalaemia, administration of diuretics.

Symptoms include:

■ muscle twitching and cramps
■ dizziness
■ lethargy
■ disorientation
■ convolutions/coma
■ nausea and vomiting.

Time out 17.4

A 30-year-old patient with a long-standing history of peptic ulceration has refused surgical intervention. He is admitted with uncontrolled vomiting. Clinically he is dehydrated. Blood profile shows potassium 2.7 mmol/litre; pH 7.59; HCO_3 43 mmol/litre; $PaCO_2$ 5.2 kPa. Discuss the intervention.

This is the most difficult disorder to treat. Again, treat the underlying cause. In severe cases IV administration of acids may be used.

In all cases, by identifying and treating indicates that these disorders are almost always a secondary problem to a primary complaint. Therefore, nurses must monitor the patient's response to intervention very carefully.

Compensation

In order to maintain homeostasis (pH 7.35–7.45) the body has to try and compensate for the abnormality. If the normal process (buffer system) fails to maintain a normal pH the renal or respiratory systems will attempt to compensate. Here, the opposite system will compensate (blood values will not be as we expect them to be, i.e. movement in the opposite direction). So, if the problem is respiratory in origin the kidneys will compensate. Equally, if the original problem is renal, the respiratory system will compensate. Respiratory compensation can occur much quicker than renal, sometimes taking as little as 10 minutes, while renal compensation may take a few days (potentially up to a week). Overcompensation does not happen.

When an acid base disorder is either uncompensated or partially compensated, the pH remains outside the normal range. Full compensation states the pH has returned within the normal range although the other values may still be abnormal.

Carbon dioxide (PaCO₂) (normal 4.5–6.0 kPa)

Carbon dioxide is produced by body cells as a waste product of metabolism and indicates the quality of alveolar ventilation. The respiratory centre in the brain stem responds primarily to the level of $PaCO_2$, but in patients with COPD it is the hypoxic drive that stimulates.

A relationship exists between the amount of ventilation and the amount of CO_2 in the blood. For example, if a patient hypoventilates CO_2 accumulates and increases above the upper parameters and produces hypercapnia ($CO_2 > 6.0$ kPa (BTS, 2002)).

Hypercapnia dilates cerebral vessels and becomes problematic with patients who have raised intracranial pressure (Malini and Wheeler, 2006). Extreme levels may induce muscular twitching and seizures. Mild forms of hypercapnia may be desirable in the acute phases of critical illness as it reduces tissue metabolism, improves surfactant function and prevents nitration of proteins (Malini and Wheeler, 2006).

Hyperventilation leads to hypocapnia (due to CO_2 being eliminated from the body), eventually causing respiratory alkalosis. Hypocapnia constricts cerebral vessels, raises neuronal pH and reduces available ionised calcium causing disturbances in cortical and peripheral nerve functioning (McCance and Huether, 2006). Light-headedness, fingertip parasthesia and muscular tetany may also occur.

Oxygen (PaO₂) (normal – 11.5–13.5 kPa)

The diffusion of O_2 is dependent upon a normal airway diameter, adequate respiratory rate/depth and a functioning nervous supply. Chemoreceptors that are located in the circulatory system and brain stem sense the effectiveness of ventilation by monitoring the pH status of the cerebrospinal fluid, oxygen content (PaO_2) and carbon dioxide ($PaCO_2$) content of the arterial blood. These respond to hypercapnia, acidaemia and hypoxaemia by sending impulses to the medulla to alter the rate of ventilation.

Oxygen is vital for the survival of cells. PaO_2 is the partial pressure of oxygen that is dissolved in arterial blood. It is less soluble than carbon dioxide and, therefore, more likely to be altered first when the patient's condition deteriorates. Hypoxaemia (Chapter 19) can occur as a result of Type 1 respiratory failure; it can also be caused by hypoventilation.

Prolonged use of high concentrations of oxygen can cause hyperoxic and toxic damage. The problem with hyperoxia is usually iatrogenic (treatment induced, i.e. oxygen therapy).

Oxygen saturation (normal – 95%)

Oxygen saturation (SaO_2) is the amount of O_2 carried in haemoglobin which is not reflected in the PaO_2 value. For example in smoke inhalation, the patient could have a normal SaO_2 and a low PaO_2 simultaneously.

Bicarbonate (normal – 24–27 mmol/litre)

Bicarbonate (HCO_3) is the main chemical buffer in plasma. It is produced mainly in the liver and kidneys. Its function is to help regulate pH. Bicarbonate levels indicate metabolic acid base status. Low levels of bicarbonate indicate extensive buffering or impaired liver failure.

Base excess

Base excess measures the number of moles of acid or base needed to return 1 litre of blood to pH of 7.4. Base indicates the amount of excess or insufficient level of the main base (bicarbonate) in the system. This is a metabolic process as the kidneys regulate this process. The normal range is between –2 to +2, with zero being a neutral score.

Therefore, too little bicarbonate in the blood indicates metabolic acidosis and produces a negative base. Too much bicarbonate indicates metabolic alkalosis and produces a positive base.

Interpreting ABG

Interpreting ABG results is a skill that can take time to develop. By examining each variable in turn, it is possible to monitor a patient's clinical condition and any response to treatment. Box 17.1 highlights certain questions to ask when interpreting results.

On occasions, venous sampling may be taken, on purpose or by mistake. Venous samples are one way of quickly measuring electrolytes. Venous blood gases have a lower pH, lower PaO_2 and slightly increased $PaCO_2$ values.

If venous samples are taken, they should be clearly labelled as such (as most machines automatically label 'arterial' unless instructed otherwise). The possible consequence is that a venous printout may be misinterpreted as arterial, therefore, too much oxygen may be administered.

Box 17.1 Questions to ask

- Look at the pH – is there acidaemia or alkalaemia?
- Look at the $PaCO_2$ – is it high, low or normal?
- Look at the PaO_2 and SaO_2 – is the patient hypoxaemic?
- Look at the HCO_3 – is it high, low or normal?
- Is there compensation occurring. Is it complete, partial or uncompensated?

Implications for practice

- Nurses should understand the need for arterial blood gas monitoring.
- Knowledge of ABG analysis is necessary in order to monitor the patient's response to treatment.
- Care when monitoring and interpretation of the patient's physiological symptoms is important as patient may necessitate transfer to ICU.

Summary

When acutely ill patients become critically ill they may require arterial blood gas analysis in order to initiate, maintain or readjust treatment. Although nurses should not be taking samples in the general ward areas, receipt of the results is part of their role. Nurses should, therefore, understand the principles of ABG analysis, to enable the prompt recognition of abnormal results and appropriate safe action.

Chapter 18

Respiratory pathologies

Philip Woodrow

Contents

Learning outcomes

After reading this chapter you will be able to:

- understand the main pathologies causing acute respiratory disease;
- provide evidence-based care for patients with these conditions;
- identify patients' needs to junior colleagues.

Fundamental knowledge

Respiratory failure; respiratory assessment (Chapter 15).

Introduction

Respiratory disease is increasing, currently being the cause of death of one in five people in the UK (BTS, 2006). This chapter describes pathologies that more often necessitate or complicate adult admission to acute wards. Gas exchange in the lungs relies on

■ ventilation (volume of air reaching alveoli)
■ perfusion (volume of blood in pulmonary capillaries) and
■ diffusion (exchange of gases between the two).

Respiratory disease can occur when one or more of these are inadequate.

Chronic disease is largely irreversible, needing prolonged (often community) care. However, people with chronic lung disease are particularly susceptible to acute exacerbations from infection or other factors. So acute care of chronic obstructive pulmonary disease (COPD), emphysema and asthma are discussed. This chapter then focuses on acute pathologies:

■ pneumothorax
■ pleural effusion
■ pulmonary embolus.

Although many diseases can cause breathlessness, hypoxia and distress, there are two types of respiratory failure:

■ Type 1 (hypoxaemia + normocapnia; $PaO_2 < 8\,kPa + PaCO_2 < 6\,kPa$)
■ Type 2 (hypoxaemia + hypercapnia; $PaO_2 < 8\,kPa + PaCO_2 > 6\,kPa$).

(BTS, 2002; see Chapter 15)

This chapter does discuss diseases, medical tests and treatments, but focus remains on nursing rather than medical aspects of care. More detailed discussion of medical aspects may be found in medical texts. Problems experienced by different patients with similar conditions will vary, so care should be individualised to each person, to meet all their needs.

Chronic obstructive pulmonary disease (COPD)

COPD is a chronic group of diseases usually caused by smoking, causing progressive permanent limitation to airflow into lungs that is usually (eventually) fatal. COPD is the sixth most common cause of death in England and Wales (Fehrenbach, 2002), causing 10–15 per cent of hospital admissions (Polkey, 2008). Incidence is rising, and expected to continue to rise (Polkey, 2008). COPD is usually either

■ chronic bronchitis (85 per cent) or
■ emphysema (15 per cent).

(Bach *et al.*, 2001)

Although respiratory disease can occur at any age, chronic limitations and disease tend to occur in later life due to changes in body tissue (airways, vasculature or interstitial) that impair gas exchange. Some changes inevitably result from ageing, but healthy ageing alone should not cause respiratory disease. Toxic damage from inhaled pollutants (cigarette smoke, environmental pollutants or other chemicals) causes nearly all chronic respiratory conditions.

COPD increases right ventricular workload, which usually causes right-sided hypertrophy (causing peaked P waves) and heart failure (*cor pulmonale*). Breathlessness often limits mobility, social life, eating and drinking. Sufferers are typically malnourished, dehydrated and emaciated. Limited airflow causes shallow breathing, making static lung bases a reservoir for developing acute chest infections. Acute exacerbations create additional problems, so care should

- maintain normal activities of living (as far as possible);
- prevent further complications;
- reverse the acute problem.

Poor quality of life may lead to depression.

Care should be individualised, but usually first-line treatments for acute exacerbations are:

- oxygen (GOLD Executive Summary, 2007), often high-flow;
- positioning upright, to aid diaphragm expansion;
- monitoring;
- providing as calm an atmosphere as reasonably possible.

Second-line treatments are:

- drugs (e.g. bronchodilators, steroids, antibiotics)
- ventilatory support (e.g. non-invasive ventilation)
- deep-breathing exercises and physiotherapy
- encouraging expectoration.

For people with hypercapnic respiratory failure, oxygen should be given to achieve target saturations of 88–92%, with an upper limit of 28% oxygen (BTS, 2008), except in emergencies or a very few specified conditions.

Arterial blood gases should be taken 60 minutes after commencing oxygen (GOLD Executive Summary, 2007), so if carbon dioxide levels increase, respiratory depression may have occurred, and oxygen may need to be replaced with non-invasive ventilation. Nebulisers should be driven with air (BTS, 2008).

Various medical tests may be performed to measure respiratory function. While spirometry is probably the most useful, peak flow monitoring is simple and widely used (Booker, 2007). With respiratory rate and depth and oxygen saturation, peak flow monitoring should form part of regular nursing observations for patients with COPD. Respiratory function (e.g. arterial blood gases, lung function tests such as FEV_1) should be assessed before discharge. People with COPD who have suffered hypercapnic respiratory failure should be given an alert card before discharge (BTS, 2008).

With acute respiratory failure from COPD the best treatment is non-invasive ventilation (NIV – see Chapter 23), which should be used before severe acidosis develops (RCP/BTS/ICS, 2008).

Stopping smoking and oxygen therapy are almost the only intervention that can prolong survival (Institute for Clinical Systems Improvement, 2006). While acute exacerbations can be treated, longer-term care for patients should include education about their disease, how to minimise further damage and exacerbations and, with advanced disease, preparation for the almost-inevitable end (Scullion, 2008). Teams treating acute admissions should consider to what extent active treatments, as opposed to palliation, are justified. For example, it may be appropriate to make non-invasive ventilation, or other interventions, 'ceiling' treatment. Each patient should, therefore, be assessed individually.

As COPD is progressive, before discharge a blood gas should be taken to assess whether long-term oxygen therapy (LTOT) is needed. For most people with COPD, NICE (2004b) and GOLD (2007) recommend LTOT if PaO_2 is 7.3 kPa or below.

Emphysema

Damage to distal airways and alveoli causes permanent distension, with loss of elasticity (compliance), severely impairing exchange of both oxygen and carbon dioxide. Acute emphysematous damage may be caused by excessive respiratory effort from diseases such as bronchopneumonia, asthma or tuberculosis. Chronic emphysema is usually caused by smoking (Hogg and Senior, 2002). Once diagnosed, damage is irreversible and usually extensive. Interventions for chronic emphysema are largely limited to alleviating acute exacerbations and supporting activities of living. Lung reduction surgery (removing the least functional quarter of the lung to allow expansion of the remaining portion) may improve function and so quality and quantity of life.

People with emphysema usually have co-existing COPD, so medical management for the two diseases is similar. However, by the time patients need hospital admission, the disease may be nearing its end-stage, so while medical management of emphysema and COPD are similar, patients with emphysema may need more psychological and social support.

Asthma

Asthma is a common condition, affecting more than five million people in the UK, one in 13 adults and one in eight children (Asthma UK, 2008), and causing 1,600 deaths each year (Wort, 2003). Although UK incidence is particularly high, worldwide rates are increasing (Holgate and Polosa, 2006). Attacks are not usually severe enough to necessitate hospital admission, but one-tenth of asthmatics seen in A&E departments are admitted to hospital, one-tenth of these needing invasive ventilation (FitzGerald, 2001).

In people with hyper-responsive airways (Borger *et al.*, 2006), triggers (e.g. smoking, pollution, cold air, pet hair, house mites, pollens, moulds, drugs, vigorous exercise) cause

■ spasm of bronchiole smooth muscle
■ oedema
■ increased mucous secretion,

resulting in narrowing and mucous plugging of small airways (Sim, 2002). One-tenth of adult asthma is occupational (Zacharisen, 2002). Drugs such as beta-blockers, aspirin and non-steroidal anti-inflammatories (NSAIDs) release mediators that cause bronchoconstriction, so may trigger asthma attacks. Although excessive excitement, fear and anxiety do not cause asthma, they may exacerbate it (Reinke and Hoffman, 2000).

Increased work of breathing (WOB) causes respiratory muscle fatigue (Sim, 2002) and distress/panic. Excessive parasympathetic stimulation on inspiration may cause pulsus paradoxus – systolic blood pressure falling more than 10 mmHg on inspiration (Sim, 2002).

BTS/SIGN (2008) define acute severe asthma (in adults) as having one of the following symptoms:

■ peak expiratory flow (PEF) 33–50 per cent of best or predicted;
■ respiratory rate ≥25/min;
■ heart rate ≥110/min;
■ inability to complete sentences in one breath.

Typically, airway responses occur on inspiration, trapping air in the lower airways and causing a distinctive expiratory wheeze as air is forced out through very constricted airways. Auscultation may reveal a 'silent wheeze'. Spirometry is the best initial test to assess severity of airflow obstruction (BTS/SIGN, 2008).

Acute asthma attacks should be treated with

■ high-concentration oxygen
■ nebulised beta-2 agonists (e.g. salbutamol)
■ steroids,

aiming to achieve oxygen saturation >92% (BTS/SIGN, 2008). If possible, nebulisers should be driven by oxygen, 6 litres/minute (BTS/SIGN, 2008). If SpO_2 is below 92%, arterial blood gas should be analysed (BTS/SIGN, 2008). Routine antibiotics should not be given, but intravenous magnesium may be effective (BTS/SIGN, 2008). Salbutamol can cause hypokalaemia, so serum potassium should be measured and if necessary corrected (BTS/SIGN, 2008). If severe asthma causes hypercapnia, urgent ICU admission is usually necessary (BTS/SIGN, 2008).

Asthma attacks are frightening, causing the person to fight for breath. Gas exchange is poor. Hypoxia may cause acute confusion. Ensuring as calm an atmosphere as possible, with information and support, can help reduce stress. Empowering patients, rather than making them passive recipients of care, can reduce distress. Sedatives which cause respiratory depression, such as morphine, may prove fatal, so should not be given. Instead of trying to treat the symptom of fear, treatment should reverse the asthma which causes the fear (Rees and Kanabar, 2000).

Perspiration and tachypnoea often cause excessive fluid loss, resulting in hypovolaemia (Sim, 2002), so fluids should be given. Sim (2002) recommends giving crystalloids, but where rapid infusion of crystalloids may exacerbate oedema, colloids may be preferred.

Asthma is often poorly controlled (Holgate and Polosa, 2006), although high-profile initiatives have significantly improved both hospital and community care. With recovery, health education may be needed to help people control their asthma and prevent further attacks (Smaha, 2001), although Paley (2000) found that some asthmatics felt guilty for 'failing' to control their asthma. Asthmatics who stop smoking show significant functional improvement in as little as six weeks (Chaudhuri *et al.*, 2006), so help and advice should be offered. Weight reduction also significantly reduces the disease (BTS/SIGN, 2008).

Pneumothorax

A pneumothorax is gas or air in the pleural space. The pleura form the two outer layers of the lung, separated by 5–10 ml of pleural fluid. Any damage to the pleura, whether from trauma or disease (spontaneous), may allow extra-pleural contents to accumulate between the pleura, resulting in severe respiratory distress. Fluids in the pleural space – blood (haemothorax) or pus (pyothorax) – cause similar problems, so although technically incorrect, in this chapter and often in practice, 'pneumothorax' refers to any abnormal volume accumulating between pleura.

Primary pneumothoraces occur in otherwise healthy people, often young, whereas secondary pneumothoraces occur in people with pre-existing lung disease (Henry *et al.*, 2003). Spontaneous pneumothorax may be identified by noticing that patients are breathing asymmetrically (see Chapter 15).

Pneumothoraces may be

- simple or
- tension.

Tension pneumothorax occurs when ruptured pleura remain open, creating a one-way valve. Each breath draws more air or fluid into the pleural space (due to negative intrathoracic pressure), but the valve (tension) prevents it leaving on expiration. Tension pneumothoraces are a life-threatening emergency.

Increased intrathoracic pressure on the side of the pneumothorax may shift the mediastinum towards the opposite side – often seen on chest x-rays, and causing cardiac tamponade and shock.

Smaller (<20 per cent) pneumothoraces may spontaneously resolve, but larger ones require needle aspiration or a chest drain (see Chapter 21). A chest drain creates an escape valve, so transforming a tension pneumothorax into a simple one.

Recurrent spontaneous pneumothoraces should be resolved by video-assisted thoracic (minimally invasive) pleurodesis, removing blebs and bullae at the lung apex to prevent further leaks progressing to a pneumothorax (Treasure, 2007). 'Talc' pleurodesis is the most widely used agent for pleurodesis (Janssen et al., 2007).

Pleural effusion

Pleural effusion is plasma-like fluid accumulating in the pleural space. It may be

- transudative or
- exudative.

Transudation is caused through either increased intracapillary pressure or reduced oncotic pressure. Exudation is caused by inflammation (pleurisy), which increases capillary permeability ('leak'). As plasma proteins accumulate, osmotic pressure draws in further fluid. The type of effusion can be diagnosed by fluid protein levels:

>30 g/litre protein = exudate

<30 g/litre protein = transudate

(Rahman et al., 2004)

Untreated pleural effusions may cause atelectasis. Pleural effusions frequently complicate severe illness. Symptoms are typically:

- severe chest pain on inspiration
- pyrexia
- non-productive cough
- hypoxia, from atelectasis.

They are usually detected by chest x-rays, providing patients are sitting up (Allibone, 2006).

Slightly more than half of pleural effusions occur in young people, usually from pneumonia causing exudative effusion (Rahman et al., 2004). Pleural effusions in older people are more often exudative, caused by malignancy (Rahman et al., 2004).

Underlying causes for pleural effusions should be reversed. Those caused by infection usually resolve with antibiotics (Rahman et al., 2004). Large (>20 per cent) effusions may be aspirated. Symptoms may require treatment, such as oxygen for hypoxia. Inflammation may be reversed with steroids. Malignant pleural effusions may necessitate long-term drains (Medford and Maskell, 2005), but are best treated with pleurodesis (Antunes et al., 2003).

Pulmonary embolism

Pulmonary emboli (PE) often occur suddenly, causing sudden severe dyspnoea. Mortality is high – up to one-fifth being fatal (Wolfe, 2003). In patients with heart failure, pulmonary emboli are the leading cause of death (Pulido *et al.*, 2006).

Without gas exchange in affected areas of the lung, blood returns to the left atrium with venous levels of gases ('shunt blood'). Ventilation/perfusion (V/Q) mismatch provokes tachypnoea and hypoxia (poor saturations). Symptoms often include:

■ pleuritic chest pain
■ haemoptysis
■ pyrexia
■ palpitations
■ cough
■ loss of consciousness.

(Khan and Movahed, 2005)

No single test diagnoses pulmonary emboli, but computerised tomographic pulmonary angiography (CTPA) is recommended for non-massive PE (BTS, 2003). Diagnosis is often based on

■ V/Q scan (Kruip *et al.*, 2003)
■ raised troponin in massive PE (BTS, 2003)
■ positive D-dimer (Kruip *et al.*, 2003)
■ unilateral wheeze (Wolfe, 2003).

ECGs may show right axis deviation, T wave inversion and other acute abnormalities caused by right ventricular strain (Khan and Movahed, 2005). Diagnosis is often missed – PEs are found in 9 per cent of post mortems, yet were only correctly diagnosed in 18 per cent of those patients before death (Owen and Gibson, 2004).

Massive PE should be treated with thrombolysis (rt-PA, also called alteplase) (BTS, 2003). Non-massive PE should be treated with low molecular weight heparin (BTS, 2003), with target INR 2.0–3.0 (BTS, 2003). High-concentration oxygen, or artificial ventilation, is often needed. Patients should be closely observed and monitored.

Pulmonary emboli usually originate from deep vein thrombosis (DVT) (Hyers, 2003; BTS, 2003). Emboli can occlude any blood vessels smaller than themselves. Hospitalised patients can easily develop DVT, so all immobile or high-risk patients should receive DVT prophylaxis unless there is a specific contra-indication. Standard DVT prophylaxis is

■ subcutaneous heparin (Lentine *et al.*, 2005)
■ knee-length anti-thrombotic stockings (TEDs) (Howard *et al.*, 2004; Morris and Woodcock, 2004; Prandoni *et al.*, 2004)
■ early mobilisation (Martinson *et al.*, 2001).

Contraindications for TEDs include:

- conditions that stockings would interfere with – e.g. dermatitis, gangrene, recent skin graft;
- severe arteriosclerosis or other ischaemic vascular disease;
- massive leg or pulmonary oedema from congestive heart failure;
- extreme leg deformity.

Psychological care

Breathing is fundamental to life, so dyspnoea causes distress. Many conditions discussed here may cause haemoptysis – distressing for both patients and their family.

Hypoxia can cause acute confusion, making the person feel vulnerable, frightened and potentially paranoid. Offering (honest) reassurance and involving relatives with their care can help patients gain confidence in their care.

Implications for practice

- Respiratory care should include respiratory observations.
- Dyspnoeic patients should sit upright and forward to optimise lung expansion (unless medical conditions contraindicate this position).
- Respiratory failure should be treated promptly and appropriately.
- Respiratory acidosis with pH between 7.25–7.35 is an indication for non-invasive ventilation.
- Severe dyspnoea usually causes an extreme stress response (panic), so good psychological support (explaining, calm atmosphere, honest reassurance) can help relieve some of the distress.
- Nurses should actively prevent or minimise complications from respiratory failure, especially encouraging breathing exercises, early mobilisation and maintenance as far as possible of normal activities of living.
- Immobile/at-risk DVT patients should receive regular subcutaneous heparin and knee-length TEDs for DVT prophylaxis.
- Chronic respiratory disease is often eventually terminal. Appropriateness of interventions should be judged by likely prognosis, with patients and their families being aware of likely outcomes.

Summary

Respiratory disease can be acute or chronic, but people with chronic respiratory diseases are more susceptible to acute exacerbations. This chapter has described the main life-threatening acute respiratory conditions. Medical intervention and tests vary according to precipitating conditions, but fundamental nursing care and monitoring can improve quality of the patient's life and detect any deterioration or complications early. Yet respiratory monitoring remains the most neglected vital sign.

In addition to fundamental care and observation, certain conditions or treatments may require specific nursing care, such as management of chest drains (see Chapter 21), non-invasive ventilation (see Chapter 23) or tracheostomies (see Chapter 22).

Clinical scenario

Jenny Franks, aged 45, is admitted to your ward with bronchopneumonia. She is known to be asthmatic and a smoker, with no history of chronic obstructive pulmonary disease. She is very anxious about her son, who left home one month ago to study at university. She is found, outside the ward, having suffered a severe asthma attack while smoking a cigarette. Her respiratory rate is now 45 bpm, blood pressure 175/95 mmHg, heart rate 128 bpm. Her oxygen saturation is 83%.

1   List your initial priorities during Jenny's attack.

Jenny is prescribed four hourly nebulisers of ipratropium and salbutamol, reducing daily doses of initially 40 mg prednisolone. Using a pharmacology text, such as the *British National Formulary*, list the expected effects and potential side effects of these medicines. What observations and other aspects of nursing care might be needed because of these drugs?

2   Drawing on your own experience, material in this chapter and any other material that you have access to, develop an evidence-based plan of care for Jenny for the first 48 hours following this attack.

3   The day following her attack, Jenny's son arrives unexpectedly on the ward, and appears very frightened and anxious. He has already seen his mother, who has given him vague information about what happened. He asks you for information. What information and other care would you give to Jenny's son? Justify your decisions.

Bibliography

Key reading

British Thoracic Society (BTS) guidelines (e.g. 2004, 2008) generally remain the UK 'gold standard' for medical management of respiratory disease, many documents including algorithms; BTS guidelines listed by author names include Henry *et al.* (2003) and Antunes *et al.* (2003). NICE (2004b) is similarly authoritative, drawing largely on the work of the BTS. NICE (2009) has recently published guidance on COPD. GOLD (2007) provides similarly authoritative US guidelines. The British Thoracic Society's journal *Thorax* regularly prints valuable articles on respiratory medicine, and has a useful website. Asthma UK also has a useful, largely patient-focused, website.

Further reading

Scullion (2008) offers useful patient-focused insights into management of COPD. Like many guidelines, those from the USA (Institute for Clinical Systems Improvement, 2006) are useful, although users should always primarily follow any guidelines from their own country. Recent nursing articles on respiratory diseases include Allibone (2006). Booker (2007) reviews peak flow monitoring.

Chapter 19

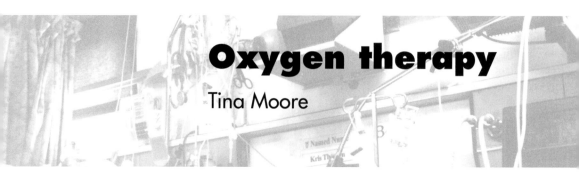

Oxygen therapy

Tina Moore

Contents

Learning outcomes

After reading this chapter you will be able to:

- identify causes of hypoxaemia;
- recognise signs of hypoxaemia (below normal oxygen content in arterial blood);
- list the different types of devices used to administer oxygen;
- illustrate knowledge and understanding of the advantages and disadvantages of each.

Fundamental knowledge

Carriage of gases; gaseous exchange; respiratory assessment (Chapter 15); pulse oximetry (Chapter 16); arterial blood gas analysis (Chapter 17).

Introduction

The administration of oxygen is used in all practice settings. In many acute situations it is the first line of treatment. Anecdotal evidence suggests that oxygen is often given without careful appraisal of its potential benefits and side effects, regularly delegated to junior staff and students. Inappropriate dosage and failure to monitor the effects of oxygen therapy can have serious consequences. This particular chapter outlines the different methods of administering oxygen, including their advantages and disadvantages.

Hypoxaemia

Air and blood both arrive at the alveoli, the aim is that the entire cardiac output should be available for exchange of gases. Adequate gas exchange requires ventilation and perfusion (blood flow) to be matched. The relationship between ventilation and perfusion in the lungs are measured by calculating the difference between the alveolar and arterial partial pressure oxygen (McCance and Huether, 2006).

At rest alveolar ventilation $(V) = 4 \, l/min$ and perfusion $(Q) = 5 \, l/min$, so the V–Q ratio (or V:Q ratio) is $4:5 = 0.8$. In a 'perfect lung' gaseous exchange will be evenly distributed (perfectly matched), i.e. all alveoli would receive an equal share of alveolar ventilation and the pulmonary capillaries would receive an equal share of cardiac output. It must be remembered that these are normal, average healthy adult values, but individual patients will not always match them, even in health.

Abnormal V:Q ratios are the most common cause of hypoxaemia (McCance and Huether, 2006). These can be caused by either inadequate ventilation of well-perfused areas of the alveoli (reduced oxygen intake) or good ventilation with poor perfusion as seen in the case of pulmonary embolism.

Time out 19.1

Before reading the next section, list the reasons why patients within your area of practice require supplementary oxygen therapy.

Causes of hypoxaemia

There is no doubt that tissues require oxygen for survival. Generally, the aim is to achieve a target saturation of 94–98% for patients aged below 70; patients aged 70 and above may have saturation levels below 94% and not require oxygen therapy (BTS, 2008). Patients with chronic pulmonary obstructive disease (COPD), and for those at risk of Type 2 respiratory failure, an initial saturation of 88–92% is suggested, pending availability of gas results (BTS, 2008). Satisfactory delivery of oxygen to the tissues depends on a number of factors: adequate alveolar ventilation; diffusion from the alveoli into the pulmonary vascular system and delivery of oxygenated blood via the circulation to cells within tissues. Failure of any of these systems could result in tissue hypoxia.

Causes of hypoxaemia include:

1   *Low inspired oxygen*: drop in atmospheric pressure associated with high altitudes.
2   *Alveolar hypoventilation*: causing hypercapnia (can occur in patients with COPD).
3   *Diffusion abnormalities*: diffusion of oxygen through the alveolar capillary membrane is impaired if the membrane is thickened or the surface area available for diffusion is decreased, e.g. pulmonary oedema.
4   *Circulatory*: cardiac output is too low, influencing oxygen haemoglobin transportation.
5   *Histotoxic or cytotoxic*: target cells are unable to utilise the oxygen which is being adequately delivered, as in the case of septicaemia, tumours.
6   *Atelectasis*: alveoli become deflated in the event of a collapsed lung (whole or partial).
7   *Low haemoglobin concentration*: for example anaemia.

Box 19.1 Patients predisposed to hypoxaemia

■ Extremes of age
■ Pregnancy
■ Obesity
■ Smoking
■ Heart disease
■ Cerebrovascular disease
■ Anaemia
■ Haemoglobinopathies
■ Head injured patient

Tolerance for hypoxaemia depends on the compensatory mechanisms available and the sensitivity of the patient to hypoxia. If the patient has no additional problems, e.g. cardiac or anaemia, no important effects will manifest until the PaO_2 falls below 6.8–7.0 kPa (Wheeler and Marini, 2006). Symptoms, e.g. malaise, light-headedness, vertigo, impaired judgement will occur (Marini and Wheeler, 2006).

Mild to moderate hypoxaemia is common in the post-operative period. It is often unrecognised and its potential to impede patient's recovery (including wound healing and an increased resistance to infection) is often underestimated. Other symptoms include: confusion, tachypnoea, dyspnoea, tachycardia (compensatory changes). Severe hypoxaemia ($PaO_2 < 4.5$ kPa) may cause bradycardia, lethargy, hypoxic drive is maximal, renal blood flow decreases.

Time out 19.2

In addition to supplementary oxygen, consider other treatments necessary to improve oxygenation.

Furthermore, tissue hypoxia occurs within four minutes of major failure of the respiratory, circulatory and cardiovascular systems (Ward *et al.*, 2006). Severe hypoxaemia can cause cyanosis, bradycardia (resulting from hypoxaemia and acidosis), hypotension, diaphoresis (sweating), coma, convulsions and possibly respiratory arrest.

Treatment for hypoxaemia

Administration of oxygen alone will not help to prevent/alleviate hypoxaemia. Every step should be undertaken to increase gas exchange:

- Patient position – upright if blood pressure/other problems allow (maximises lung expansion).
- Maintenance of adequate fluid balance.
- Maintenance of adequate blood pressure.
- Slow, deep breaths – hyperventilation decreases the amount of oxygen inspired (increases tidal volume and thus gas exchange).
- Physiotherapy may be useful.
- Supplementary oxygen.
- Patient compliance is essential as oxygen needs to be given continuously. If the patient is confused it may be a symptom of hypoxia.
- Non-invasive ventilation – if no response to the above.

Indications for giving oxygen therapy

The need for supplementary oxygen should be determined through evaluation of the patient's arterial blood gas and clinical assessment. Oxygen is a drug and requires care and attention, following procedures for administering drugs. Nurses are encouraged to consult the BTS (2008) guidelines as there is an extensive list of clinical situations complete with guidance on the administration of oxygen. It is beyond the remit of this chapter to include such detail.

Administration of oxygen

Outside of the resuscitation situation, oxygen should always be prescribed by a doctor, stating the flow rate, delivery system, duration and monitoring of treatment. When oxygen is being administered, the patient should be positioned upright if possible, to maximise lung expansion. If using nasal cannulae, the flow rate of oxygen must not exceed 4 l/min. This prevents discomfort and damage to the nasal mucosa (refer to manufacturer's guidance). A full respiratory assessment should be undertaken and the patient closely monitored.

Guidelines produced by NICE (2004b) of oxygen therapy provides guidance in relation to long-term oxygen therapy but these guidelines fail to provide such direction in acute situations. The long-awaited BTS guidelines should be considered gold standard practice in acute/critical care.

Time out 19.3

1   List the different types of administration devices you have observed/used to administer supplementary oxygen.
2   What have been the advantages of using such devices?
3   What problems have you encountered?

Oxygen-delivering devices are usually classified into to two general categories: low-flow systems and high-flow systems. Whether a system is low or high flow does not determine its capability of delivering low versus high concentrations of oxygen (Pierce, 2007). Dosage should be adjusted in accordance with ABG results if available/appropriate.

Low-flow systems

Low-flow systems do not provide all the gas necessary to meet the patient's total minute ventilation. It requires patient to entrain (draw in air) while gas enriched on oxygen is also inspired from a reservoir (mask or reservoir bag), making it difficult to estimate exactly how much inspired oxygen a patient is receiving.

Simple face mask

A simple face mask (see Figure 19.1) has ventilation holes on the sides for entrainment of room air and the release of exhaled gases and is calibrated to deliver a flow of up to 60% of oxygen delivery. During inspiration the patient

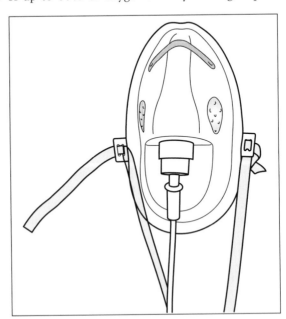

Figure 19.1 **Simple face mask**

draws in air around the sides of the mask, and so is variable in performance. Face masks should be well fitting, failure to do so will result in an increase in entrained room air further reducing the inspired oxygen concentration.

These masks are not considered suitable for patients who are vigorously breathing, drawing larger amounts of air around the sides of the mask (diluting the inspired oxygen concentration). Patients who are hypopnoeic will cause less air to dilute producing a higher concentration of oxygen. Limitations of access for expectoration of sputum, vomiting, eating and drinking can also be problematic. Patients may develop drying or irritation of the eyes.

Partial rebreathing bag and mask

By adding a reservoir bag (see Figure 19.2) an extra supply of oxygen will be provided, resulting in the patient's peak inspiratory flow rate having a larger amount of oxygen, i.e. greater than 60%. The oxygen flow rate should be adjusted so that the bag deflates by only about one-third on inspiration (Pierce, 2007). During inspiration the patient draws air from the mask, bag and through the holes in the side of the mask. During exhalation the first third of exhaled gases flows back into the reservoir bag. This portion of exhaled gases comes from anatomic deadspace, still being rich in oxygen, humidified and warmed and containing little CO_2. If the oxygen flow to the system is high enough to keep the bag from deflating more than one-third during inhalation, then exhaled CO_2 does not accumulate in the reservoir bag (Pierce, 2007).

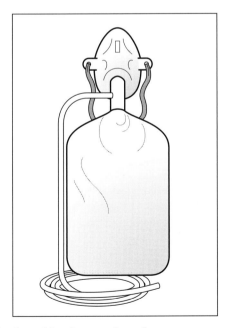

Figure 19.2 Partial rebreathing bag and mask

Non-rebreathing bag and mask

All patients with shock, major trauma, sepsis or other critical illnesses should be managed initially with high concentrations of oxygen therapy from a reservoir mask at 10–15 litres (BTS, 2008). This includes those who are severely hypoxic. A reservoir bag can be used.

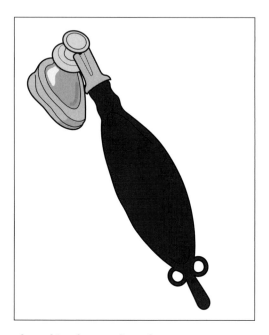

Figure 19.3 Non-rebreathing bag and mask

The non-rebreathing mask contains valves which prevent exhaled gas from entering the reservoir bag, therefore, eliminates the rebreathing of expired gas. During inspiration the side port valves (mask) close and the valve between the bag and mask connection opens allowing for inspiration of 100% oxygen. During expiration the exhalation port valves open and the valve between the bag and mask closes, promoting the release of exhaled gases into the room and preventing entry into the bag (Pierce, 2007).

The reservoir bag should not collapse during inspiration as this suggests flow rates that are insufficient to meet the patient's ventilatory demands. This can increase the patient's work of breathing as the patient struggles against the one-way valve to entrain room air (Agarwal, 2006), making continual respiratory observations essential.

Nasal cannulae

Nasal cannulae are the preferred devices for use in medium dosage oxygen administration (BTS, 2008): simple, unobtrusive and useful for patients unable to tolerate a mask or who are eating and drinking, or coughing, expectorating copious amounts of sputum and vomiting. They are capable of delivering a flow of oxygen ranging from 24–44% depending on the amount of flow in litres. However, it is advised that manufacturer's guidelines are always followed. Limitations include discomfort caused by crusting and drying of the nasal cavity due to dry oxygen.

High-flow systems

Flow of gas is sufficient to meet all of the patient's minute ventilation requirements and provides a consistent flow of oxygen. Delivery of oxygen concentration is more accurate and is not altered by variations in ventilation, thus making blood gas analysis more meaningful.

Venturi masks are most commonly used. These masks have a jet adapter (often colour coded) placed between masks and tubing to the oxygen source. At this point kinetic energy (speed of movement) of flowing gas is increased permitting variable flow of oxygen through the mask.

This device is useful in patients with hypoxaemic COPD (BTS, 2008) where delivery of excessive oxygen could depress the respiratory drive. It is also viewed as useful for patients with variable, deep, irregular, shallow ventilatory patterns (Pierce, 2007). Caution needs to be taken when administrating oxygen with patients who have COPD, due to the hypoxic drive. Normally carbon dioxide levels influence the respiratory centre to increase the rate and depth of breathing, resulting in increase in the excretion of carbon dioxide. Patients with COPD retain carbon dioxide (raised $PaCO_2$ levels) thus depending upon hypoxia to stimulate their respiratory drive.

If these patients are severely hypoxic they should still receive appropriately higher dosages of oxygen. It is well understood that hypoxaemia is highly dangerous and is responsible for many cardiorespiratory arrests and thus a sudden and profound risk to life. Failure to correct hypoxaemia for fear of causing hypoventilation and carbon dioxide retention is an unacceptable clinical practice.

Treatment guidelines should be based on achieving target PaO_2 and SpO_2 rather than administering predetermined concentrations or flow rates of inspired oxygen as determined by the BTS (2008). Trust guidelines should reflect these recommendations, which provide useful guidance for a variety of acute and critical problems.

Monitoring the patient

Oxygen is a drug and so should always be prescribed (flow rate, delivery system and duration) and monitored for signs of deterioration or improvement. Despite receiving supplementary oxygen, patients can and do deteriorate, sometimes rapidly, requiring more invasive intervention. It is essential that patients are closely monitored for signs of deterioration as well as improvement.

Monitoring should include:

- Clinical signs – a comprehensive respiratory (Chapter 15) and cardiovascular (Chapter 24) assessment.
- Cardiac monitoring if patient's PaO_2 is low.
- Oxygen saturation within the first 5 minutes of initiating oxygen therapy (BTS, 2008). This also provides continuous monitoring and indicates when to take an arterial blood gas reading. This should be considered the fifth vital sign (BTS, 2008).
- Arterial blood gas.

Risks of oxygen therapy

- *Combustibility* – oxygen supports combustion of other fuels. Extreme care should be taken, particularly during advanced CPR.
- *Absorbed atelectasis* – prolonged administration of high concentrations of oxygen may cause the alveoli to collapse due to the absorption of gas into the bloodstream. Nitrogen, a relatively insoluble gas, normally maintains a residual volume within the alveolus. During the breathing of high concentrations of oxygen, nitrogen may be replaced or 'washed-out' of the alveolus (Pierce, 2007). When the alveolar oxygen is then absorbed into the pulmonary capillary, the alveolus partially to totally collapses.
- *Hyperoxia* (known as oxygen toxicity) may be harmful to some patients. Pathological changes within the lung occur depending upon the amount of exposure and oxygen tension of inspired air. Generally a flow of oxygen of more than 50 per cent is considered toxic (Pierce, 2007). Symptoms include early to mild tracheobronchitis; depression of mucocilliary function (leading to impaired mucous clearance); prolongation of non-productive cough; substernal pain and nasal stiffness. More prolonged exposure to high tension may lead to damages that mimic ARDS. Oxygen replacement of nitrogen eventually causes collapse of poorly ventilated units, leading to atelectasis and diminished lung compliance (Marini and Wheeler, 2006).
- *Carbon dioxide necrosis* – carbon dioxide is normally the primary stimulant driving the respiratory system. However, in patients with chronic hypercapnia (as in COPD) hypoxaemia becomes the major respiratory stimulus. Generally, patients receiving low dosages of <30% oxygen should be observed for signs of respiratory depression.
- *Discomfort* – oxygen is a dry gas that can dehydrate exposed membrane resulting in a dry mouth. Oral fluids and mouth care can help. Humidification will also reduce this.

Checklist for the safe administration of oxygen

- How can inadequate tissue oxygenation be recognised?
- When is acute oxygen therapy appropriate and at what dose?
- How is oxygen best delivered? Is humidification necessary?

- What are the dangers of oxygen therapy?
- What assessment and monitoring are necessary?
- Is outcome of the disease improved?
- When should oxygen therapy be stopped?

(Bateman and Leach, 1998)

Implications for practice

- Oxygen should be administered by staff who are trained in oxygen administration (BTS, 2008).
- A comprehensive respiratory assessment is vital before, during and after administering oxygen.
- Nurses need to be aware that despite receiving oxygen therapy patients could deteriorate very quickly, often developing Type 2 respiratory failure.
- The dosage of oxygen administered should be regularly reviewed and titrated according to the BTS guidelines.
- Patients require education and support to ensure their co-operation with treatment.

Summary

A large number of acute/critically ill patients will require supplementary oxygen therapy. Nurses need to be conversant with the correct administration techniques. Extreme competence is required in the careful monitoring of such patients, particularly for signs of deterioration.

Clinical scenario

Mary O'Brien has been admitted to your ward with an acute exacerbation of her COPD. Pulse oximetry analysis shows a saturation of 86% and oxygen therapy is prescribed.

1   How would you explain to Mary that she needs oxygen therapy?

2   What type of device would you use? Explain the reasons why. How would you evaluate its effectiveness?

3   Identify complications of oxygen therapy that specifically affect Mary.

Bibliography

Key reading

BTS guidelines – together with essential guidance to practice, this document provides useful algorithms for the administration and dosage of oxygen.

NICE – useful for guidance on long-term oxygen therapy (which some acute/critically ill patients have experience of).

Chapter 20

Suctioning

Tina Moore

Contents

Learning outcomes

After reading this chapter you will be able to:

- identify the indications for suctioning;
- demonstrate the ability to select an appropriate route for suctioning;
- demonstrate the correct suctioning procedure;
- outline the dangers/complications of suctioning;
- discuss appropriate strategies to prevent complications.

Fundamental knowledge

Anatomy and physiology of upper and lower airways; gaseous exchange, pulse oximetry (Chapter 16); principles of asepsis; respiratory assessment (Chapter 15).

Introduction

For the acutely/critically ill patient during their illness there may be periods when normal respiratory function cannot be maintained; this includes the cough reflex (which aids the removal of secretions). As a result retention of secretions and altered gaseous exchange will occur, thus interfering with normal respiratory status. If this continues over time the secretions retained may damage cilia and interfere with their mucus-raising properties, thus leading to atelectasis (collapse of the alveoli) and infection. If non-invasive interventions, such as educating the patient to cough, deep-breathing exercises, postural drainage fail, then patients may require the artificial removal of secretions via suctioning. This procedure is necessary for the management of open airways.

Inconsistencies in its practice (Thompson, 2000; Day *et al.*, 2001) and dangerous practices (Day *et al.*, 2002) exist. Current literature reviews continue to highlight inconsistencies among the evidence (Pedersen *et al.*, 2008), and a lack of clear protocols or guidelines related to clinical practice (Day *et al.*, 2001). Nonetheless, it has been seen that despite some knowledge, nurses continue to deliver outdated modes of practice (Day *et al.*, 2001). Nurses are accountable for giving safe and correct care and need to adopt an evidence-based approach to guide practice. Ritualised approaches could be detrimental to the patient. The suctioning procedure is associated with complications, e.g. bleeding, infection, hypoxaemia, atelectasis, cardiovascular instability (arrhythmias, elevated intracranial pressure (Thompson *et al.*, 2000)).

This chapter aims to improve the nurse's knowledge in assessing the need for suctioning the adult patient; the suctioning procedure and the overall care of the patient together with its management. A systematic review of current literature by Pedersen *et al.* (2008) revealed little new evidence.

Time out 20.1

1 Revise the anatomy and physiology of the upper and lower airways. Read and understand the physiology of gaseous exchange.
2 Draw and label a diagram of the upper and lower airways. Describe the function of each structure labelled. Now check your answers referring to an anatomy and physiology book.

Routes for suctioning

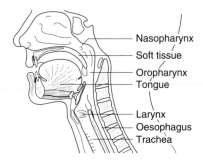

Nasopharynx
Soft tissue
Oropharynx
Tongue

Larynx
Oesophagus
Trachea

Figure 20.1 **Routes used for suctioning**

Box 20.1 Routes for suctioning

Suctioning is the mechanical aspiration of pulmonary sections with an artificial airway in position (AARC, 1993). However, in the acutely/critically ill patient the normal protective mechanisms aiding the removal of debris from the lungs are often compromised and therefore require artificial removal via suctioning.

Suctioning can be performed via various routes. Nurses need to select the most appropriate one in order to minimise/prevent trauma. The following routes are available:

- *Oral* – removes secretions from the mouth, usually performed by a yankeur suction catheter.
- *Oropharyngeal* – can be performed for patients who are breathing spontaneously but are unable to keep an open airway. Requires the insertion of a suction catheter through the mouth and pharynx into the trachea. An airway adjunct, e.g. guedel airway may be indicated.
- *Nasopharyngeal* – airway adjuncts may also be used if the patient is unable to tolerate suction without them.
- *Nasotracheal* – route requires the insertion of a suction catheter through the nasal passage and pharynx into the trachea. As the tube bypasses the body's normal protective functions (warming and filtering air), this may result in dry and tenacious secretions (Blackwood, 1999).
- *Tracheal* – suctioning usually occurs through an artificial opening in the trachea, i.e. tracheostomy. An airway adjunct, being a foreign object, increases the production of secretions. Therefore, suctioning is required to ensure patency of the airway. Contraindications for using nasopharyngeal/nasotracheal suctioning are included in Box 20.2.
- Some patients may be unable to maintain spontaneous respirations and, therefore, require artificial mechanical ventilation, which is a means of ensuring an open airway and facilitating adequate gaseous exchange – *endotracheal* (ET) suctioning can be performed through an endotracheal tube or tracheostomy tube.

> **Box 20.2 Contraindications to nasopharyngeal and nasotracheal suctioning**
>
> ■ Nasal bleeding
> ■ Epiglottis or croup (absolute)
> ■ Acute head, facial or neck injuries
> ■ Bleeding disorders
> ■ Laryngospasm
> ■ Irritable airway
> ■ Upper respiratory tract infection

Time out 20.2

1 Reflect on the patients whom you may have performed this procedure on.
2 What were the reasons for them requiring suctioning?
3 What criteria did you use to make this judgement?
4 What route did you select for this procedure? Give reasons for your decision.

Indications for suctioning

The ultimate aim of suctioning is to remove pulmonary secretions in order to maintain a patent airway and thus facilitating ventilation and oxygenation. Common indications for suctioning are included in Box 20.3.

> **Box 20.3 Indications for suctioning**
>
> ■ Audible secretions (i.e. 'rattling'/'bubbling' sounds heard with or without a stethoscope)
> ■ Feeling secretions in chest (by the patient)
> ■ Cough
> ■ Deteriorating arterial blood gas values
> ■ Altered chest movement (however, this may indicate other ailments, e.g. pneumothorax)
> ■ Restlessness in association with other indicators
> ■ Decreased oxygen saturation levels (desaturation)
> ■ Altered haemodynamics (increased blood pressure, tachycardia) in association with other indicators
> ■ Diminished air entry
> ■ Change in skin colour
> ■ Tachypnoea
> ■ For the assessment of airway patency, cough reflex stimulation and sputum specimen collection

Assessment

Prior to suctioning an appropriate assessment of the patient should be performed to establish the need for this intervention. This particular aspect of the procedure has not done particularly well (Day *et al.*, 2001), possibly as a result of nurses' lack of knowledge and confidence in noting the patient's signs and symptoms. A comprehensive respiratory assessment, including auscultation should be performed (Chapter 15).

Post-suctioning assessment should include the type, tenacity, consistency and amount of secretions. Normal secretions (if produced, as most is swallowed) are white and mucoid. If the secretions are loose, copious in amount, pink, frothy and possibly blood-stained this may indicate fluid overload (pulmonary oedema); yellow/green may be indicative of infection; rusty sputum indicative of pneumonia. In the presence of pulmonary disease, infection or dehydration, respiratory secretions may become thick and tenacious, making removal by suctioning difficult. If the patient becomes dehydrated, the mucosal membranes will be drier, mucocilliary transport will decrease and there will be retention of secretions. Additional fluid replacement and/or humidification may be required.

Any deteriorating changes in the patient's physiological status (including bradycardia – detected if the patient is attached to a cardiac monitor) during suctioning, may require termination of the procedure, hyperoxygenation and appropriate intervention. This is also a painful procedure (Puntillo *et al.*, 2008; Arroyo-Novoa *et al.*, 2008), so close monitoring of the patient is required.

Suctioning procedure

Time out 20.3

1 Before reading further, discuss with your colleagues the procedure of suctioning.
2 Write down practices that you have been involved in/observed.
3 Make a note of any consistencies or inconsistencies of this practice.

Box 20.4 provides a list of suctioning equipment required for all routes. Generally, the same procedure is adopted apart form the length of catheter inserted, which will depend on the route selected for suctioning.

Box 20.4 Equipment required (for all routes)

- Suction machine (wall mounted or portable)
- Suction catheter (a selection of appropriate sizes)
- Clean disposable gloves (Dougherty and Lister, 2008)
- Sterile water for irrigation
- Disposable plastic apron

- Sterile disposable container
- Bactericidal alcohol handrub
- Tissues
- Goggles (Day *et al.*, 2002; nurses should consult their Trust's infection control policy)

The suctioning procedure is outlined in Box 20.5.

Box 20.5 Suctioning procedure (not oral)

- Communicate with patient and gain verbal consent (if able).
- Explain the procedure to the patient.
- Check that the suction machine is on.
- Set at appropriate suction pressure (discussed later).
- Calculate appropriate catheter size – for endotracheal and tracheostomy tubes the catheter size should not be larger than one-half of the tube diameter (ICS, 2008).
- Some patients may require hyperoxygenation and hyperinflation prior to suctioning.
- If possible the patient should be sitting upright.
- Clean hands with alcohol rubs.
- Use a clean disposable glove on the other (Dougherty and Lister, 2008; DOH, 2007).
- Withdraw catheter from sleeve.
- Insert the suction catheter via the selected route. Do not apply negative pressure on insertion.
- On withdrawing the catheter slowly apply suction pressure (by placing the thumb over the suction port control).
- Withdraw catheter gently without rotating the catheter. Multiple-eyed catheters have holes around their diameters making the rotating method unnecessary.
- Monitor oxygen saturation levels and heart rate levels for any decrease indicating hypoxaemia throughout the procedure.
- On completion wrap catheter around gloved hand, then pull back glove over soiled catheter and discard safely (Dougherty and Lister, 2008).
- Rinse connection by dipping its end in the jug of sterile water (Dougherty and Lister, 2008) and discard other glove.
- Clean hands with bactericidal alcohol handrub.
- If further suctioning is required start the procedure again with another sterile catheter and glove. Cross-infection can become a problem if nurses do not adhere to the correct procedure for suctioning and as a result hands become contaminated. Patients who require suctioning are usually very ill and are often debilitated and susceptible to colonisation by the hands of staff during suctioning (Cobley *et al.*, 1991).

- Repeat until the airway is clear (auscultate post-suctioning). However, no more than a total of three suction passes are suggested (Glass and Grap, 1995). Smith (1993) suggests that pre-suctioning oxygen saturation parameters should be returned to before suctioning again.
- The patient must be allowed to rest between each suction pass.
- Reconnect oxygen apparatus as soon as possible.
- Evaluate effectiveness by conducting a comprehensive post-suctioning procedure – respiratory assessment (Glass and Grap, 1995).
- Wash hands post-suctioning.
- Clean patient's oral cavity.
- Document findings.

Particular attention should be given to patients who have chronic obstructive pulmonary disorder (COPD) or those who desaturate very quickly for whatever reason. Pulse oxymetry monitoring is advisable. Pre-oxygenation may be required.

Frequency of suctioning

This procedure should be performed in response to clinical signs and symptoms rather than on a routine basis (Blackwood, 1999; Day et al., 2002; Van de Leur et al., 2003), therefore reducing the risk of associated complications.

The exact timing to carry out this procedure cannot be identified. However, by withholding suctioning until the patient's condition changes is dangerous practice. Retained pulmonary secretions become a medium for bacterial growth with the risk of potential problems including dyspnoea, atelectasis and hypoxaemia. Therefore, patients require continuous assessment to establish the need for suctioning.

Hyperoxygenation and hyperinflation

Hyperoxygenation is performed by increasing the intake of oxygen immediately prior to suctioning and when appropriate after suctioning (Pedersen et al., 2008) and helps reduce the occurrence of hypoxaemia (Oh and Seo, 2003). Hyperoxygenation (pre-oxygenation) before suctioning offers some protection from a drop in arterial blood oxygen. In practice hyperoxygenation (via face mask) is the delivery of between 75–95% of oxygen; patients are encouraged to take three to five deep breaths before, between and after passes of the suction catheter. Hyperoxygenation provides some protection from a drop in arterial blood oxygen, but is most effective when combined with hyperinflation (Stone et al., 1991).

For self-ventilating patients hyperoxygenation and hyperinflation can be achieved by increasing their oxygen intake and educating them to breathe deeply. Its success will be dependent on the patient's ability to increase lung capacity. Patients with COPD may require hyperinflation without the increase in oxygen (as this may reduce the hypoxic drive).

Hyperinflation involves inflating the lungs with a larger tidal volume (Wood, 1998). Hyperinflation volume of 100–150 per cent is normally recommended (Grap *et al.*, 1994).

Suction catheters

Insertion of a suction catheter into the trachea often initiates a cough reflex, which may be enough to dislodge and expel the sputum. The function of coughing alters the intrathoracic pressures to aid mobilisation of secretions. Often the degree of cough is not forceful enough to complete expulsion of secretions through the mouth, resulting in secretions being left in the trachea. Nurses need to suction secretions mobilised by coughing. Suction pressure should be applied to aid removal of secretions.

If the patient is unconscious and unable to cough it may be necessary to advance the catheter to the carina (a point of resistance felt). If this resistance is felt then the catheter should be withdrawn 1 cm before suctioning (Pedersen *et al.*, 2008).

There is a general consensus in the literature that suction catheters should be as small as possible but large enough to facilitate removal of secretions (Pedersen *et al.*, 2008). Suction catheters are available in different sizes. Size 12 (French Gauge) is most commonly used for the adult. The size of the suction catheter is dependent on the tenacity and volume of secretions, i.e. the thicker the secretions and the larger the volume, the greater the bore of the tube (Dougherty and Lister, 2008), but should not occlude more than half of the catheter diameter. The larger the size, the greater risk of mucosal contact and trauma.

All suction catheters now used have multiple eyes which cause less damage than the single-eyed catheters (Fiorentini, 1992). Multiple-eyed catheters dissipate the focus of suction pressure resulting in a less likely chance of the mucosa being sucked into the side holes, thus minimising the need to rotate the catheter on removal. Still, this may create a false sense of security. All suction catheters will cause trauma when pushed against the tracheal wall.

Yankeur suction catheters provide the easiest and safest way to remove oral secretions and vomit, particularly if patients with tracheostomies can cough the secretions to the end of the tube. Many of them are able to use the yankeur themselves. However, they are rigid and not as flexible as suction catheters, and may cause trauma of the oral cavity if not used with care.

Suction pressure

Negative pressure should be sufficient to clear secretions, although the amount of suction pressure used can affect the amount of secretions removed. Too low a suction pressure can result in the patient's airway not being cleared. If the suction pressure is too high, the suction catheter can adhere to the tracheal wall causing mucosal damage and atelectasis (Burglass, 1999). The suction catheter is also more likely to collapse (Czarnik *et al.*, 1991).

Generally, the lowest amount of suction pressure needed to remove secretions should be used. This reduces the risk of atelectasis, hypoxia and tracheal mucosal damage (Wood, 1998; Day *et al.*, 2002). Suction pressures should be between 80–120 mmHg (ICS, 2008). Sputum that is more tenacious will require more powerful suction, the maximum level being 200 mmHg (Oh and Seo, 2003; Dougherty and Lister, 2008). It has been found that no more secretions are removed at 200 mmHg than at 100 mmHg (Czarnik *et al.*, 1991). However, Pedersen *et al.* (2008) suggest that a negative pressure of 200 mmHg may be applied if the appropriate suction catheter is used. This suggestion should be treated with caution.

Measures that could reduce the tenacity of secretions are:

- ensuring patients are well hydrated (Blackwood, 1999; Akgul, 2002);
- ensuring airway heat and humidity (Blackwood, 1999; Akgul, 2002);
- using mucolytic agents and nebuliser treatments (Blackwood, 1999).

Negative suction pressure should only be applied when removing the catheter; if pressure is applied during insertion, the catheter will adhere to the mucosal wall. When withdrawing the suction catheter continuous pressure should be applied (Glass and Grap, 1995) as intermittent release of negative pressure causes damage to the tracheal wall (Czarnik *et al.*, 1991).

Length of time spent suctioning

Suctioning the patient should take no longer than 10 seconds (ICS, 2008). Alternative methods, such as nurses holding their breath is unreliable and potentially dangerous, as this approach does not take into consideration patient's non-healthy lung status (a person who is healthy can hold their breath for up to 25–30 seconds without difficulty). The *whole* suctioning procedure should take no longer than 15 seconds (Celik and Elbas, 2000).

Before suctioning the patient should (if possible) be encouraged to take a deep breath. At least two full minutes of recovery time is needed for adult patients with closed head injury to return to baseline oxygen saturation values after suctioning (Crosby and Parsons, 1992). Indeed, this principle could be applied to the majority of patients requiring suctioning. The patient's susceptibility to hypoxaemia should be monitored (i.e. bradycardia and hypotension – this is caused by the negative pressure removing oxygen from the lungs during withdrawal). Therefore, post-suctioning, nurses should check the patient's pulse, if the pulse is significantly slowed, then check BP, if this has significantly dropped, then a 12-lead ECG should be taken.

Tracheal suctioning

A systematic review of this procedure in adults concluded that the quality of evidence available was lacking in rigorous research design, consequently affecting the validity and reliability of findings (Thompson, 2000). Although the Intensive Care Society (ICS, 2008) has attempted to provide some guidance it is still insufficient.

The presence of a tracheostomy causes cool, dry air to react with the bronchi and lungs as the trachea is ill equipped to warm and humidify air (Jackson, 1996), resulting in drying of secretions, therefore, making patients susceptible to pulmonary infections and atelectasis. Retention of secretions can be caused by lack of humidification. Systemic dehydration will complicate this further.

In order to prevent hypoxaemia occurring during suction, the size of the catheter selected should not occlude more than half of the diameter of the artificial airway (Wood, 1998; Day *et al.*, 2002). For patients requiring suction via a tracheostomy tube, calculate the size of the suction catheters by multiplying the tracheostomy tube's internal diameter by two; this gives the external diameter of the suction catheter, then minus this number by 4 to obtain the FG size (Day *et al.*, 2002). So, if the tracheostomy tube is size 8 – multiply by $2 = 16$, then minus $4 = 12$ FG catheter (ICS, 2008). Fenestrated tracheostomies must have an unfenestrated inner cannulae placed before suctioning (Chapter 22).

Special needs: patients with head injuries

Prior to, during and after the procedure, assessments should include neurological, cardiovascular and respiratory. When performing suctioning on patients with head injury, caution has to be adopted. Neuronal viability is threatened due to sudden and acute increases in intracranial pressure (ICP) (Crosby and Parsons, 1992).

Hyperventilation can result in hypocapnia leading to induced cerebral vasoconstriction, thus reducing the potential of increased intracranial pressure that occurs during end tracheal suctioning when used long term (Ropper, 1993).

For patients who have sustained traumatic brain injury even a moderate increase in ICP will increase cerebral ischaemia and oedema. It is inadvisable to suction patients who have sustained a fracture base of their skull, as the suction catheter could accidentally pass through the fracture.

Psychological care

Patients dreaded the procedure as they endured a great deal of pain after coughing (Jablonski, 1994). During the procedure, patients felt a choking sensation and felt the need to cough (Thompson, 2000). Suctioning is an invasive procedure and can also initiate anxiety (Thompson, 2000). Wherever possible, patients should be informed of the procedure and consent gained. Nurses should not assume that because patients have experienced this procedure before, that they know what to expect or have complete knowledge of it, and, therefore, omit information. Patients who are acutely ill often suffer problems with concentration, due to the intensity of their illness, influences of medication, e.g. powerful analgesia. Informing patients and encouraging participation helps to reduce the patient's stress (Fiorentini, 1992).

The use of invasive techniques and therapies can result in patients experiencing a feeling of being 'tied down' (Clifford, 1985), further producing sensations of fear, anxiety and helplessness (Granberg *et al.*, 1996). Effective communication is a key strategy in minimising anxiety.

Complications of suctioning

Suctioning is an important and necessary aspect of care but may be wrongly viewed as a routine skill. This procedure is full of potential dangers. The following list provides identification of the associated complications (some have already been discussed):

- hypoxaemia;
- contamination of airway leading to nonocomial infection;
- mucosal trauma;
- pneumothorax;
- bradycardia and hypotension (Wainright and Gould, 1996): syncope, ventricular irritability, ventricular tachycardia and asystole (Flynn and Bruce, 1993), attributed to mechanical stimulation of the vagus nerve;
- prolonged coughing during the procedure;
- paroxysmal cough caused by stimulation of the tracheal and carinal reflexes which may in turn affect venous return and cardiac output and also cause infection (Flynn and Bruce, 1993);
- bleeding (possibly more common when higher suction pressures used).

Implications for practice

- Nurses should be competent in assessing the need for performing suctioning.
- Suctioning should be performed on the basis of clinical evidence (patient's signs and symptoms).
- Nurses should take particular care when suctioning patients who have additional medical problems (e.g. COPD or head injury).
- Continuous monitoring of the patients for signs of complications during and after the procedure is essential.

Summary

The procedure of suctioning is a necessary part of nursing intervention. This intervention can and does induce problems. The correct procedure, which is also based on evidence, needs to be adhered to throughout. Nurses should be competent in assessing the need for performing this skill. The decision to perform this procedure should be based upon the patient's clinical signs and symptoms and not as a matter of routine.

Bibliography

Further reading

There appears to be little new material available on the procedure/effects of suctioning. However, the literature review conducted by Pedersen *et al.* (2008) provides a systematic account of 'current' available literature.

Chapter 21

Intrapleural chest drains

Philip Woodrow

Contents

Learning outcomes

After reading this chapter you will be able to:

- understand benefits and problems of intrapleural chest drains;
- identify nursing care of patients with chest drains.

Fundamental knowledge

Anatomy of pleura.

Introduction

Chest drains can remove any abnormal collection of fluid or air from thorax. As there are two main organs in the chest (the heart and lungs), chest drains are almost always used to treat problems with either of these organs. Cardiac drains are widely used following cardiac surgery, but this chapter describes chest drains used to treat pulmonary problems.

Intrapleural chest drains, more often just called 'chest drains', are used to treat:

- pneumothorax
- pleural effusions (see Chapter 18).

Although chest drains have been used for over a century, there is surprisingly little research-based evidence. Most literature remains largely anecdotal (Godden and Hiley, 1998) and is often based on rituals and dated ideas, providing limited evidence for practice (Charnock and Evans, 2001) and leaving many unanswered questions for practice. There are British Thoracic Society guidelines for insertion (2003, currently being revised), and there has been a National Patient Safety Alert about insertion (NPSA, 2008), but insertion is a medical role; there are no national guidelines about nursing management (Sullivan, 2008), and little literature has appeared since the previous edition of this book. This chapter reviews current nursing management of chest drains, but practice may develop once more extensive research-based evidence becomes available. While this chapter focuses on management of chest drains, care of patients should meet all their needs. For example, diseases necessitating chest drainage usually make patients breathless and hypoxic, so their respiratory function (rate, depth, saturations) should be closely monitored, and they often need supplementary oxygen both before and following insertion of drains.

Physiology

Breathing uses negative pressure – the diaphragm, intercostal and (sometimes) clavicular muscles move outward, increasing intrathoracic space, making intrathoracic pressure negative compared with atmospheric (air) pressure. The parietal pleura is attached to tissues surrounding the lungs, so is drawn outward on inspiration. A small volume (about 50 ml) of fluid between the pleura creates sufficient *surface tension* to draw the visceral (or pulmonary) pleura outward, expanding lung volume, and so drawing air from the atmosphere into alveoli.

In health, intrapleural pressure remains slightly negative, ranging between -2 to $-6 \text{cmH}_2\text{O}$ (Hough, 2001). This constant negative pressure helps keep alveoli patent and prevents atelectasis. If intrapleural pressure equalises with intrapulmonary or atmospheric pressure, the pleura collapse, resulting in loss of lung volume and, usually, respiratory distress.

Pneumothorax

A pneumothorax is a collection of gas or air in the pleural space, which may be caused by trauma or be spontaneous (see Chapter 18). Equalisation of pressure across the pleura causes lung collapse, but the pneumothorax remains *simple* if pressure can equalise. If tension exists between the two sides of the hole, the pneumothorax acts as a one-way valve, drawing more air or fluid into the space with each breath, which cannot escape on expiration. This creates positive, instead of negative, pressure within the thorax, resulting in a life-threatening emergency requiring urgent removal of the air or blood. If the pneumothorax is small (<20 per cent of the lung) it may be removed through needle aspiration, but larger pneumothoraces necessitate insertion of a chest drain. The chest drain will enable air to escape, so turning a tension pneumothorax into a simple pneumothorax.

Chest drains

Drains inserted high in the pleural space (2nd–4th intercostal space; apical) remove air, while lower drains (5th or 6th intercostal space; basal) remove fluid. Small 'pig-tail' (10–14 FG) drains are usually used, being replaced with larger ones if leaks persist (Henry *et al.*, 2003; Liu *et al.*, 2003). For longer-term use, such as with malignant pleural effusions, containers with 'flutter valves' help patients mobilise (Davies, 2007).

The end of the drain is inserted into water. This creates an underwater seal drain (UWSD), preventing air returning to the thorax as long as the bottle is below the patient's chest. A second tube leading out of the collection chamber will either remain open to air or be connected to low suction.

If moving the bottle above the patient's chest level is unavoidable (e.g. during transfer), tubing should be temporarily clamped. While healthcare staff are usually aware of this danger, Gallon (1998) warns that some patients have placed their chest-drain bottles on lockers to make room for their visitors. Therefore, patients with chest drains should also be told why they should never raise the bottle up to their chest level.

Water levels in bottles affects suction exerted within the pleural space (Carroll, 2000). Most manufacturers mark the water level, recommended volume typically being 500 ml or less.

Suction

Davies *et al.* (2003) recommend −20 cmH$_2$O suction for drains with small tubes, although Henry *et al.* (2003) and Davies (2007) recommend commencing without suction, adding −10 to −20 cmH$_2$O after 48 hours if air leaks persist (= persistent bubbling) or pneumothoraces fail to re-expand. Excessive negative pressure may damage the delicate pleural tissue.

Tubing

Drainage relies on a siphon, so tubing must be air-tight to prevent atmospheric air being siphoned into the pleura. Graham (1996) warns that an inadequately tied drain 'will' fall out. Godden and Hiley (1998) advise taping connections, although they warn that tape will mask any disconnection. Should the system become disconnected, the pneumothorax will re-collapse, so the drain should be clamped or occluded. Where clamps are not immediately available, a bio-occlusive dressing is probably the best 'first aid' measure, although in emergencies even a finger (Gallon, 1998) may prove life-saving until help arrives. Loops in drainage tubing might cause air pockets, reducing or preventing further flow (Davies, 2007).

Changing bottles

There is no consensus about whether bottles should be changed as indicated, daily or when full (Godden and Hiley, 1998). Practice is increasingly to change only when full (O'Hanlon-Nichols, 1996; McMahon-Parkes, 1997), remembering that bacteria may enter once closed circuits are broken (Godden and Hiley, 1998).

Dressings

Dressings should be as airtight as possible, comfortable, and prevent disconnection. Roskelly (2008) recommends dry gauze dressings around the insertion site, and avoiding heavy strapping which would prevent chest wall movement. Bio-occlusive dressings, preferably transparent so insertion sites can be seen, are often used. Patient allergies should be considered, and should they occur, be recorded.

Pain management

If deep breaths and coughs cause pain, a natural response is to breathe shallowly and minimise coughing, both of which increase the risk of chest infection (Gray, 2001). Good pain control is, therefore, an important part of chest drain management (Carroll, 2002). Patients' needs vary, and should be individually assessed, using available services such as acute pain teams, but options include:

- patient-controlled analgesia (PCA)
- local nerve block
- non-steroidal anti-inflammatories
- transcutaneous electrical nerve stimulators.

(Roskelly, 2008)

Inflammation around the site often occurs, so anti-inflammatory drugs are also useful (Gray, 2001).

Observations

In addition to 'basic' respiratory observations, such as rate and depth of breathing and oxygen saturation, nurses should observe whether chest drains are

- swinging (between inspiration and expiration)
- bubbling (on expiration)
- draining.

If frothing is present, fluid level may be difficult to measure; adding 5–10 ml of a silicone-based defoamer can resolve the problem (Davies, 2007). If audible sucking is heard at the insertion site, the drain has probably become displaced (Gallon, 1998).

Swinging

Without suction, swinging should be visible, as intrapleural pressure changes between inspiration and expiration. Swing will vary depending on depth of breathing. Loss of swinging indicates blockage (Sullivan, 2008). Suction creates a constant negative pressure, and so drains on suction will not swing.

Bubbling

If no air is in the pleural space, bubbling should not be seen. Basal drains or drains for pleural effusions may not bubble. Otherwise, cessation of bubbling indicates either that all air has been removed or the tube has become blocked (e.g. with blood clots, lung tissue or fat). If bubbling ceases, ask the patient to cough (Gallon, 1998), which may dislodge any occlusion. Normally, chest drains will not be removed until 24 hours after bubbling has ceased, or draining <100 ml/day (Davies, 2008). If suction is used, excessive turbulence indicates excessive negative pressure (Bar-El *et al.*, 2001).

Draining

Although enough blood will almost always drain to stain water in the bottle, volume will only significantly increase if fluid is drained. The water level should, therefore, be marked with the time and date each shift (if possible) so volume of drainage can be assessed. Drainage may be blood, plasma or pus (or any combination of these), so colour and type of drainage should be noted.

Rapid drainage is both painful and may cause fatal pulmonary oedema (Hall and Jones, 1997), as loss of protein causes hydrostatic shifts of fluid into interstitial spaces. If initial drainage exceeds more than 1 litre in the first 30 minutes, the drain should be clamped.

Oxygen

Although oxygen may be needed for hypoxia, high concentration oxygen absorbs air from the pleural cavity. The British Thoracic Society (BTS, 2008), therefore, recommends aiming for 100% saturation, using 10–15 litres via a reservoir facemask.

Mobility

Immobility can provoke many problems, including:

- muscle wasting
- deep vein thromboses
- chest infection.

Early mobilisation reduces mortality (Martinson *et al.*, 2001) so, like all other patients, those with chest drains should be encouraged to mobilise. Chest drain bottles are now made of durable plastic, so can be safely carried provided patients are taught to

- never raise the bottle up to their chest;
- keep the water level reasonably horizontal;
- always keep the end of the drain below the water level.

Flushing

Small-bore flexible catheters are prone to blockage (Medford and Maskell, 2005). Regular flushing with 30 ml saline every 6 hours via three-way tap (Davies *et al.*, 2003; Medford and Maskell, 2005), with additional flushes of 20–50 ml saline if blocked (Davies *et al.*, 2003), may prevent blockage, but evidence is poor (Medford and Maskell, 2005) and as flushing necessitates breaking a closed circuit, it is probably best avoided.

Clamping

Clamping can convert a simple pneumothorax into life-threatening tension pneumothorax. Drains should only be clamped

- if drains become disconnected;
- when moving the drain above the patient is unavoidable;
- for changing bottles;
- if excessive drainage (see above).

Pneumothoraces may recur following removal (Gupta, 2001); Gallon (1998) suggests that first-time pneumothoraces recur in 30 per cent of young people and 50 per cent of older people, with higher recurrence rates, such as 70 per cent in young people, in the case of second pneumothoraces. Many (e.g. McMahon-Parkes, 1997; Gupta, 2001) recommend clamping drains for up to 24 hours before removal. Should pneumothoraces recur, removing clamps is preferable to inserting a new drain. However, Laws *et al.* (2003) suggest clamping drains before removal is not beneficial.

To ensure sealing the often rigid tubing of chest drains, two clamps should be used, one clamped from the left and the other from the right (O'Hanlon-Nichols, 1996). Clamps should only remain in place for the minimal time necessary (Gallon, 1998). If respiratory distress (e.g. dyspnoea, cyanosis) occurs, clamps should be released immediately (O'Hanlon-Nichols, 1996).

Removing chest drains

Once pneumothoraces have healed, drains are normally removed, although this is a medical rather than a nursing decision. With acute pleural effusions, drains are often removed when drainage is below 200 ml/day (Younes *et al.*, 2002). Malignant pleural effusions are likely to recur, so drains may be left in longer to reduce dyspnoea (Medford and Maskell, 2005). Removal is painful (Owen and Gould, 1997; Gray, 2001), so patients should be given analgesia. Gallon (1998) recommends entonox, although the manufacturers (BOC) state that entonox is contraindicated for patients with a pneumothorax.

Removal often needs, and is safest with, two people, preferably a doctor who can reinsert a drain if necessary. Patients are usually asked to hold their breath out (end expiration) while the drain is removed (Godden and Hiley, 1998; Gallon, 1998), or to use the Valsalva manoeuvre (breathing out against a closed glottis, like straining at stool) (McMahon-Parkes, 1997), which again ensures breath is held at the end of expiration. Both ensure intrapleural pressure is equal to or above intrapulmonary pressure. Bell *et al.* (2001) found similar rates of recurrent pneumothoraces with end-inspiration and end-expiration removal. Although physiologically illogical, they concluded that both were, therefore, equally safe. The site should be covered with an occlusive dressing, such as a hydrocolloid.

Following removal, lung re-expansion should be checked with a chest x-ray. Close respiratory observations should be maintained for 24 hours (O'Hanlon-Nichols, 1996).

Implications for practice

- If suction is used, limit negative pressures between –10 and –20 cmH$_2$O.
- Patients with chest drains usually need strong analgesics, and usually also benefit from anti-inflammatory medicines.
- Dressings should be secure and air-tight.
- Observe for swinging, bubbling, draining.
- Listen for airleaks at the insertion site.
- Tubing should be examined at least each shift for patency.
- Patients should be encouraged to mobilise, having been taught how to safely manage their drain bottle.

- Clamping drains is not recommended, except for very brief times during emergency, to change bottle or to move the bottle over patient.
- During removal, give additional analgesia.

Summary

Intrapleural chest drains are a useful medical solution to a large (>20 per cent) pneumothorax. However, much nursing and medical practice is based on tradition rather than reliable evidence. Sound research is needed into almost all aspects of management. However, in the absence of adequate evidence, nurses are still expected to deliver care.

Clinical scenario

Marion Janes has been admitted following a road traffic accident. She is very breathless, with oxygen saturation of 83% on 60% oxygen. Chest x-ray reveals a large pneumothorax, which needs both apical and chest drain insertion. She has been given a bolus of intravenous morphine, which is currently keeping her pain under control.

1   With the help of colleagues from work, list the items that will be needed for insertion of a chest drain.

2   You are asked to assist the doctor inserting the drain. Identify what is expected of you, both by the doctor and to care safely for your patient.

3   Devise a plan of care to manage Marion's chest drain for the first 12 hours following insertion.

Bibliography

Key reading

Sullivan (2008) provides a nursing review of chest drain management.

Further reading

Miller and Harvey (1993) remains the most widely followed medical review of chest drains. Pain management is reviewed by Gray (2001).

Chapter 22

Temporary tracheostomies

Philip Woodrow

Contents

Learning outcomes

After reading this chapter you will be able to:

- identify why temporary tracheostomies may be used;
- understand problems and risks they may cause patients;
- list emergency equipment, and checks that should be performed at least once every shift;
- to develop an evidence-based plan of nursing care for a patient with a temporary tracheostomy.

Fundamental knowledge

Tracheal anatomy; respiratory failure.

Introduction

A tracheostomy (= stoma in the trachea, created by a *tracheotomy*) may be

■ temporary
■ permanent
■ a minitracheostomy.

Patients with acute severe respiratory disease or who are being weaned from invasive ventilation may benefit from formation of a temporary tracheostomy to reduce *deadspace*. In practice, most ward patients with temporary tracheostomies are transferred from intensive care units (ICUs), where the stomas were created. Permanent tracheostomies are usually formed when part of the airway has been removed due to cancer. Minitracheostomies are currently rarely used. This chapter, therefore, discusses only temporary tracheostomies.

Tracheostomies may be surgical or percutaneous. Most are percutaneous, being safer and easier to perform, so exposing patients to fewer risks. However, percutaneous stomas may not 'mature' for 7–10 days (Broomhead, 2002), so emergency reintubation may create a false and fatal passage.

Reducing deadspace

Exchange of gases only occurs in alveoli. Air remaining between where it enters the airway (normally mouth or nose) and the alveoli forms the first part of the next breath to reach alveoli. This air, remaining from the last breath, is relatively oxygen poor (often about 15%) and carbon dioxide rich (often about 6%). This volume is called deadspace.

Normal adult deadspace is about 150 ml. Healthy adult breaths (at rest) are 300–500 ml, so deadspace air forms a relatively small part of air reaching the lungs. But with shallow breathing, a greater proportion is deadspace air. If breath size is reduced from 450 ml to 200 ml, oxygen-rich air is reduced from 300 ml to 50 ml. This disproportionately large reduction provokes severe respiratory distress/failure. For people in respiratory distress, such as acute exacerbation of chronic obstructive pulmonary disease (COPD), this change may make the difference between breathing adequately and suffering respiratory failure.

Tube sizes

Normal adult tracheostomy sizes are: 7.0, 7.5, 8.0 and 8.5 mm internal diameter. Sizes are printed on the external bladder and neckplate. Tube size should be recorded clearly in patients' notes, but nurses caring for patients with tracheostomies should also check the tube size each shift.

Inner cannulae

Temporary tracheostomies usually have (two) inner tubes. These should be changed initially two hourly, so that any build-up of secretions can be removed.

Inner tubes are single patient use, but not single use, so should be cleaned (with water) and dried after removal. If secretions are minimal, and tube patency maintained, specialist staff (e.g. Critical Care Outreach) may advise less frequent changing of inner tubes.

Problems

Tracheostomies may create various problems for both patients and staff.

Box 22.1 Tracheostomies: problems

- Communication
- Nutrition
- Impaired cough reflex
- Ulceration
- Infection
- Loss of normal airway functions (humidification, warming, filtering of air)

Communication

Speech is created by air passing through vocal cords. Tracheostomy tubes are inserted below vocal cords, so if cuffs are inflated they usually prevent sound being formed. Loss of speech isolates patients, so nurses should explain that the tube causes loss of speech, and that voice will return following its removal.

Alternative ways to communicate may include:

- mouthing words and lip reading
- writing boards and pens
- sign/alphabet boards
- speaking valves/tubes.

Speaking valves (see Figure 22.1) or tubes necessitate cuff deflation, so patients will be able to protect their own airway (cough, swallow). Speech therapists should be included in the multidisciplinary care team.

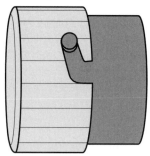

Figure 22.1 **Speaking valve**

Some patients with deflated cuffs or with sufficient cuff-leak find placing fingers over their tube restores their voice. However, human skin is covered with commensals which, in the respiratory tract, could become pathogens. So finger occlusion should be discouraged.

Tubes with fenestrations (holes in the side) allow air to pass through vocal cords. Fenestrated tubes should have both fenestrated and unfenestrated inner tubes. Fenestrated inner tubes normally remain in place to enable speech. For suction, unfenestrated inner tubes should be inserted to prevent catheters passing through fenestrations and damaging delicate tracheal tissue (NHS Quality Improvement Scotland, 2007).

Nutrition

The oesophagus and trachea being virtually adjacent, tracheal tubes can make swallowing difficult (ICS, 2008). Swallowing should be assessed before commencing oral fluids/diet, ideally by a speech and language therapist. Nurses should observe patients when eating or drinking in case aspiration occurs. Nutrition should be monitored, supplementing with liquid or nasogastric feeding if necessary, and involving dieticians.

Impaired cough reflex

Effective coughs rely on closure of the glottis creating sufficient pressure in lungs to force the glottis open and rapidly expel mucus. Tracheostomy tubes prevent complete glottis closure, often making cough reflexes weak. Deep suction may be needed to clear secretions.

Although suction catheter size should be chosen according to the size of the tracheostomy, the only suction catheter sizes that should be available on most adult wards are:

- FG10
- FG12
- FG14.

Suctioning (see Chapter 20) can cause mechanical damage to the delicate airway tissue. For most adult tracheostomies, the FG10 should adequately clear secretions while minimising trauma. If secretions are thick, an FG12 may be needed. FG14 catheters are not recommended for use with tracheostomies.

Suction causes trauma, so pressure should be limited to 13–16 kPa (ICS, 2008) and passes should be limited, generally to two (Docherty and Bench, 2002). If further suction is needed, then either copious secretions need help to mobilise, such as saline nebulisers/physiotherapy, or suction technique is ineffective, needing someone more experienced at suctioning. In either case, nurses should re-evaluate the patient's needs after two passes.

Ulceration

Pressure sores, usually associated with visible skin near bony prominences, can develop wherever sustained pressure exceeds perfusion pressure of capillaries supplying oxygen and nutrients to that tissue. Most tracheostomies on wards have deflated cuffs, but if cuffs are inflated they place continuous pressure on very delicate tracheal epithelium. When pressure sores heal, scar tissue remains, which, being inelastic, could cause chronic respiratory limitation.

Cuff pressure can be measured with a simple manometer (similar to tyre pressure gauges) which attaches to the external bladder. Cuff pressures should not exceed 20–25 cmH$_2$O. Pressure should be checked each shift and whenever air is removed from or added to the cuff.

Infection

Like most surgical wounds, tracheal stomas should be kept clean and redressed. Dressings should usually be changed daily, or more frequently if soiled, but nurses should check surgical/medical notes before performing the first dressing.

Changing tracheostomy dressings *always* requires two people, to prevent loss of the tracheostomy and possible respiratory arrest. The second person, standing on the other side of the patient, assists by holding the tube, so acts under supervision and need not be a qualified nurse.

Redressing tracheostomies requires

- standard dressing pack (including sterile swabs)
- sterile normal saline (0.9%)
- sterile tracheostomy dressing
- clean tracheostomy tapes.

Dressing is easiest if patients lie supine, which makes them less likely to cough.

Tracheostomies can damage skin and other body tissue. Sores may develop around the site of the stoma. These are most likely to be caused by

- pressure
- irritant fluids

and may form a source for infection from micro-organisms colonising the respiratory tract.

The warm moist area underneath neckplates can easily be colonised by micro-organisms. A swab may need to be sent for culture (MC+S). Excessive secretions may necessitate a soft suction catheter to remove them. The stoma should be cleaned thoroughly with saline. Current medical practice varies about whether or not neckplates are stitched to the skin. If stitches are used, sterile cotton buds or forceps and gauze may be needed. Buds with loose cotton may leave fibres which could be inhaled, so should be avoided.

Once clean and dry, stomas are covered with a commercially produced dressing (e.g. Lyofoam®), which has a cross-shaped incision to fit around tracheostomy tubes. If stitched in, forceps may be needed to draw the dressing fully under the neckplate. Dressings have foam and a matt side; the matt side should be placed against the skin.

Two unequal lengths of tape/tube-holder should now be used to secure the tube. The shorter length is fixed on the side of the nurse performing the dressing, the longer one on the side of the assistant, then drawn behind the patient's neck and fixed to the shorter holder. Holders should be tight enough to allow two fingers to slide beneath them (Docherty and Bench, 2002), adequately supporting the tracheostomy tube without being uncomfortably tight for the patient.

Dressing changes should be recorded together with relevant observations:

- How clean is the site?
- Colour and amount of secretions.

Loss of normal airway function

The human airway

- warms
- humidifies
- filters

inhaled air. Most of these functions take place in the deadspace (discussed above). Reducing deadspace by up to half significantly impairs all three functions, so artificial alternatives are needed to replace them.

Heat/moisture exchanger humidifiers (e.g. 'Swedish nose' – see Figure 22.2) reflect warmth and moisture back into the airways, and filter inspired air. Heated water humidification is more effective for the patient, but can cause burns and infection, so is not recommended unless it can be closely supervised.

Inadequate humidification can cause airway obstruction/arrest from dry, sticky mucus plugs. Saline (0.9%) nebulisers (e.g. 2 ml every 2–6 hours) may help mobilise secretions (ICS, 2008), but instilling bolus saline with a syringe into the tracheostomy is not recommended (Cook, 2003).

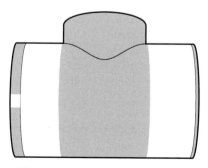

Figure 22.2 **HME humidifier ('Swedish nose')**

Occlusion

As with any arrest situation, help should be summoned urgently. If suction fails to clear the airway, the tracheostomy cuff should be deflated with a syringe to allow some air to bypass the tube. As much oxygen as possible should be given, preferably 100%.

The tracheostomy tube should now be removed, so cut/remove tapes and any stitches, using scissors – there is not usually time to fetch a stitch cutter. The tracheostomy tube should be easy to remove. Stomas are usually well formed by 7 days (Bodenham and Barry, 2001), so should provide the patient with a reasonable airway, although a replacement tube should be inserted as quickly as possible. New stomas may collapse quickly, necessitating more rapid insertion of a replacement tube.

Two spare tubes (one the same size as the patient's, and one a size smaller) should be kept near the patient's bedside, together with a pair of tracheal dilators. With a well-formed stoma, a new tube of the same size should be easy to insert. If the stoma is newly formed, appears to be collapsing or if there is any difficulty with trying to insert a tube of the same size, there are two options:

- inserting the smaller tube (which can be replaced later in a planned, controlled procedure);
- using tracheal dilators to enlarge the stoma.

In an emergency, it is usually quicker, and so safer, to opt for the smaller tube.

Now the patient has a patent airway, a doctor (preferably an anaesthetist) should urgently review the patient.

Should tracheostomies occlude, removal of the inner tube usually restores patency. If removing the inner tube fails to establish a patent airway, suction should usually be attempted. If this fails, the old tube should be removed and replaced, ideally with a tube of the same size. If a similar size tube cannot be inserted, either the stoma may be dilated with tracheal dilators, or a tube a half-size smaller should be inserted.

Emergency equipment

The tracheostomy is the patient's only airway, so emergency equipment needs to be quickly and easily accessible, mainly by the patient's bedside. Items which could be dangerous (e.g. stitch-cutters) should be stored in some other easily accessible place, such as at the nurses' station.

Emergency equipment near the bedside should include:

- tracheal dilators
- spare tubes (one the same size and one a size smaller)
- suction (working and ready to use)
- suction catheters
- gloves

- rebreathing bag and tubing
- syringe
- artery forceps
- resuscitation equipment.

(ICS, 2008)

Much of the kit may be included with a 'tracheostomy box' supplied by ICU/Outreach.

Remembering individual professional accountability (NMC, 2008), staff caring for patients with a tracheostomy should ensure emergency equipment is easily accessible at the start of their shift, including that suction equipment is working.

Planned removal

Removing tracheostomies significantly increases work of breathing, by up to one-third (Chadda *et al.*, 2002). This may cause dyspnoea. Traditionally, literature recommends deflating cuffs one day before removal (Serra, 2000), occluding the tube, and closely monitoring respiratory function. If the patient can breathe satisfactorily past the deflated cuff, the tube can then be removed after 24 hours. If respiratory distress occurs, the occluder should be removed.

However, the occluded tube leaves a very small airway around the deflated cuff, so most practitioners prefer to remove the tube and monitor function.

Implications for practice

- Temporary tracheostomies reduce airway deadspace, so can significantly reduce work of breathing.
- The upper airway warms, moistens and filters air; bypassing most of the upper airway creates potential risks and problems.
- Although the cough reflex normally remains, tracheostomies weaken the strength of coughs, so patients often need suction to clear airway secretions.
- Thick, dry secretions can occlude the tracheostomy, causing respiratory arrest.
- Staff caring for patients with temporary tracheostomies should know how to re-establish an airway as quickly as possible.
- Emergency equipment should be checked each shift.
- Unless the patient is adequately clearing their own airway secretions, suction should also be performed at least once each shift, as near the start to enable individualised planning of care for that shift.

Summary

Temporary tracheostomies can provide a useful medical treatment for severe acute respiratory limitations, but they create many actual and potential problems for patients. Nurses should, therefore, know the potential risks created and how to minimise the problems created by tracheostomies. Critical Care Outreach services should usually be involved in the team caring for patients with tracheostomies (Lewis and Oliver, 2005).

Clinical scenario

Thomas Fraser was admitted to hospital three weeks ago with a severe acute exacerbation of COPD, initially requiring artificial ventilation in ICU, where a percutaneous temporary tracheostomy was inserted. He is now self-ventilating, but still has the tracheostomy, and has now been transferred to a step-down unit.

1   From reading this chapter, and your own experiences, list actual and potential problems the tracheostomy might cause Thomas. Identify any equipment that will be needed. Where it is not stocked in your own workplace, identify where you could obtain this equipment.

2   Identify nursing observations that should be performed in relation to Thomas' tracheostomy. Include frequency of observations. From this book, and any other available sources, identify the evidence-base for this aspect of care.

3   Over the following week Thomas' condition slowly deteriorates. Without non-invasive or invasive ventilation it is unlikely that Thomas will survive. But if ventilation is started, his chances of discharge home without it are slim. Unfortunately Thomas is hypoxic and appears frightened, so the multidisciplinary team consider that his ability to make an informed decision is limited. Note down your own thoughts about the advantages and disadvantages of whether more aggressive treatment should be initiated. As Thomas' nurse, decide whether, on balance, how far, if at all, you would advocate any escalation of treatment.

Bibliography

Key reading

NHS Quality Improvement Scotland (2007) and the ICS (2008) provide guidelines. Recent nursing reviews of tracheostomies include Serra (2000) and Docherty and Bench (2002). Lewis and Oliver (2005) include a useful chart for practical ward care.

Further reading

General texts, such as Dougherty and Lister (2008) provide useful supplementary material. Recent nursing reviews include Russell (2005) and St George's Healthcare Trust (2006).

Chapter 23

Non-invasive ventilation

Philip Woodrow

Contents

Learning outcomes

After reading this chapter you will be able to:

- identify which patients are likely and unlikely to benefit from non-invasive ventilation (NIV);
- understand the main differences between continuous positive airway pressure (CPAP) and bilevel NIV;

■ explain the main options offered by most bilevel non-invasive ventilators;

■ identify safe nursing care of patients being supported by NIV.

Fundamental knowledge

Respiratory anatomy and physiology; respiratory failure.

Introduction

Ventilation is the movement of air in and out of the lungs. Failure of ventilation is, therefore, life-threatening, often necessitating ventilatory support. Two decades ago, this usually necessitated admission to intensive care units (ICUs) for invasive artificial ventilation, but rapid progress in bilevel NIV since then enables many patients with ventilatory failure to be cared for both in the community and in acute hospital wards.

Before widespread availability of NIV, CPAP was developed from supports originally available on invasive ventilators. Technically, CPAP is not ventilation, as it hinders, rather than helps, expiration. However, as both useful respiratory support and a means to understand bilevel NIV, it is included. This chapter frequently refers to the authoritative RCP/BTS/ICS guidelines for NIV, which updates the classic 2002 BTS guidelines.

NIV is used in community settings mainly to treat

■ sleep apnoea.

In acute hospitals, non-invasive ventilation is usually used to treat

■ acute exacerbations of chronic obstructive pulmonary disease (COPD)

although other uses include to treat

■ pulmonary oedema
■ neuromuscular disease, such as Guillain–Barré Syndrome
■ chest wall deformity, such as scoliosis
■ severe pneumonia
■ weaning from invasive ventilation
■ pre-surgical optimisation.

NIV for neuromuscular disease and chest wall deformity may need to be continued in the community.

Respiratory failure

Respiratory failure is either Type 1 (oxygenation failure) or Type 2 (ventilatory failure, or hypercapnic respiratory failure) – see Chapter 15. British Thoracic Society (BTS, 2002) definitions are:

Type 1:
- arterial oxygen (PaO$_2$) below 8.0 kPa
- arterial carbon dioxide (PaCO$_2$) below 6.0 kPa

Type 2:
- arterial oxygen (PaO$_2$) below 8.0 kPa
- arterial carbon dioxide (PaCO$_2$) above 6.0 kPa

The difference can be easily remembered as: Type 1 affects one gas, Type 2 affects two gases. Type 1 failure therefore needs support for oxygenation (such as CPAP); Type 2 needs support for ventilation, such as bilevel NIV.

CPAP

CPAP originated as an adjunct to invasive ventilation, where a resistance valve was placed over the expiratory port – positive end expiratory pressure (PEEP). When force (pressure) near the end of expiration becomes too weak to keep the valve open, it closes, trapping the last bit of breath in the circuit, which includes the patient's lungs. Air trapped in alveoli

- prevents collapse (*atelectasis*);
- enables oxygen exchange to continue,

while the positive pressure in airways before collapsed alveoli helps reinflation (reverses atelectasis). CPAP, therefore, improves oxygenation, so is useful for treating Type 1 respiratory failure. CPAP is also useful for treating pulmonary oedema (see p. 219).

While improved oxygenation makes CPAP useful for Type 1 failure, so the same pressure that supports inspiration inhibits expiration. Carbon dioxide clearance from lungs depends on expired volume. The 'gas trapping' caused by CPAP may inhibit carbon dioxide removal, worsening hypercapnia. This limits the usefulness of CPAP for treating hypercapnic respiratory failure, such as from acute exacerbations of COPD.

Some hospitals use positive pressure ventilators intermittently for physiotherapy, usually to reverse atelectasis, especially post-operative. Modes include intermittent positive pressure breathing (IPPB; the 'Bird®'), CPAP and bilevel NIV. Negative pressure cuirasses are sometimes used to mobilise sputum. Pryor and Prasad (2008) devote a chapter to NIV, but elsewhere include only passing mention of intermittent interventions.

High-flow nasal oxygen

High-flow humidified nasal oxygen (e.g. Vapotherm®, Fisher&Paykell®) effectively provides a low-pressure CPAP (about 2–3 cmH$_2$O), although many CPAP machines could be used with nasal masks. In acute care nasal masks are not generally used, and nasal masks usually prevent humidification. High-flow systems can achieve about 95 per cent humidity. Anecdotal reports are encouraging, with good tolerance and high success rates.

Bilevel NIV

Bilevel non-invasive ventilators essentially provide two alternating levels of CPAP – a higher one on inspiration, and a lower one on expiration:

- IPAP = inspired positive airway pressure;
- EPAP = expired positive airway pressure.

The higher pressure of IPAP assists inspiration, delivering larger volumes for less effort by the respiratory muscles. In addition to inhaling larger volumes, and so more oxygen, reducing the *work of breathing* (respiratory muscles use less oxygen and energy) leaves more oxygen for other parts of the body. The lower pressure of EPAP enables more of the inhaled volume to escape, compared with CPAP. This, therefore, assists more carbon dioxide clearance. Increasing the gap between IPAP and EPAP (sometimes termed 'pressure support') increases carbon dioxide clearance. Bilevel NIV is, therefore, useful for treating Type 2 respiratory failure – in practice, in acute hospitals, this usually means acute exacerbations of COPD.

Most bilevel machines include a *trigger*. This senses respiratory effort, causing the machine to change from EPAP to IPAP. Machine cycles normally follow patient's own breaths, rather than imposing their cycle on the patient.

Bilevel NIV is sometimes called by the brand name of whatever system is used within the hospital (e.g. NIPPY®, BiPAP®). Many bilevel machines can also deliver CPAP.

Contraindications

CPAP and bilevel NIV are useful supports for people with respiratory failure, but being non-invasive, they do not protect the airway. Although most bilevel NIV machines include a back-up apnoea mode, this is a safety feature to overcome short periods of apnoea, and is not intended for prolonged use. Contraindications for NIV are:

- life-threatening hypoxaemia;
- severe co-morbidity;
- confusion/agitation/severe cognitive impairment;
- facial burns/trauma/recent facial or upper airway surgery;
- vomiting;
- fixed upper airway obstruction;
- undrained pneumothorax;
- upper gastrointestinal surgery;
- inability to protect the airway;
- copious respiratory secretions;
- haemodynamically unstable requiring inotropes/pressors (unless in a critical care unit);
- patient moribund;
- bowel obstruction.

(RCP/BTS/ICS, 2008)

Settings

Positive airway pressure compromises various body systems (see p. 219), so the ideal pressure is one that achieves the therapeutic aim with minimal side effects. Pressures are usually commenced low, increasing incrementally until optimal therapy and minimal complications are achieved. CPAP is often commenced at $5\,cmH_2O$, while bilevel NIV is commenced at IPAP $8–10\,cmH_2O$ and EPAP $4\,cmH_2O$, although Chapman and Davies (2003) suggest typical starting pressures are 12/4.

Equipment is variable, but most modern CPAP machines autoregulate most aspects, leaving users little to set beyond CPAP pressure and oxygen percentage. If equipment contains a gas flow setting, this should be sufficiently high to ensure that the exit valve, which creates the positive pressure, always 'hovers' open (on many modern CPAP machines, the valve is not visible).

Bilevel NIV machines offer various ways to adjust breath patterns. Some common adjustments are included here, but various others may be available, so users should be familiar with machines used locally – see the manufacturer's handbook. Usual features include:

- *Ramp/rise time* is the time taken for IPAP to reach full pressure. Middle settings are usually best, but with tachypnoea (>30 breaths/minute), shorter rise time helps ensure full IPAP, and so lung volume, is reached in the relatively short inspiratory phase. With obstructed airways, slower rise time is likely to cause less distress.
- *Rate*. Most machines usually follow the patient's own breathing pattern. Rate settings usually only determine time machines allow for IPAP. Rate should be half the patient's own rate, and adjusted downwards when tachypnoea subsides.

Most bilevel non-invasive ventilators deliver air, and so if supplementary oxygen is needed it usually has to be added through ports directly into the face mask or earlier into the circuit.

Masks

For both CPAP and bilevel NIV, masks should be accurately fitted. Most CPAP circuits rely on a near-complete seal around the face, making masks tight and uncomfortable, and often causing pressure sores. Many bilevel ventilators compensate for leaks, so masks are less tight. Leaking of air upwards into eyes should be avoided, as this may cause conjunctivitis (Hillberg and Johnson, 1997; Kannan, 1999). Condition of facial skin should be observed and recorded both before

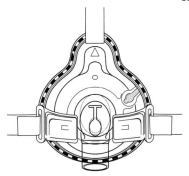

Figure 23.1 Full-face mask

starting NIV and during use. Some discomfort may be unavoidable, but whenever possible nurses should relieve or reduce discomfort, for example, by repositioning the mask.

Usually, full-face masks are used. However, most manufacturers supply other options, such as

- total face mask
- helmet
- nasal mask
- mouth-piece.

Patients unable to tolerate face masks may comply with other options. Nasal masks should only be used if patients breathe through their nose, while mouth-pieces necessitate mouth-breathing.

Deterioration

Many patients benefit from NIV, but about one-quarter deteriorate further, necessitating intubation (or withdrawal/limitation of treatment). Which patients will deteriorate is unpredictable (Poponcik et al., 1999), so NIV should be attempted (Jolliet et al., 2001), monitored closely, and if necessary be replaced by invasive ventilation within four hours of commencing NIV (RCP/BTS/ICS, 2008). If intubation is necessary, delay can be fatal (Esteban et al., 2004).

Failure rate for NIV is high (Squadrone et al., 2004), either from patients refusing the treatment or it not being effective, so plans to commence NIV should also include clear plans for action if NIV fails (Telfer et al., 2007; RCP/BTS/ICS, 2008) – including whether NIV is 'ceiling treatment', and whether resuscitation or palliative care are appropriate. If NIV fails, there are two broad options:

- escalation of treatment to invasive ventilation;
- terminal care.

ICU admission and invasive ventilation with sedation may merely prolong death. Terminal, compassionate care may be a better option. The ICU/Critical Care Outreach team should, therefore, be involved in planning. If NIV fails, Squadrone et al. (2004) suggest the delay to intubation caused by NIV may not be detrimental, although Esteban et al. (2004) found mortality was higher in patients if intubation was delayed by NIV.

Pathologies

COPD

Bilevel NIV significantly improves survival from acute exacerbations of COPD (Plant et al., 2001; Girou et al., 2003; Plant et al., 2003), making this the most common indication for its use in acute hospitals. Bilevel NIV should be the first-line intervention with respiratory failure in COPD (Lightowler *et al.*, 2003), so should be initiated as soon as respiratory acidosis occurs (arterial pH < 7.35, $PaCO_2 > 6\,kPa$), rather than used when other options fail. Underlying causes should also be treated concurrently – for example, suspected infection should be investigated (sputum specimen) and treated with antibiotics.

Pulmonary oedema

Positive pressure within alveoli encourages return of interstitial oedema into pulmonary circulation. NIV (CPAP or bilevel) speeds resolution of dyspnoea, respiratory distress and metabolic abnormalities, although does not improve survival (Gray *et al.*, 2008). Combined with diuretic therapy to remove the fluid from the body, treatment times often need to be limited to a few hours.

Pneumonia

Jolliet *et al.* (2001) and Baudouin (2002) recommend using NIV for severe pneumonia. While few other studies address this issue, bilevel NIV is widely used for Type 2 respiratory failure, and is an effective treatment for severe hypoxaemia (Ferer *et al.*, 2003), which could be caused by severe pneumonia.

Sleep apnoea

Sleep apnoea causes poor sleep for both sufferers and carers, and tissue hypoxia to sufferers. Overnight positive pressure ventilation (CPAP or bilevel) significantly improves sleep, so enabling more daytime activity (Patel *et al.*, 2003). It may also restore hypercapnia as the main respiratory drive. While normally managed in the community, these people may be admitted to acute hospital for respiratory crises or non-respiratory problems, so need overnight NIV.

Complications

Physiological

Hypotension

Positive intrathoracic pressure reduces ventricular filling and so, unless compensatory mechanisms occur, reduces blood pressure. Problems from reduced perfusion pressure may be offset by improved oxygenation, including to the myocardium. For some patients, NIV improves cardiac function (Nelson *et al.*, 2001; Sin *et al.*, 2000; Yin *et al.*, 2001).

At low pressures, this effect is usually insignificant, but CPAP above $10\,cmH_2O$ can cause significant hypotension (Kiely *et al.*, 1998). Bilevel NIV does not appear to cause significant hypotension (Somauroo *et al.*, 2000). However, when commending positive pressure NIV, blood pressure should be closely monitored, such as setting automated non-invasive blood pressure monitors on 5- or

10-minute cycles for 30 minutes, and using appropriate alarm settings to warn staff about hypotension.

Renal

Hypotension may compromise all systems but kidneys are at high risk from

- acute kidney injury
- ischaemia (acute tubular necrosis).

Hydration should, therefore, be optimised. Renal failure can also cause toxicity from drug or drug metabolite accumulation.

Endocrine

Stress increases hormone release

- renin–angiotensin–aldosterone cascade (hypertension; see Chapter 28)
- anti-diuretic hormone (oliguria)

while positive intrathoracic pressure reduces plasma atrial natriuretic peptide (oliguria). Together, these hormones can cause various problems, including oedema – systemic and pulmonary. Pulmonary oedema worsens hypoxia.

Gut

With swallowing, some air enters the stomach. Because both the trachea and the oesophagus lead off the oropharynx, positive pressure in the upper airway causes more air to be swallowed, impeding its escape. Air accumulating in the stomach causes

- gastric distension;
- splinting of the diaphragm (reducing breath size and making breathing more difficult); and
- discomfort, nausea and/or vomiting;

and if not removed

- flatus (Parsons *et al.*, 2000).

If gastric distension is problematic a nasogastric tube should be passed and left on free drainage. The bag may need frequent emptying. Anti-emetics and peppermint should be prescribed to relieve discomfort.

Psychological

Many people find NIV, especially CPAP, uncomfortable and distressing. While some patients may overtly refuse it, others may covertly resist its use by removing, or attempting to remove, it frequently. Like many other respiratory interventions, little or no benefit is gained until about 20 minutes. Frequent removal is not therapeutic, but also indicates patients are not willing to consent to treatment, and are becoming distressed. The stress response causes detrimental physiological effects, including tachypnoea, tachycardia, hypertension, hyperglycaemia and fluid retention (see Chapter 13). So to prevent harmful distress, and potential claims of assault, frequent removal should be recognised as an indication for discontinuation.

Approaching patients with face masks and NIV headgear may provoke fear. Having explained what NIV can offer, whenever possible patients should be offered the mask to hold in their hands and place it against their own face. Slowly building up the gas flow may also help tolerance. If patients are comfortable with the treatment, they are more likely to accept it (Jarvis, 2006); if patients reject the treatment, they are unlikely to consent to further attempts. As nurses usually commence NIV, and adjust equipment, success or failure of NIV largely depends on nursing management (Jarvis, 2006).

Like many respiratory interventions, commencing NIV relies largely on inspired guesses, using close monitoring and subsequent adjustments to achieve optimal effect. Not all treatments will succeed. NIV in the community for people with sleep apnoea has a one-third failure rate (Russo-Magno *et al.*, 2001). Using NIV for acute respiratory failure, with less time and fewer options, should, therefore, be considered successful if two-thirds of attempts are successful.

Observation

NIV is usually commenced because patients cannot adequately breathe by themselves. Therefore, patients receiving NIV should be closely observed. Observation should include:

- respiratory rate, heart rate;
- level of consciousness, patient comfort;
- chest wall movement, ventilator synchrony, accessory muscle use.

(RCP/BTS/ICS, 2008)

Pulse oximetry indicates oxygenation, so should be continuously monitored for at least the first 12 hours of NIV (RCP/BTS/ICS, 2008). Hypoxia may cause

- confusion, drowsiness or agitation;
- compensatory tachycardia.

But oximetry does not measure carbon dioxide or haemoglobin levels (see Chapter 16). Visual observations indicating poor ventilation (hypercapnia) include:

■ very slow or fast respiratory rate (<10 or > 30 breaths per minute);
■ shallow chest wall (or accessory muscle) movement.

The mainstay of carbon dioxide measurement in clinical practice remains blood gas analysis (see Chapter 17):

■ arterial
■ capillary
■ transcutaneous.

Transcutaneous gases, usually measured on the ear, differs slightly from arterial, but generally have close correlation (Cox *et al.*, 2006), so provide a useful means for continuous or frequent monitoring of trends. Recent developments in technology (e.g. Tosca®) have reduced both times to obtain readings and temperature applied to the skin, making it more practical for adult use (Chhajed *et al.*, 2005). Attempts to develop pulse co-oximeters (pulse oximeters that also measure carbon dioxide) have so far not yielded reliable technology (Bolliger *et al.*, 2007). BTS (2008) recommend earlobe capillary sampling, citing recent studies supporting its reliability with carbon dioxide levels.

RCP/BTS/ICS (2008) recommend arterial gas sampling within one hour of commencing NIV, within one hour of subsequent changes, and within 4 hours if the patient is not clinically improving. NIV has failed so should be replaced by invasive ventilation (RCP/BTS/ICS, 2008) or terminal care.

Weaning

Chronic respiratory disease usually necessitates weaning rather than suddenly stopping NIV. Kramer *et al.* (1995) recommend weaning criteria of:

■ respiratory rate <24
■ heart rate <110
■ pH > 7.35
■ SpO_2 > 90% on 4 litres of oxygen.

However, with severe COPD normal respiratory rate may exceed 24, and normal SaO_2 be below 90%. Assessing comfort and mental state are potentially subjective. So although each of these signs may indicate respiratory distress, they do need to be individualised.

Implications for practice

■ CPAP is useful for Type 1 respiratory failure.
■ Bilevel NIV is useful for Type 2 respiratory failure.

- NIV should be a first-line treatment for Type 2 respiratory failure.
- Respiratory acidosis causing blood pH of 7.25–7.35 is an indication for NIV.
- Patients receiving NIV should be closely monitored and observed, which necessitates sufficient numbers of staff with sufficient knowledge and skills of using NIV to safely care for the patient.
- When commencing NIV, plans should be made for treatment options if NIV fails. There are usually only two options:

  – invasive ventilation (usually in ICU)
  – palliative care.

- If six hours of treatment has not resulted in significant improvement, treatment should be changed to one of the above options.

Summary

NIV has significantly improved outcome from respiratory failure, so is now used in various wards specialising in respiratory care, and sometimes elsewhere. Patients with chronic respiratory disease may have previously experienced successful treatment with NIV, expecting nursing staff to be as familiar with the treatments as they are. CPAP, although technically not ventilation, can be a useful respiratory support for Type 1 respiratory failure, especially when caused by pulmonary oedema. Bilevel NIV is useful for ventilatory (Type 2) respiratory failure. However, NIV will not be successful for all patients, so patients should be closely observed, monitored and reviewed.

Clinical scenario

Jack Adams, aged 74, is admitted with an acute exacerbation of COPD. On arrival in A&E he was breathless and cyanosed. Arterial blood gas analysis showed pH 7.27, PaO_2 7.2 kPa, $PaCO_2$ 8.3 kPa. Bilevel NIV is commenced and he is transferred to the medical assessment ward for further observation.

1   List the nursing observations that should be made. Identify which observations should be continuous, and suggest an initial frequency for observation which will be intermittent.

2   Identify problems that Jack is likely to, or may experience as a result of NIV. Suggest ways these problems could be resolved or minimised.

3   After two days of NIV support and other medical treatments, Jack's condition improves sufficiently to consider removing ventilatory support. Make a list of criteria that you would use before removing or to wean NIV. Identify the rationales for these criteria. Analyse the evidence on which these are based, and how reliable you consider that evidence to be.

Bibliography

Key reading

RCP/BTS/ICS (2008) guidelines are the single most important resource for all UK staff using NIV. Readers should be familiar with NIV and other relevant protocols of their own hospital.

Further reading

Recent useful articles include Cox *et al.* (2006), Jarvis (2006), Masip *et al.* (2005) and Telfer (2007).

Part 4

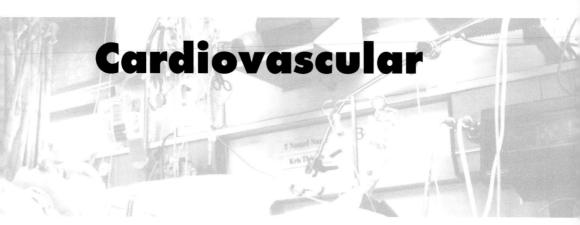

Cardiovascular

Chapter 24

Haemodynamic assessment

Philip Woodrow

Contents

Learning outcomes

After reading this chapter you will be able to:

- understand the significance of haemodynamic assessment;
- recognise causes of inaccurate measurement;
- understand the significance of mean arterial pressure and pulse pressure;
- identify main causes of high and low central venous pressure measurements;
- apply knowledge of haemodynamic assessment to patient care.

Fundamental knowledge

Cardiac physiology.

Introduction

Acute illness often either originates or compromises cardiovascular function, so assessing and monitoring cardiovascular function is important when caring for sicker patients. Automated non-invasive devices are generally used to measure pulse and blood pressure and, provided they are calibrated regularly (most hospitals check equipment annually), are useful and reliable (Jones *et al.*, 2003). But they only provide some of the haemodynamic information that can easily be assessed. With sicker patients, central venous pressure (CVP) may be used to guide fluid management. Although more advanced methods of haemodynamic monitoring, such as arterial lines and cardiac output studies, are available on critical care units, these are rarely used in ward areas, so are not discussed here but are included in *Intensive Care Nursing* (Woodrow, 2006).

Pulse

Pulse rates are frequently recorded from automated blood pressure monitors. While this is generally acceptable, pulse should be felt to assess

- strength
- regularity.

Irregular pulses are usually caused by atrial fibrillation (AF), the most common dysrhythmia (see Chapter 25). Newly detected irregularities should be reported, and an ECG recorded. With AF apex-radial deficit should be measured – one person using a stethoscope to count the rate at the apex of the heart over a whole minute, while a second person counts the radial pulse over the same minute. Pre-scribed digoxin should only be omitted if the *apex* rate is below 60 bpm.

Feeling pulse strength provides an indication of pulse volume (cardiac stroke volume). Most readers should have normal strength pulses and stroke volume (about 70 ml at rest), but to get used to feeling normal strength pulses, it is also advisable to ask to feel colleagues' pulses. Strong, bounding pulses indicate stroke volumes over 100 ml, while weak, thready pulses indicate stroke volumes below 40 ml. Abnormalities should be recorded and reported.

Assessing peripheries

Looking at and feeling feet, and hands, for colour and warmth indicates perfusion, or lack of it. Mottled, cold peripheries are poorly perfused. Excessive dilation (e.g. from sepsis) causes peripheries to be abnormally warm and appear flushed. Inspecting peripheries may also reveal oedema, ulceration or other symptoms of haemodynamic compromise.

Capillary refill

Pressing on a finger tip for five seconds compresses capillaries. In health, initial blanching should disappear within two seconds (Ahern and Philpot, 2002) of releasing pressure. Delayed capillary refill indicates poor perfusion (Lima and Bakker, 2005), usually from hypovolaemia/dehydration, but may occur with vessel disease (e.g. atherosclerosis), or arterial hypotension.

Arterial blood pressure

Blood pressure is the pressure exerted on vessel walls. All blood vessels have a blood pressure, but 'blood pressure' usually refers to *arterial blood pressure.* Most cuffs display marks to show how to place them on arms, and the range of arm circumferences they can be used on (see Figure 24.1). Using cuffs which are too small causes over-readings, while cuffs that are too large under-read. Most adult wards only need to stock small, medium (also called 'average') and large-sized cuffs.

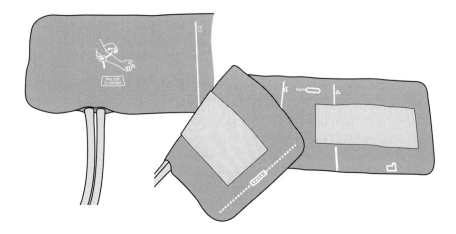

Figure 24.1 NIBP cuff, with markings

Systolic pressure

Peak transient pressure occurs when flow through vessels is at its greatest. Very high systolic pressure can cause bleeds, strokes or other problems. Hypotension can cause inadequate perfusion, and so cell death. Sustained systolic pressure above 140mmHg should be actively treated (see Chapter 28). Systolic blood pressure below 100mmHg is generally a cause for concern, and widely used by many early-warning scores. Shock is often defined as <80mmHg for more than one hour. However, a few people normally have very low blood pressure, and may be healthy with surprisingly low figures, while people who are normally hypertensive may suffer perfusion failure with pressures above these figures. So target blood pressure should be assessed for each patient.

Mean arterial pressure (MAP)

MAP is calculated by most automated blood pressure devices. Averaging (mean) pressure across the whole pulse cycle provides a more valuable indication of whether perfusion is adequate, so in patients who are hypotensive MAP is the most valuable pressure to monitor. Minimum perfusion pressure is often cited as a MAP of 65 mmHg (Dellinger *et al.*, 2004), although patients who are normally very hypertensive may need higher minimum mean pressures (e.g. 70–80 mmHg). Pressures can be clearly charted by using arrows for systolic and diastolic pressures, and a cross for mean pressures (see Figure 24.2).

Diastolic pressure

The lowest arterial pressure occurs between pulses. Diastolic pressure is arguably the least important of the three pressures discussed so far, although very high (rule of thumb >100 mmHg) diastolic pressures increase the risk of strokes, while very low diastolic pressures (possibly <60 mmHg), may indicate shock, probably from vasodilatation (distributive shock).

Pulse pressure

Pulse pressure is the pressure created by each pulse – the difference between diastolic and systolic. For example, blood pressure of 140/90 creates a pulse pressure of 50. Pulse pressure increases as more pressure is exerted on vessel walls. Although hypervolaemia could widen pulse pressure, in practice wide pressures are almost invariably from lack of vessel stretch (e.g. atherosclerosis). Narrow pulse pressures indicate hypovolaemia, which may be caused by cardiac failure or systemic hypovolaemia. Pulse pressure is visibly obvious on charts – the greater the distance between systolic and diastolic marks, the greater the pulse pressure.

CVP

Central lines, or central venous catheters (CVCs), are placed in one of the two central veins: superior or inferior vena cava. CVP measures pressure of blood returning to, or filling, the right atrium. This indicates

- blood volume
- vascular tone
- cardiac function.

CVP, sometimes called 'filling' pressure or right atrial pressure (RAP), is therefore useful to guide fluid management in sicker patients.

CVP is usually measured by digital transducers (see Figure 24.3), although can also be measured by the largely obsolete water manometers (see Figure 24.4). Skills of using each are different, and readers should be shown how to use equipment with which they are unfamiliar.

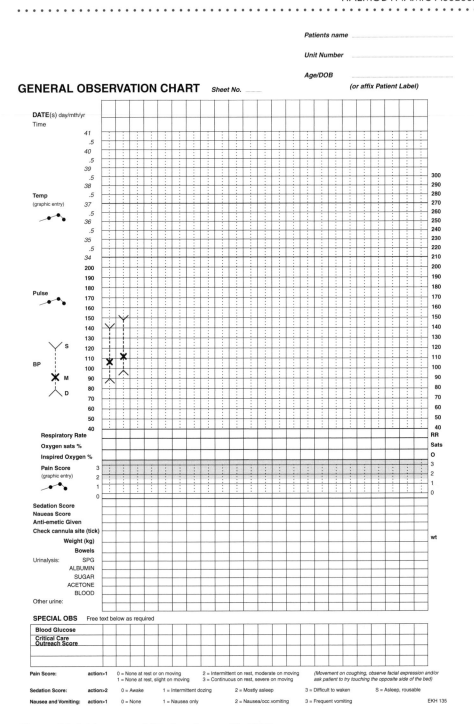

Figure 24.2 **Diagram of BP charting, with MAP**

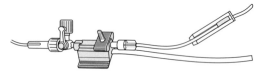

Figure 24.3 **Transduced system**

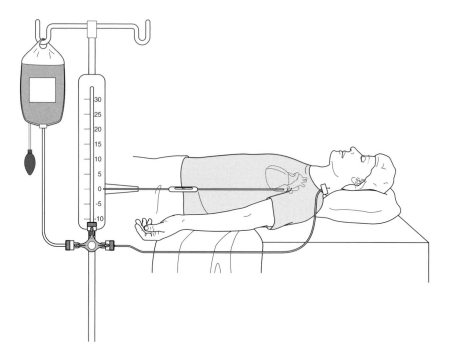

Figure 24.4 **Water manometer**

Measurement

CVP should be read from mid-axilla (right atrial level). A small ink mark on skin may help ensure consistency of site.

To reflect RAP, patients should ideally lie supine. However, many breathless patients become distressed in this position, so if measured semi-recumbent or in an upright position, the position should be recorded on charts so that future measurements can, whenever possible, be made in the same position. The more upright the patient, the lower CVP will read.

Any infusions running through the same lumen of the central line should be stopped during the time of measurement (infusions through other lumens will not significantly affect readings). 'Zeroing' the CVP ensures that atmospheric pressure at the point of measurement is read as zero. Water manometers are zeroed by placing the '0' at mid-axilla. This usually necessitates a spirit level. Transducers should also be placed at mid-axilla level, but the 'zero' button on the equipment will also need to then be activated.

Digital monitors display a trace and reading. Provided the scale is sufficiently large, traces should show clear waveforms (see Figure 24.5). There will usually be a respiratory 'swing' – the whole trace moving up and down with breathing. Digital equipment without monitors usually only display CVP measurements.

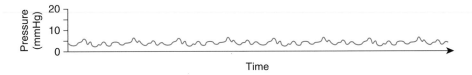

Figure 24.5 CVP trace

After zeroing, the chamber of water manometers should be almost filled with fluid without getting the air filter at the top wet – wet filters resist air entry, giving falsely high readings. The tap should then be turned to open the chamber to the patient. Gravity makes the fluid fall until resistance from central venous pressure matches gravity. Slight changes in pressure from the patient's respiratory pattern (usually about 1 cm) makes the fluid fall in a 'swinging' pattern, until it oscillates between two figures. Intrathoracic pressure, and so fluid level, falls on inspiration (except with positive pressure artificial ventilation). The higher figure of the swing is recorded.

Pressures

Transducers normally measure CVP in millimetres of mercury (mmHg). Water manometers measure centimetres of water (cmH_2O). $1 cmH_2O = 0.74 mmHg$, a negligible difference at low pressures, but significant as pressures rise. Table 24.1 shows equivalents between 0–20 for both scales. Users should clarify which scale any medical targets are intended for.

In health, CVP is normally 2–6 mmHg/5–10 cmH_2O (mid-axilla). Sicker patients often have abnormally high or low pressures. Treatment usually aims to maintain slightly higher than normal CVP to ensure sufficient blood return to the heart (*preload*).

Low CVP almost invariably indicates hypovolaemia, either from fluid loss by

- haemorrhage (e.g. trauma, surgery)
- excessive diuresis (e.g. diabetes, diuretics)

or from

- poor return (e.g. shock).

High CVP may be from

- cardiac failure;
- hypervolaemia (e.g. renal failure);

Table 24.1 Comparison of mmHg and cmH₂O

cmH₂O	mmHg (exact)	mmHg (rounded)
1	(0.74)	1
2	(1.48)	1
3	(2.22)	2
4	(2.96)	3
5	(3.70)	4
6	(4.44)	4
7	(5.18)	5
8	(5.92)	6
9	(6.66)	7
10	(7.40)	7
11	(8.14)	8
12	(8.88)	9
13	(9.62)	10
14	(10.36)	10
15	(11.10)	11
16	(11.84)	12
17	(12.58)	13
18	(13.32)	13
19	(14.06)	14
20	(14.80)	15

mmHg	cmH₂O (exact)	cmH₂O (rounded)
1	(1.36)	1
2	(2.72)	3
3	(4.08)	4
4	(5.44)	5
5	(6.80)	7
6	(8.16)	8
7	(9.52)	10
8	(10.88)	11
9	(12.22)	12
10	(13.60)	14
11	(14.96)	15
12	(16.32)	16
13	(17.68)	18
14	(19.04)	19
15	(20.40)	20
16	(21.76)	22
17	(23.10)	23
18	(24.44)	24
19	(25.82)	26
20	(27.20)	27

- increased intrathoracic pressure (e.g. non-invasive ventilation);
- portal hypertension/liver cirrhosis;
- lumen occlusion/obstruction (e.g. cannula against vein wall; thrombus);
- artefact (e.g. viscous drugs/fluids remaining in the line);
- user error (e.g. wet air filter in water manometers, or running infusions through the same lumen).

Blocked lines

Lines should be kept patent by running a slow drip through the line. Transduced systems should include a pressure bag inflated to 300 mmHg to maintain transducer calibration. Water manometers should be kept patent with a slow drip – as slow as possible unless IVIs are needed therapeutically. The RCN (2003b) recommend flushing blocked catheters with 10 ml saline, but this might dislodge thrombi or biofilm to form an embolus (Hadaway, 2005) in blood soon to flow into pulmonary circulation. Thrombus obstruction may be dissolved with small doses of urokinase, a thrombolytic agent (Polderman and Girbes, 2002). Stewart (2001) reports successfully using a percussive technique to break up and remove thrombi.

Implications for practice

- Trends are more significant than absolute figure.
- If readings appear abnormal, recheck (e.g. within 15 minutes).
- Mean arterial pressure is the best indicator of perfusion pressure – maintain above 65 mmHg.
- Wide pulse pressure indicates cardiovascular disease.
- Central venous pressure indicates blood volume and cardiac function:

  - low CVP indicates hypovolaemia;
  - high CVP has more causes, but heart failure or hypervolaemia are the most common.

Summary

For many acutely ill patients, monitoring blood pressure and heart rate provide sufficient information for medical management. Blood pressure is a vital sign. Problems with blood pressure (hyper- or hypo-tension) are, however, symptoms of underlying problems. Nurses caring for highly dependent patients therefore need to consider factors causing abnormal pressure. Capillary refill, pulse pressure and MAP provide further useful information about cardiovascular function. CVP can indicate fluid status.

Clinical scenario

Hugh Barton has been admitted following recent episodes of dizziness. He has a history of hypertension, and despite taking his daily 10 mg of Atenolol this morning, his blood pressure is 173/86 and he feels tingling in his fingers. His heart rate is 65 (regular).

1 Comment on this information, identifying what it indicates. Include comments on his systolic, diastolic and pulse pressures. What other haemodynamic assessments would be useful, and why?

2 His mean arterial pressure is 115. What does this indicate?

3 Would central venous cannulation be beneficial for Hugh? Evaluate risks and benefits.

Bibliography

Key reading

Jevon and Ewens (2007) is a useful handbook, while the *Marsden Manual* (Dougherty and Lister, 2008) reviews evidence.

Further reading

Readers should be familiar with handbooks and manuals for equipment used in their workplace. Nursing journals frequently publish review articles, such as Kisel and Perkins (2006) and Cole (2007).

Chapter 25

ECGs and common dysrhythmias

Philip Woodrow

Contents

Learning outcomes

After reading this chapter you will be able to:

- understand how normal cardiac conduction relates to electrocardiogram (ECG) traces for normal sinus rhythm;
- recognise common dysrhythmias;
- recognise difference between, and implications of, broad and narrow complex tachycardias;
- identify main treatments for common dysrhythmias.

Fundamental knowledge

Cardiac anatomy (including coronary arteries); basic electrophysiology, including normal conduction pathways (SA node, AV node, Bundle of His, Branch Bundle, Purkinje Fibres) and how this is 'viewed' in the six limb leads.

Introduction

ECGs are the most commonly conducted cardiovascular diagnostic procedure (Kligfield *et al.*, 2007) used to diagnose, or exclude, cardiac dysrhythmias and cardiac disease. Acutely ill patients may have chronic dysrhythmias, or develop acute dysrhythmias in response to disease or treatments. For example, about 7 per cent of general surgical patients develop new dysrhythmias post-operatively (Walsh *et al.*, 2007). Level 2 patients may need continuous ECG monitoring or 12-lead ECGs. Although primarily used for medical diagnoses, nurses in acute care should be able to recognise most dysrhythmias, and know what, if any, treatments are likely to benefit their patients to enable earlier and optimal intervention. Monitoring, without staff able to interpret monitoring, induces a dangerous false sense of security. The appendix lists some commonly used drugs to treat dysrhythmias. The chapter begins with 'basics'; if these are unfamiliar, further descriptions can be found in texts such as Hampton (2008a).

All qualified nurses should be able to record a 12-lead ECG and attach bedside monitors. Yet simple errors, such as lead misplacement, can cause erroneous diagnosis. 12-lead ECGs should be reviewed by doctors, but nurses should summon help for urgent problems. Nurses should be able to interpret common rhythms and problems. This chapter, therefore, provides a framework for ECG interpretation, describes common dysrhythmias and key interventions/treatments. Drugs listed are those commonly used; other drugs may also be effective. Like any skill, ECG interpretation needs repeated practice.

The graph

When no electrical activity is recorded, the graph is horizontal (isoelectric). A line upward from the isoelectric line is a *positive deflection*, while a line downward is a *negative deflection*. ECGs represent three-dimensional electrical activity of cardiac conduction on a two-dimensional graph.

With standard settings:

■   height represents voltage: 1 cm = 1 millivolt (2 large squares, or 10 small squares);
■   length represents time: 1 small square = 0.04 seconds, 1 large square = 0.2 seconds.

Figure 25.1 shows a normal sinus rhythm complex.

Cardiac muscle contraction follows electrical activity, except with pulseless electrical activity (PEA). With PEA, whatever rhythm is displayed does not produce a pulse.

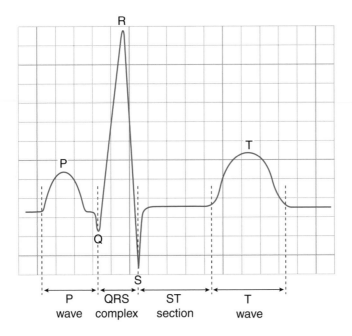

Figure 25.1 **Normal sinus rhythm**

Electrodes

The six limb leads use three electrodes:

- right arm (red)
- left arm (yellow)
- left leg/hip (green).

Positions can be memorised as 'traffic lights'. Electrical 'pictures' are unchanged along each limb, so electrodes may be anywhere between the hand/foot and the shoulder/hip.

These produce the six limb leads ('views'):

- I: right arm to left arm
- II: right arm to left leg
- III: left arm to left leg
- aVR: right arm
- aVL: left arm
- aVF: left leg (foot)

12-lead ECGs use a fourth limb electrode on the right leg (black) (see Figure 25.2).

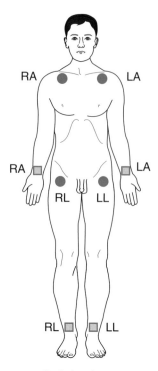

***Figure 25.2* Electrode placement: limb leads**

Five-electrode limb-lead monitors also use the 4th intercostal space to right of sternum, like C1 (white).

The six chest lead (precordial) traces each use a single electrode (see Figure 25.3):

- C (or V) 1: 4th intercostal space (right of sternum) – red;
- C2: 4th intercostal space (left of sternum) – yellow;
- C4: 5th intercostal space, mid-clavicular line – brown;
- C6: 5th intercostal space mid-axilla – purple;
- C3: between C2 and C4 – green;
- C5: 5th intercostal space between C4 and C6 – black.

With normal (healthy) hearts:

- C1 = right atrium
- C2 = right ventricle
- C3 = sternum
- C4 = left ventricle

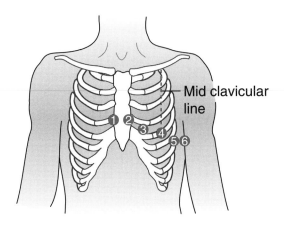

Mid clavicular line

Figure 25.3 **Electrode placement: chest leads**

- C5 = left ventricle
- C6 = left atrium

so 12-lead ECGs indicate different views of impulses (see Figure 25.4).

I	aVR	C1	C4
lateral		*anterior*	*anterior*
II	aVL	C2	C5
inferior	*lateral*	*anterior*	*lateral*
III	aVF	C3	C6
inferior	**inferior**	*anterior*	*lateral*

Figure 25.4 **Areas of the heart represented by standard 12-lead ECGs**

Reading ECGs

ECGs contain much information in a small graph, so are best deciphered in logical stages, using a framework such as Box 25.1.

Box 25.1 Reading ECGs

Reading the ECG
Regularity:

- Is the rate regular?
- If not, is the rate:
  - regularly irregular (is there a pattern)?
  - irregularly irregular (no pattern)?

P wave:

- Does the P wave appear before the QRS?
- Is there one P wave before every QRS?
- Is the shape normal?
- Is the P wave missing? (check for pacing spikes)

PR interval:

- Is the PR interval 3–5 small squares?

QRS complex:

- Is QRS width within 3 small squares?
- Is the QRS positive or negative?
- Is the axis normal?
- Does the QRS look normal?

ST segment:

- Does the isoelectric line return between the S and the T?
- If not, is it:
  - elevated?
  - depressed?

T wave:

- Does the T wave look normal?
- Is the QT interval < half preceding R–R interval?

Tachycardia (>100 bpm):

- narrow complex (usually with P waves) = atrial (supraventricular);
- wide complex (without P wave) = ventricular.

When analysing 12-lead ECGs, start with one lead, usually the 'rhythm strip' – a single lead usually running the whole printout length, usually II or C1.

Regularity

Begin by looking at regularity of rhythms. Using scrap paper, mark two R waves (peaks), then move the paper to see if all R–R intervals are the same. If they are, the rhythm is

■   regular.

Regular rhythms can be pathological (e.g. ventricular tachycardia). If the rhythm is irregular, is it

■   regularly irregular (is there a pattern)?
■   irregularly irregular (no pattern)?

P wave

This represents atrial depolarisation.

■   Is there a P wave?

It should be followed by ventricular depolarisation, so:

■   Does the P wave appear before the QRS?
■   Is there one P wave before every QRS?

Atrial muscle mass is small, so voltage (height) is limited. The shape should, however, be rounded, above the isoelectric line:

■   Is the shape normal?

Abnormal P waves, with normal QRSs, indicate atrial (supraventricular) problems.

PR interval

Atria have no specialised conduction pathway, so impulses are conducted from one muscle fibre to another. This makes conduction across atria relatively slow in proportion to muscle size. Impulses are then normally delayed at the atrioventricular (AV) node. So PR intervals, from the beginning of P wave to the beginning of QRS, should be 3 to 5 small squares (0.12–0.2 seconds):

■   Is the PR interval 3–5 small squares?

Prolonged PR intervals, often from atrioventricular node disease, delays conduction (see First degree block, p. 251).

Q wave

The first negative deflection represents septal depolarisation. Normally, Q waves are either small or absent. Deep (>2 small squares) Q waves indicate myocardial infarction, although not all myocardial infarctions cause deep Q waves. Where deep Q waves do occur (30-day) mortality is higher (Wong *et al.*, 2006). So although largely useful for retrospective diagnosis, for example, in community settings, Wong *et al.* (2006) suggest deep Q waves may be an indication for more aggressive therapy.

QRS complex

From the atrioventricular node, impulses pass down the Bundle of His, which divides into left and right branches, the left bundle further dividing into anterior and posterior hemibranches (or fascicles). From these three branches, impulses spread through Purkinje fibres to ventricular myocytes.

The QRS represents ventricular depolarisation. Although tall (due to the large muscle mass of ventricles), it is narrow (less than 3 small squares). It should be positive (mainly above the isoelectric line), except in right-sided leads (aVR, C1, C2).

- Is QRS positive or negative?
- Is its width within 3 small squares?
- Does it look normal?

ST segment

After the QRS, the trace should return rapidly to the isoelectric line.

- Does the isoelectric line return between the S and the T?

Ventricular conduction abnormalities can cause ST segments to be depressed or raised. Elevation, with chest pain, indicates infarction – ST elevation myocardial infarction (STEMI). Depression is often caused by ischaemia, but can have other causes.

- If not, is it:
  - elevated?
  - depressed?

T wave

This represents ventricular repolarisation. Slightly asymmetrical, T waves are normally larger than P waves. T wave abnormalities are 'non-specific', but common causes are

- high Ts = high serum potassium
- low Ts = low serum potassium
- inversion = ischaemia

- Does the T wave look normal?

QT interval

QT interval should be less than half the distance between the preceding two R waves. Prolonged QT intervals increase risk of sudden cardiac death (Straus *et al.*, 2006). A few people are genetically prone to long QT syndrome. In those affected, this is often caused by drugs containing sodium. Many drugs contain sodium, including salbutamol, so seek pharmacist advice about which drugs are safe to give.

Artefact

Electrocardiographs record any electrical activity they detect. All muscle conduction uses electricity, so skeletal muscle activity, such as shivering or tremors, may be detected. External electrical activity, such as electrical equipment or mobile phones, may also be recorded. Artefact usually creates constant interference ('fuzz').

Dysrhythmias and blocks

Dysrhythmias are symptoms, only treated if causing, or are likely to cause, problems. Frequently seen dysrhythmias are identified below. Acute dysrhythmias are often triggered by myocardial hypoxia, so oxygen is usually needed, and should be viewed as 'first aid' for new dysrhythmias. Underlying causes/triggers for dysrhythmias should be resolved if possible; for example, blood chemistry (especially potassium and calcium) should be optimised. Optimal serum potassium for cardiac conduction is 4–5 mmol/litre, slightly higher than normal physiological levels. Optimal serum total calcium is 2.0–2.5 mmol/litre; nb arterial blood gas analysers usually measure *ionised* calcium (normal 1.0–1.5).

Sinus arrhythmia

Sinus arrhythmia is where two rates alternate with breathing. Some young, usually athletic, adults normally have sinus arrhythmia. It is rare in hospitalised

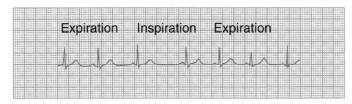

Figure 25.5 Sinus arrhythmia

patients, but may indicate respiratory distress. Sinus arrhythmia should not be treated, although any respiratory distress should.

Sinus bradycardia

Sinus bradycardia is sinus rhythm below 60 bpm. If very slow (<40), it is usually caused by a block, so positive chronotropes (e.g. atropine) are given to increase rate. Underlying causes (e.g. hypothermia) should be resolved.

Sinus tachycardia/supraventricular tachycardia

Sinus tachycardia/supraventricular tachycardia is sinus rhythm above 100 bpm. Check the tachycardia is not ventricular:

- narrow (QRS) complex tachycardia = supraventricular
- broad (QRS) complex tachycardia = ventricular.

Tachycardias reduce diastolic time, so reducing myocardial oxygenation while increasing myocardial oxygen consumption. Very fast rates (especially >140, usually called 'supraventricular tachycardia' – SVT) can be slowed by drugs:

- adenosine (if regular);
- beta-blocker, digoxin or amiodarone (if irregular – see Resuscitation Council Tachycardia algorithm.

Ectopics

Ectopics are isolated beats from abnormal pacemakers, so complexes differ from underlying rhythms. Their origin may be

- atrial
- junctional or
- ventricular.

Atrial ectopics have abnormal P waves and possibly different PR intervals, but normal QRS (see Figure 25.6). Junctional impulses usually have no visible P waves, but normal QRS. Ventricular impulses have no P wave, but wide and bizarre QRS complexes. If all ventricular ectopics have the same shape, they are

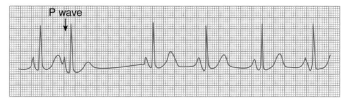

Figure 25.6 Atrial ectopic

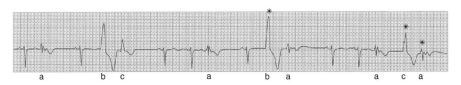

Figure 25.7 Ventricular ectopics

from the same focus ('unifocal'). If shapes vary, each shape is from a different focus ('multifocal') (see Figure 25.7).

Ectopics are

■ premature

if they occur before the expected complex, and

■ escape

if they appear after a missing expected complex, the ectopic 'escaping' into the gap. Premature ectopics indicate over-excitability (the problem). Escape ectopics indicate conduction failure, so the problem is failed conduction, not the ectopic. Isolated ectopics are not usually treated, but may indicate underlying problems, such as hypokalaemia, which require treatment.

Dysrhythmias and ectopics may be caused by electrolyte imbalances, especially potassium. So if not immediately life-threatening, check potassium and other electrolytes (calcium, magnesium). Mild hyperkalaemia (5.0–6.0 mmol/litre) may resolve with enteral calcium resonium, provided the gut is functioning. Higher levels (>6.0 mmol/litre) may cause life-threatening dysrhythmias (Humphreys, 2002), needing intravenous insulin and glucose (50 iu actrapid in 50 ml 5% glucose, usually over 1 hour), which transfers potassium into cells. Intravenous calcium gluconate/chloride is often given to stabilise myocardial conduction. Hypokalaemia (physiologically <3.5 mmol/litre, but <4.0 is often treated with cardiac disease) requires potassium supplements. Potassium loss largely correlates with urine volumes, so diuresis should also be considered before treating potassium levels.

Atrial kick

In sinus rhythm, atrial contraction precedes ventricular contraction, ensuring optimisation of ventricular volume to create a good-volume pulse. Almost all rhythms not originating from the sinoatrial node lose sequential filling. Loss of 'atrial kick' typically reduces stroke (pulse) volume by one-fifth, compromising blood pressure.

Atrial fibrillation (AF)

AF is the most common dysrhythmia, occurring in one-tenth of the UK population aged 65 and above, with incidence doubling each subsequent decade of life. Multiple rapid impulses were traditionally explained as atria muscle 'quivering', causing characteristically chaotic wavy baselines to ECG of 'coarse' AF – with fine AF usually only ventricular activity (QRS complex, T wave) is seen. It is now thought that ectopic foci originating from pulmonary veins may initiate AF (Adgey and Walsh, 2004). Whatever the cause, timing between impulses conducted by the AV node is erratic, causing the typical 'irregularly irregular' rate of AF. Ventricular conduction is normal (normal QRS). Irregularly irregular ECGs are usually AF, although other possibilities are:

- multiple dysrhythmias superseding each other;
- multiple ectopics;
- intermittent AV block.

Various classifications for AF exist, but one claiming consensus, and widely used, is:

- initial event;
- paroxysmal: spontaneous termination, recurrent (<7 days, often <48 hours);
- persistent: not self-terminating;
- permanent ('accepted'):
    - not terminated
    - terminated but relapsed
    - no cardioversion attempted.

(Levy *et al.*, 2003; RCP/NICE, 2006)

The first three types may also be termed *acute*, whereas permanent AF is *chronic*. Management of acute AF aims to restore sinus (or original) rhythm, whereas permanent AF cannot be reversed, but does need to be controlled. Pharmacotherapy, mentioned below, is reviewed comprehensively in RCP/NICE (2006).

Acute AF is triggered by disease (such as hypovolaemia), and is especially likely to occur if pulse pressure is wide (Mitchell *et al.*, 2007) (see Chapter 24). AF is the most common acute post-operative dysrhythmia (Walsh *et al.*, 2007).

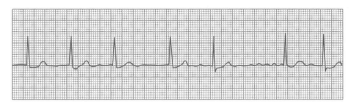

Figure 25.8 Atrial fibrillation

Treatable underlying causes should be reversed – patients should be normovolaemic, with electrolyte and other blood chemistry optimised. Acute AF causing life-threatening hypotension should be treated by urgent electrical cardioversion or intravenous amiodarone (RCP/NICE, 2006). Otherwise, drugs such as flecainide are often used (RCP/NICE, 2006). Pulmonary vein ablation has a high (80 per cent) success rate (Oal *et al.*, 2006), although is only available at specialist centres.

Passive atrial blood flow during fibrillation may have caused thrombi, so thrombotic events (e.g. stroke, pulmonary embolus) may follow if sinus rhythm is restored – Alchaghouri (2004) cites risk incidence being up to 7 per cent. Electrical cardioversion while cardioactive drugs (e.g. digoxin, beta-blockers) remain in circulation may cause asystole. Anticoagulation should be maintained for at least four weeks following successful cardioversion (RCP/NICE, 2006). Permanent (chronic) atrial fibrillation should not prevent people living relatively healthy lives, provided it is controlled:

- rate <100 bpm
- thrombus formation prevented.

People with AF have a six-fold risk of strokes unless adequately anticoagulated (Hart *et al.*, 2003). Control usually necessitates life-long drug therapy with

- rate-controlling drugs
- anti-coagulants.

Rate, rather than rhythm, control improves survival (Roy *et al.*, 2008). Digoxin, a rate-control drug, is often used, although is the best drug only for a minority of patients (RCP/NICE, 2006); beta-blockers or calcium channel blockers are better rate-control drugs (RCP/NICE, 2006; Musco *et al.*, 2008). Zimetbaum (2007) and Musco *et al.* (2008) suggest amiodarone is the most effective rhythm-control drug.

Warfarin is a most effective anticoagulant for AF (Mant *et al.*, 2007; Waldo, 2008). Both digoxin and warfarin have narrow therapeutic ranges, necessitating frequent monitoring of levels – in-patients on warfarin will usually have levels measured daily before doses are prescribed, with target INR of 2–3 (RCP/NICE, 2006). Patients receiving digoxin should only normally be given a dose if their apex rate is above 60 bpm. If brachial rate (measured by blood pressure monitors) is 60, apex rate must also be above 60, but lower brachial rates can occur with fast apex rates. Both apex and radial rates should be measured simultaneously over a full minute to measure apex-radial deficit. Significant deficits suggest poor rate control.

Atrial flutter

Atrial flutter is caused by an ectopic atrial pacemaker firing very rapidly – typically 300 times each minute (= one flutter wave every large ECG square). This

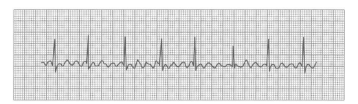

Figure 25.9 Atrial flutter

ectopic focus creates 'saw-tooth' or 'shark's tooth' *flutter* waves instead of P waves. The AV node cannot conduct 300 impulses each minute, so imposes a block, usually even-numbered (e.g. 2:1, 4:1, 8:1). Normal ventricular conduction pathway makes QRS complexes and T waves normal.

Atrial rates of 300 each minute and 4:1 AV block cause 75 ventricular responses (pulses). But AV blocks can rapidly change, usually to another even number. 4:1 blocks may suddenly become 2:1 (ventricular response 150 bpm) or 8:1 (ventricular response 35–40 bpm).

Atrial flutter is, therefore, sinister. If acute, rapid reversal is necessary, with

- (urgent) electrical cardioversion.

If this fails, chemical cardioversion may be attempted with

- flecainide
- calcium antagonists.

Radiofrequency catheter ablation is increasingly a first-line treatment (Sawhney and Feld, 2008).

Nodal/junctional rhythm

Nodal/junctional rhythm originates in or near the atrioventricular node (junction). Rates are usually 40–60 bpm, which can often be tolerated. Slower rates usually necessitate pacing. Causes for failed atrial conduction should be investigated and treated.

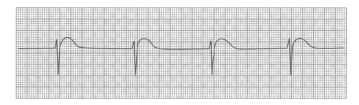

Figure 25.10 Nodal/junctional rhythm

Blocks

Blocks can occur anywhere in conduction pathways, but often occur at the atrioventricular junction:

- first degree block (delayed atrioventricular conduction)
- second degree block (incomplete heart block)
- third degree block (complete heart block)

or in one of the bundle branches:

- bundle branch block.

A block in conduction may be caused by

- infarction
- oedema
- ischaemia.

Oedema or ischaemia can be reversed, resolving the block, but infarction usually creates permanent block. Following infarction, an ischaemic area surrounds dead myocardium. This ischaemic area will either reperfuse or infarct ('extend').

First degree block

First degree block is *delay* in atrioventricular conduction, causing prolonged PR intervals and sometimes bradycardia. First degree block is usually caused either by

- age-related thickening of the AV node; or
- by anti-hypertensive or other cardiac drugs (e.g. digoxin, beta-blockers, calcium channel blockers).

Provided cardiac output and blood pressure remain adequate, first degree blocks are not usually treated, although underlying causes should be reversed if possible. Symptomatic bradycardia may necessitate treatment (e.g. pacing).

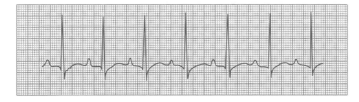

Figure 25.11 First degree block

Second degree block

Second degree heart block is *incomplete heart block*, where at regular intervals P waves are not conducted. The block is regular (e.g. 5:1 = 5 P waves conducted, one unconducted), so ECGs have a pattern (*regularly irregular*). There are two types of second degree heart block:

- type 1 (Wenkebach phenomenon; Mobitz type 1): PR intervals progressively lengthen until a P wave remains unconducted (see Figure 25.12);
- type 2 (Mobitz or Mobitz type 2): PR intervals remain constant.

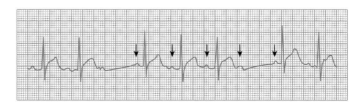

Figure 25.12 Second degree block type 1

Second degree heart block type 1 occurs more frequently, is usually asymptomatic and resolves spontaneously. Type 2 is more serious, so more likely to require treatment:

- oxygen
- atropine
- pacing if unresponsive.

Figure 25.13 is probably second degree heart block type 2, although without consecutive PR intervals type 1 could not be excluded.

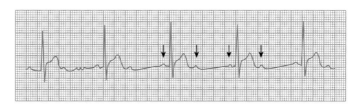

Figure 25.13 Second degree block type 2 (probably)

Third degree block

Third degree block is *complete heart block*, causing complete dissociation between atrial and ventricular activity. P waves may be present and regular, but do not initiate QRS complexes (some P wave may be 'lost' in QRS complexes or T wave). The QRS, originating in ventricular muscle, is wide and very slow

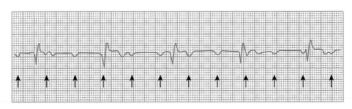

Figure 25.14 Third degree block

(30–40 bpm), necessitating urgent pacing. 'First aid' is 100% oxygen and atropine.

Bundle branch block

Bundle branch block is a block in either the left or right branch bundle. Impulses pass normally through the intact branch, creating a normal QRS. The side of the block receives the same impulse after it has crossed the septum, causing a second, wider QRS. ECGs show the two QRS complexes by a biphasic, or RSR, shape.

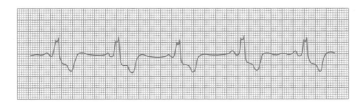

Figure 25.15 Bundle branch block

M- or W-shaped complexes are usually seen in many leads. To distinguish left from right branch bundle blocks, check the chest leads. Left bundle branch blocks (LBBB) have Ws in early chest leads (C1, C2) and Ms in late chest leads (C4–6). Right bundle branch blocks (RBBB) have Ms in early chest leads (C1, C2) and sometimes Ws in late chest leads (C4–C6). Bundle branch blocks may be differentiated by the mnemonics MaRRoW and WiLLiaM.

Chest pain, with a new left bundle branch block (i.e. not on the last ECG) indicates STEMI (see Chapter 26), necessitating urgent

■ revascularisation with percutaneous coronary intervention (PCI) – angioplasty; or
■ reperfusion with thrombolysis.

Ventricular dysrhythmias

Impulses originating in ventricular muscle do not use normal conduction pathways, instead spread from muscle fibre to muscle fibre. This causes absence of P waves and wide QRS. Ventricular dysrhythmias are life-threatening, requiring urgent treatment.

Ventricular tachycardia (VT)

VT is a regular, but life-threatening, rhythm, showing only ventricular (wide) complexes without P waves. Cardiac output and blood pressure will be very poor. Ventricular tachycardia usually progresses rapidly to ventricular fibrillation.

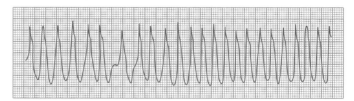

Figure 25.16 Ventricular tachycardia

Ventricular tachycardia with a pulse should be cardioverted with drugs:

■ amiodarone.

Pulseless VT is treated with

■ external cardiac compressions
■ defibrillation
■ drugs (e.g. adrenaline).

Ventricular fibrillation (VF)

VF is an irregularly irregular rhythm, with little or no cardiac output. Untreated, it is almost invariably fatal within 2–3 minutes. It is an arrest situation, and should be treated according to current resuscitation protocols. European Resuscitation Council (2005) guidelines for pulseless VT and VF use the same algorithm.

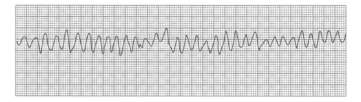

Figure 25.17 Ventricular fibrillation

Asystole

Asystole, also called 'ventricular standstill', is where there is no cardiac electrical activity. ECGs show only an isoelectric line. An arrest situation, it should be treated according to current resuscitation protocols. However, before putting out an arrest call, staff should look at the patient, in case electrodes have become disconnected. Defibrillation is not used for asystole, as the heart is not fibrillating. Although resuscitation should normally be attempted, few patients survive asystole.

Pulseless electrical activity (PEA)

PEA is when there is no pulse despite complexes (usually abnormal) on the ECG. PEA is an arrest situation. The European Resuscitation Council (2005) list the eight causes of PEA in a 'consider' box below the VT/VF algorithm:

1 hypoxia
2 hypovolaemia
3 hyper/hypokalaemia/metabolic
4 hypothermia
5 tension pneumothorax
6 tamponade, cardiac
7 toxins
8 thrombosis (coronary or pulmonary).

Underlying causes of PEA should, therefore, be resolved as part of resuscitation.

Time out 25.1

1 List the main reasons patients, having their ECG recorded, may be anxious. Identify where 12-lead ECGs may cause more or less anxiety than continuous monitoring. Using this list, what explanations would you normally give to patients before recording their ECG?
2 Find a printout of an ECG from a patient that you have cared for. Cover any printed analysis, and using the framework in Box 25.1, analyse the ECG. At the earliest opportunity, discuss your analysis with a nursing or medical colleague skilled in ECG analysis.
3 Reflecting on your experience over the last year, list the dysrhythmias you have seen. What treatments can you remember being used for each dysrhythmia? What dysrhythmias were not actively treated, and why?

Implications for practice

- ECGs contain much information in a small graph. Understanding normal cardiac electrophysiology and how this translates onto ECGs assists interpretation. Analyse one lead at a time, using a framework such as Figure 25.1.
- Interpreting ECGs is a skill that requires practice. Take every possible opportunity to study ECGs of patients cared for, interpreting information holistically.

- Most dysrhythmias are only treated if they cause, or are likely to cause, problems.
- Underlying causes for dysrhythmias (e.g. electrolyte imbalances) should be resolved.
- Readers should be familiar with current resuscitation protocols (at the time of writing: European Resuscitation Council (2005)), attend annual updates, and have posters of current resuscitation algorithms displayed prominently in clinical areas.

Summary

ECGs can provide useful information for monitoring and treating acutely ill patients. However, ECG monitoring is only effective if staff have the knowledge and skill to interpret what they see. Like most skills, interpreting ECGs improves with practice, so use the framework provided here to analyse ECGs of patients you care for.

Bibliography

Key reading

Readers should know resuscitation protocols (currently, European Resuscitation Council (2005)). Hampton (2008a) and Houghton and Gray (2008) are two useful pocket-sized books on ECGs. RCP/NICE (2006) provide national guidelines for atrial fibrillation, although focusing on management outside acute hospitals.

Further reading

Readers ready to develop skills beyond this level will find more detail in Hampton (2008b), while Hampton (2008c) provides exercises for readers to test and develop interpretation skills. Other useful ECG books include Morris *et al.* (2003) and Jevon (2003).

Chapter 26

Acute coronary syndromes

Noirin Egan

Contents

Learning outcomes

After reading this chapter you will be able to:

- recognise priorities for managing acute ST segment elevation myocardial infarction (STEMI) and its common complications;
- appreciate the critical nature of other acute coronary syndromes (ACSs) and their management.

Fundamental knowledge

Cardiovascular anatomy and physiology; basic ECG interpretation.

Introduction

Coronary heart disease (CHD) is the commonest cause of premature death in the developing world, the predominant underlying cause being atherosclerosis of coronary arteries. The disease is associated with many risk factors, including cigarette smoking, diabetes mellitus, hypertension, dyslipidaemia and family history. Coronary atherosclerosis is a chronic disease process with stable and unstable periods. During unstable periods a myocardial infarction (MI) may occur.

ACS, an umbrella term used to describe acute complications of atherosclerosis of coronary arteries, has three clinical presentations:

- acute ST segment elevation myocardial infarction (STEMI) also known as acute myocardial infarction – AMI (Grech and Ramsdale, 2003; Jones, 2003; Peters *et al.*, 2007);
- unstable angina (UA);
- non-ST segment elevation MI (NSTEMI).

Implementation of the National Service Framework for CHD (DOH, 2000b) heralded major changes in prevention and management of CHD in the UK. These changes have been rapidly evolving to bring prevention and management of CHD in line with that of other countries. More recently the American Heart Association (AHA), American College of Cardiology (ACC), European College of Cardiology (ESC) and World Heart Federation (WHF) produced a new expert consensus document on a universal definition of AMI based on evidence of myocardial cell death detected by different techniques and tools (Thygesen *et al.*, 2007). These include sensitive and specific biomarkers such as Troponin and imaging techniques which allow detection of very minor degrees of myocardial necrosis.

Early diagnosis is important, and can be provided by specially trained paramedics who can interpret ECG and initiate treatment such as aspirin. Patients with STEMI, who were traditionally admitted to coronary care units (CCUs), are increasingly 'blue-lighted' to specialist centres for critical intervention. Other ACSs will either be admitted to CCUs or may overflow into less acute areas such as clinical decision units (CDUs). Some of these will still be high risk and will require close monitoring by nursing staff.

This chapter focuses on STEMI: the pathophysiological processes and critical management within the first 12 hours. Potential complications will be highlighted. Other acute coronary syndromes will then be discussed as they often require a high dependency focus. Nurses working in high dependency areas may not experience caring for patients diagnosed with ACS on a regular basis, but need to be conversant with current approaches to caring for them.

Pathophysiology

Although ACS has three different clinical presentations, there is a common pathophysiological process – atherosclerotic plaque rupture or erosion with differing degrees of superimposed thrombosis and distal embolisation.

Atherosclerosis is a chronic process initiated by lipid deposition which in turn leads to vascular wall injury and increased endothelial permeability. Inflammatory cells accumulate oxidised lipids to form macrophages and foam cells which migrate into intima and ingest lipids. In an attempt to contain this, lipid core vascular smooth muscle cells then migrate from the media to intima, where they proliferate and change to form a fibrous cap (Grech, 2003; Newby and Grubb, 2005).

ACS arises when an atheromatous plaque becomes unstable and either ruptures or becomes eroded. Plaque rupture exposes the lipid core, which is highly thrombogenic, and surface-binding glycoproteins. Platelets adhere to the surface around ruptured plaque, releasing vasoactive substances. Glycoprotein 11b/111a receptors change configuration to bind fibrinogen and form a complex platelet linkage (Watson et al., 2002). This creates a platelet-rich thrombus at the site of plaque rupture, resulting in partial or total occlusion of the coronary artery (Peters et al., 2007). Both UA and NSTEMI are associated with a platelet-rich thrombus, leading to acute reduction in vessel patency, and worsening of angina symptoms (Grech and Ramsdale, 2003).

NSTEMI is associated with more persistent occlusion. Thrombi may embolise to downstream vessels, causing vasospasm and microinfarcts. Extent of myocardial damage depends on the site and duration of occlusion, as well as presence of collateral circulation which may develop in preceding weeks as a response to repeated attacks of ischaemia.

In contrast STEMI results from a red fibrin-rich thrombus which is more stable and occlusive (Grech and Ramsdale, 2003; Jones, 2003). This restricts myocardial perfusion, causing myocardial necrosis. This wavefront of myocardial necrosis begins within minutes of occlusion and progresses from sub-endocardium to epicardial surface – full-thickness transmural area of infarction. Rapid reopening of the infarct-related artery salvages more myocardium.

STEMI

For patients presenting with features of STEMI, initial assessment aims to establish diagnosis, assessing haemodynamic function, determining suitability for reperfusion, and most importantly relieving symptoms. Determining the nature of chest pain and distinguishing it from other causes is a priority, although atypical presentations are not uncommon (Bertrand et al., 2002).

Patients presenting with features of STEMI may not have diagnostic ECG changes and ECG recordings may be required at 15-minute intervals to assess for ongoing changes. Diagnosis of STEMI is based on the following ECG criteria:

- 1 mm of ST segment elevation in standard leads;
- 2 mm of elevation in one or more of chest leads;
- presumed new left bundle branch block;
- ST segment depression V1–V3 suggesting potential posterior MI.

(Johnson and Rawlings, 2007)

Patients with clear clinical history and diagnostic ECG changes follow the management pathway for STEMI. Priorities in care include ECG monitoring, cannulation, pain relief and cardiac and vital sign monitoring. Diagnosing STEMI involves critical decision-making and a clear defined time-dependant pathway of management. Pain is usually retrosternal, possibly radiating to neck, arms and sometimes the back. There may be numbness or tingling in arms or fingertips. Other clinical features are:

- pain, often with nausea/and or vomiting;
- sweating, from release of toxins from injured myocardial cells and increased autonomic activation;
- blood pressure and heart rate may be slightly increased;
- profound hypotension and dysrhythmias if severe myocardial damage has already occurred;
- shortness of breath – often an indication of the extent of myocardial damage.

Pain control

Pain relief is the first priority, as uncontrolled pain increases sympathetic stimulation, which leads to increased myocardial oxygen consumption. This can further aggravate ischaemia and increase the threshold for cardiac dysrhythmias. Intravenous morphine and an antiemetic should be given. Unrelieved pain may require intravenous beta-blockers, which dramatically reduce myocardial oxygen demand and prevent myocardial rupture (Newby and Grubb, 2005). Limiting infarction may preserve more left ventricular function. Intravenous nitrates can also optimise blood flow to ischaemic myocardium. Blood pressure should be monitored to detect hypotension.

Supplemental oxygen is important for managing STEMI with normal saturations, as optimising oxygen delivery to the cardiomyocytes may limit ischaemia. Initially, vital signs may need to be monitored every 15 minutes to detect hypotension and cardiac dysrhythmias. This also helps monitor response to treatment. Monitoring of respiratory rate and oxygen saturations may identify left ventricular failure (LVF). The importance of reassuring the patient throughout the critical aspect of care cannot be understated. Anxiety is a major feature, and may cause further ischaemia if not acknowledged and managed. Reassurance can be given by the calm and confident manner with which their care is managed.

Thrombolysis

Thrombolytic therapy is used to restore patency of occluded vessels, reperfusing the myocardium under threat of necrosis. Used within the 'golden hour' after STEMI, it significantly reduces mortality. Patients eligible for it have almost doubled in the last few years (Saab, 2005). Thrombolytic therapy should not be used without ST segment elevation (Bertrand et al., 2002; Connolly et al., 2002). Clot lysis occurs by activating plasminogen to form plasmin, which in turn degrades fibrin threads which bind the clot.

Suitability for thrombolysis needs careful and quick assessment. Risks and benefits should be explained and informed consent obtained. Stroke in the last six months, recent GI bleed or surgery are definite contraindications to thrombolysis. Other contraindications are relative and need careful consideration against benefits of administration.

Agents commonly used include recombinant tissue plasminogen activator (rt-PA; Alteplase) and Tenecteplase (a single bolus). Prior to administration of thrombolytic therapy, aspirin 300 mg is administered orally to inhibit platelet aggregation. Vital signs should be observed for 15–30 minutes to detect adverse reaction to therapy, such as hypotension, dysrhythmias and bleeding.

Dysrhythmias during thrombolysis can be multiple and varied, caused by reperfusion of the infarcted area with a surge of oxygen-rich blood which can cause electrolyte imbalance and microhaemorrhage. Such dysrhythmias may be transient and not cause adverse haemodynamic response. They may indicate successful reperfusion. Other indicators of successful reperfusion may be:

- pain relief;
- ST segments return to baseline – an ECG recorded 90 minutes later is required to determine this.

Patients who fail to reperfuse and have ongoing symptoms are suitable for rescue percutaneous coronary intervention (PCI). Although thrombolysis is still the prevailing treatment in many countries, mechanical reperfusion is rapidly becoming the treatment of choice where available.

Primary PCI

PCI involves insertion of a balloon-tipped catheter which is guided via the groin or arm to the blocked artery. It is then inflated, pushing the atheromatous plaque against the artery wall (angioplasty) and deflated, often leaving a 'stent' in its place to maintain patency. Primary PCI (PPCI) is PCI as the primary strategy for reperfusing acute STEMI. In some areas patients are transported straight to the cardiac catheterisation laboratory, bypassing the A&E department.

Many now believe this technique to be superior to thrombolysis. Compared with thrombolysis, PCI reduces rate of reinfarction, and to a lesser extent reduces stroke and death (Keely et al., 2003; Kristensen et al., 2004). Although primary PCI has advantages, it cannot always be delivered rapidly, depending on availability of experienced PCI operators and other trained personnel, and geographical location. Whereas thrombolysis needs to be administered within 20 minutes of arrival in A&E ('door to needle time'), PCI is less time-dependent, and thought to be effective within 4 hours ('door to balloon time'). Success of PCI is strongly linked to how quickly it can be performed, so an emerging strategy is to combine use of thrombolytic and/or other antithrombotic agents such as glycoprotein 11b/111a inhibitors as an adjunct to PCI (facilitated or rescue PCI) within 24 hours.

Patients with diabetes or those non-diabetic patients who present with hyperglycaemia require sliding-scale insulin to maintain normoglycaemia. Glucose is a major energy source for ischaemic myocardium and insulin enhances its uptake. Hyperglycaemia is associated with increased mortality in this group of patients (Newby and Grubb, 2005; Zarich and Nesto, 2007) and tight glycaemic control is imperative.

Complications following STEMI

LVF

Acute LVF and pulmonary oedema are common complications following STEMI, caused primarily by extensive infarction of the left ventricular wall. Both complications are characterised by sudden acute onset of breathlessness, tachycardia and hypotension. Compensatory mechanisms are initiated in an effort to maintain cardiac output, which can be explained by the principles of preload and afterload.

According to Starling's Law, cardiac output and the force of contraction are directly related to the amount the muscle-fibres stretch during contraction. Preload, the filling phase of the cardiac cycle, refers to passive stretching of myofibrils. It is determined by blood volume in the ventricle at the end of diastole, and influenced by venous return to the heart and ability of the heart to fill. After-load is the resistance to left ventricular emptying and an increase in systemic vascular resistance.

Extensive left ventricular damage reduces ability of myofibrils to stretch. The heart thus compensates by increasing heart rate in an effort to maintain cardiac output. This further increases systemic vascular resistance and a viscous cycle begins. When left ventricular emptying is restricted, back flow to pulmonary capillaries causes pulmonary hypertension and can lead to pulmonary oedema. The patient, therefore, becomes breathless and hypoxic. This constitutes an acute emergency situation. Priorities of management are:

- sit patient upright;
- give high-flow oxygen and monitor oxygen saturations;
- intravenous morphine: morphine not only has a sedative effect but also veno-dilates, which decreases venous return;
- antiemetic;
- furosemide – this may be ineffective if the patient is profoundly hypotensive, as there may be insufficient renal flow to achieve diuresis.

Inotropes may improve blood pressure, but should be used very cautiously as they may induce further tachydysrhythmias.

If blood pressure allows, intravenous nitrates can reduce preload and afterload through their biphasic action of venous and arterial dilation. Bilevel non-invasive ventilation (NIV) is commonly used – positive pressure in the alveoli at the end of expiration not only increases oxygen delivery to pulmonary capillaries but also decreases venous return to the heart and, therefore, influences preload (see Chapter 23).

Left ventricular remodelling can begin in early stages, leading to a downward spiral of events: stretching and thinning myocardium, dilatation compensatory hypertrophy tachycardia and exacerbated ischaemia. Use of drugs such as ACE inhibitors prevent remodelling, and are started very soon after the initial event in order to prevent long-term occurrence of chronic heart failure.

Cardiogenic shock

Cardiogenic shock is a serious complication following STEMI, usually presenting within the first 24 hours. Acute and sustained failure of the heart to maintain adequate tissue perfusion may cause multiple organ failure. Hypotension initiates and sustains a viscous cycle of reduced coronary artery perfusion leading to further ischaemia and infarct extension, thereby worsening ventricular dysfunction.

Lactic acidosis, from tissue hypoxia, further suppresses myocardial contractility and blunts the response to inotropic and other vasopressor agents. A downward spiral of events ensues unless this cycle is interrupted at an early stage (see Chapter 27).

Dysrhythmias

In the acute phase of STEMI, dysrhythmias are primarily from a combination of electrolyte imbalance and ischaemia. Ischaemia precipitates anaerobic metabolism, and so acidosis. Acidosis increases stimulation of the sympathetic nervous system and an increase in the automaticity of myocytes through release of catecholamines (e.g. noradrenaline). So resting membrane potential of cells decreases, increasing rate and frequency of depolarisation, which leads to tachydysrhythmias.

Increased heart rates increase oxygen demand, decrease diastolic filling pressure, which in turn is detrimental to an already struggling heart. Anterior wall MI often displays such sympathetic effects and tachydysrhythmias are most common with large anterior wall MI. The most serious are ventricular tachycardia (VT) and ventricular fibrillation (VF). Both pulseless VT and VF are rapidly fatal unless the patient is defibrillated within 90 seconds. Introduction of semi-automated defibrillators has meant that more personnel can influence survival.

Ischaemia can increase extracellular potassium and levels of adenosine, which can slow impulses in the conducting system. Slow heart rates often complicate inferior wall MI (IFWMI), which may accompany right coronary artery occlusion. The right coronary also supplies the conductive tissue, which explains why bradycardia and heart blocks may be more common with IFWMI. Heart blocks which compromise the patient's condition require insertion of a temporary transvenous pacing wire.

With transfer of STEMIs to specialist centres, nurses in general hospitals are more likely to encounter patients with other acute coronary syndromes, and their management is equally critical. Management of ACS in recent years has shifted its emphasis from relief of ischaemic pain to relieving the ischaemia itself (Schulman and Fessler, 2001). Heparin and other antithrombotic agents, such as aspirin and Clopidogrel®, help stabilise patients' symptoms.

Unstable angina and NSTEMI

Unlike STEMI, presenting symptoms for UA and NSTEMI are not as easily recognisable, and rely on a triad of clinical indicators which include clinical history, ECG changes and biochemical markers.

For both, presenting symptoms may be undistinguishable. Pain is usually recent in onset, worsening in frequency, and there may be symptoms of pain at rest. Symptoms may be new or may present on a background of chronic stable angina. The ECG in both instances may be normal or have some ST segment depression or minor T wave abnormalities. UA and NSTEMI are associated with unstable lesions caused by platelet-rich thrombus cardiac biomarkers. Troponin I and Troponin T are very sensitive markers of myocardial necrosis, and diagnosis of MI requires evidence of myocardial necrosis (Peters *et al.*, 2007). NSTEMI is detected by raised Troponin, whereas UA is not. Because the underlying lesion is a platelet-rich thrombus, patients with UA and NSTEMI would not benefit from thrombolysis. Antithrombotics, such as unfractionated heparin, and antiplatelet agents, such as aspirin and Clopidogrel® are important for managing acute coronary lesions. Aspirin alone may substantially reduce the rate of intra-coronary thrombus formation (Connolly *et al.*, 2002). Despite adequate treatment with antiplatelet agents, platelet activation may still continue along the other pathways not blocked by these agents. In patients with ongoing chest pain and evidence of ongoing ischaemia the use of glycoprotein IIb/IIIa inhibitors (e.g. Tirofiban) can block the final common pathway of platelet aggregation, and are primarily indicated in patients scheduled for PCI.

Implications for practice

- Nurses caring for patients with ACS play a pivotal role in identifying significant changes in their condition.
- Monitoring for new ECG changes and careful assessment of the nature for chest pain are vital.
- The emphasis of care is also on preventative measures, through pharmacological management and/or health promotion.

Summary

Nurses caring for patients with ACS play a pivotal role in flagging up significant changes in condition. Monitoring for new ECG changes and careful assessment of the nature of chest pain are vital, as is having confidence in monitoring the administration of new adjunctive therapy.

Clinical scenario

John Taylor is admitted with STEMI and has been thrombolysed in A&E. He has continuous unresolved pain and his ECG has failed to show evidence of reperfusion.

1 Identify his immediate priorities on admission.

2 Discuss other possible complications that may ensue.

3 What drugs intervention may be used to manage a complication of LVF in this instance?

Bibliography

Key reading

Newby and Grubb (2005) and Johnson *et al.* (2007) provide useful texts on cardiac nursing.

Further reading

Staff should be familiar with local guidelines for managing ACS.

Chapter 27

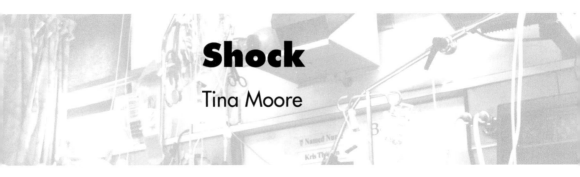

Shock

Tina Moore

Contents

Learning outcomes

After reading this chapter you will be able to:

- understand the physiological changes during shock;
- recognise the different types of shock and the management for each;
- demonstrate knowledge and understanding of how shock affects other organs;
- identify the nursing responsibilities when caring for a patient in shock.

Fundamental knowledge

Baroreceptors and chemoreceptors; renin–angiotensin–alsdosterone cascade; normal inflammatory response.

Introduction

Generally, shock is defined as acute circulatory failure resulting in reduced tissue perfusion and general hypoxaemia. Many definitions fail to capture its complexity. Irrespective of the cause of shock, the resultant features are the same, i.e. inadequate tissue perfusion and impairment of homeostasis. Each type can equally be life-threatening, requiring quick and aggressive management. Shock can develop in any patient, in any clinical setting. Thus, it is imperative that nurses recognise clinical manifestations of shock early and initiate early appropriate intervention.

This chapter provides an explanation for the physiological changes occurring in each stage of shock. Different types of shock are examined, together with the nursing and medical management.

Time out 27.1

1 Reflect on the patients you have nursed who have been diagnosed in a shock state.
2 What were the clinical manifestations?
3 What type of shock was diagnosed?
4 Describe the intervention for each patient.

Stages of shock

There are four identified stages. Each stage is progressive and interrelated. Table 27.1 lists the stages of shock.

Table 27.1 Stages of shock

1. Initial stage	Clinical features are not apparent, often unrecognised
2. Compensatory stage	Occurs if the cause persists
3. Progressive stage	Compensation
4. Refactory stage	Multi-organ dysfunction syndrome

Types of shock

Hypovolaemic shock

Hypovolaemic shock, the most common type, is a clinical condition in which tissue perfusion is inadequate due to a loss of blood or plasma. Fluid loss of approximately 750 ml will cause compensatory changes (McLuckie, 2003). Hypovolaemic shock develops when the intravascular volume decreases to the point that compensatory mechanisms cannot maintain homeostasis. Inadequate ventricular pre-load is usually manifested by a reduction in circulatory blood volume leading to decreased cardiac output and mean arterial pressure (MAP). There is general agreement that shock begins to develop when intravascular volume has decreased by about 15 per cent, but this would depend on the person's ability to compensate (e.g. baroreceptor response).

Causes include:

- haemorrhage – loss of whole blood, e.g. trauma, gastrointestinal bleed;
- plasma – severe burns (increased capillary permeability leading to a shift in plasma from the vascular space into the interstitial space);
- third-space shifts – permeability causes movement of fluids enabling water, electrolytes and albumin to flow into the interstitial space;
- interstitial fluid loss – promotes diffusion of plasma from the intravascular to the extravascular space, e.g. diabetic ketoacidosis.

Compensatory changes lead to alterations in both regional blood flow and the distribution of fluid between body compartments. Acute fluid volume loss does not allow for the normal compensatory mechanism. Many older patients and those with chronic diseases may have subtle compensatory responses (Cassel *et al.*, 2003; Meldon *et al.*, 2003).

Pathophysiological changes include a reduction in venous return to the heart; baroreceptors sense this decrease in blood volume causing fluid and sodium retention and increases in the heart rate and force of contraction. Vasoconstriction shunts blood to vital organs resulting in a reduction in cardiac output. Persistence causes diversion of blood to vital organs (heart, lung, brain) leading to hypoperfusion of other organs.

Compensatory stage (occurs if the cause persists)

This stage is designed to preserve cellular function, the responses are first activated by reduced circulating blood volume and decreasing cardiac output. If prolonged, baroreceptor reflexes are initiated, causing stimulation of sympathetic nervous activity. Catecholamines (adrenaline (epinephrine) and noradrenaline (norepinephrine)) are released, increasing cardiac output and myocardial contractility (stimulating feelings of fear and anxiety with increased ventricular and muscle tremor, sweating and vomiting). Catecholamines also stimulate the liver to convert glycogen to glucose, causing hyperglycaemia.

Adrenaline produces an adrenoceptor effect, causing general vasoconstriction and increased metabolic rate. Relaxation of bronchial smooth muscles raises respiratory rate and minute volume, improving gaseous exchange. Symptoms include tachypnoea and metabolic acidosis.

Chemoreceptors relay signals to the hypothalamus, stimulating the release of adrenocorticotrophic hormone (ACTH), growth hormone (GH) and antidiuretic hormone (ADH). The combined effects of ACTH and GH increase blood glucose and expands circulating blood volume through sodium and water retention, resulting in oliguria.

Aldosterone is secreted, aiding fluid retention. Increased cortisol production also increase fluid retention and antagonises the effects of insulin, leading to further hyperglycaemia. Generalised symptoms are seen in Box 27.1

Box 27.1 General symptoms during compensatory stage

- Tachypnoea
- Tachycardia
- Hypertension
- Oliguria
- Hyperglycaemia
- Altered level of consciousness
- Sweating

During this particular stage physiological changes may be very subtle. Hence, it is important nurses monitor the patient's vital signs very carefully, making clinical interpretations about the trend of observations rather than comparing the most recent with the previous one. Even the most subtle of changes should be noted.

Progressive stage

Failure of compensatory mechanisms (decompensation) to restore adequate circulatory volume causes prolonged vasoconstriction, cellular hypoxia and eventual organ damage. Cellular hypoperfusion and the inability to meet oxygen consumption (VO_2) requirements causes cellular anaerobic metabolism in a worsening acidotic state. There is also a depletion of adenosine triphosphate (ATP) and failure of the cell membrane sodium-potassium pump. This influx of sodium and water will cause cellular swelling again worsening metabolic acidosis.

Respiratory acidosis is also likely to occur. Further vasoconstriction makes tissues ischaemic and causes arteriolar vasodilatation, causing pooling of blood in the capillary bed (Mattson Porth, 2005). Increased hydrostatic pressure (causes capillary leakage), peripheral oedema also occurs. Decompensation processes further aggravate hypovolaemia with resultant altered cellular metabolism (initiating acidosis; cardiac depression; intravascular coagulation; increased capillary permeability and release of vasoactive mediators).

Box 27.2 General symptoms during progressive stage

- Skin cold and clammy
- Increasing tachycardia
- Further tachypnoea
- Hypotension
- Signs of hypoxaemia
- Confusion/restlessness
- Hyperkalaemia

Refractory stage

When compensatory mechanisms fail irreversible cellular necrosis takes place. Increased vasoactive metabolites, released by the damaged cells causes localised vasodilatation of the pre-capillary sphincters. This causes further hypoperfusion. Histamine released by damaged endothelium increases the permeability of the capillaries, resulting in proteins leaking into extracellular spaces. Changes, as the result of tissue ischaemia, can cause disseminated intravascular coagulation (DIC) (Chapter 32). Further appearance of hypoperfusion, hypercapnia, increased hydrogen ions and bacteraemia lead to multiple organ failure and eventual death.

Symptoms of hypovolaemic shock

Early clinical features of hypovolaemic shock include:

- Dizziness.
- Weakness.
- Nausea/vomiting.
- Anxiety/apprehension.
- Blood pressure can appear normal due to compensatory mechanisms. This may prevent a significant decrease in systolic blood pressure, until the patient has lost 30 per cent of the blood volume (Kolecki, 2008).
- Attention should be paid to pulse, respiratory rate and skin perfusion.

Severe volume depletion causes the following:

- Dehydration: dry mucous membranes, dry furred tongue, sunken eyeballs, thirst.
- Cardiovascular changes: decreased central venous pressure, decreased cardiac output, rapid and thready pulse (NB: patients on beta-blockers may have a decrease in pulse (Kolecki, 2008)), decreased mean arterial pressure (MAP), and increased systemic vascular resistance. Blood pressure is initially increased due to catecholamine release then decreases after sustained volume depletion.
- Increased respiratory rate and depth.
- Decreased oxygen saturation.
- Cool clammy skin.
- Agitation, an indicator of inadequate cerebral blood flow.
- Reduced urine output.

Severe blood loss causes bradycardia. However, with more haemorrhaging the heart rate rises again (Ganong, 2005). Bradycardia may be due to unmasking of mediated depressor reflexes of the vagus nerve, whose response is possibly a way of stopping the bleeding (Ganong, 2005).

Management of hypovolaemic shock

The answer to successful management is the early detection, minimising fluid loss and prevention (where possible) (Woodrow, 2006). The goal is for pre-load optimisation and stabilisation, and a possible eradication of the cause. The type

Table 27.2 Types of fluids used in hypovolaemic shock

Balanced crystalloid solutions

Isotonic saline (0.9% normal saline) – mainly expands extracellular fluid (ECF)

Hypotonic saline (0.45% saline) – expands ECF and provides some free water for the cells (could overload the patient)

Glucose and water – provides free water only and will be distributed evenly through both intracellular fluid (ICF) and ECF – used to treat water deficit

Mixed saline and electrolyte solutions – provides additional electrolytes.

Colloids

Plasma substitutes (albumin etc.)

Gelatins (e.g. Gelofusine®, Volplex® or rarely used Haemaccel®)

Starches (e.g. Hetastarch®, Pentastarch such as HAES-steril® Tetrastarch such as Voluven®)

Dextrans (e.g. Dextran 40® or Dextran 70® rarely used)

of fluid loss will determine the form of fluid replacement. Fluid replacement continues to be an area of strong debate and opinions.

Immediate restoration of effective circulating blood volume and correction of acid base and electrolyte disturbances via one or more wide-bore intravenous cannulae is a priority. The aim of a MAP of 70 mmHg (Cottingham, 2006) to 80 mmHg is considered sufficient. Fluid resuscitation can be both complex and controversial. Patients (particularly the older person) should be monitored closely for signs of fluid overload (Chapter 29). Electrolyte monitoring is also recommended.

In recent years there has been much debate about the use of colloids and crystalloids. A systematic review by Alderson *et al.* (2004) found no evidence to support the use of one over the other, making the choice individual, dependent upon the patients' requirements. Crystalloids (cheaper than colloids) are rapidly distributed across the intravascular and interstitial spaces. However, two to four times more volume is required than with colloid and, therefore, pulmonary oedema may occur.

Fluid balance and vital signs need to be closely monitored (including central venous pressure (CVP)). Blood products and other colloid solutions are used to assist in acute blood loss. Inotropic support may be indicated if volume replacement attempts fail, necessitating admission to the ICU. High flow supplementary oxygen should also be given (BTS, 2008).

Cardiogenic shock (pump failure)

Cardiogenic shock results from a loss of critical contraction of the heart (left ventricle) causing a reduction in cardiac output and reduced circulatory perfusion. Unlike hypovolaemic shock causes are restricted. The most common cause is following acute myocardial infarction (AMI) where greater than 40 per cent of the myocardium has been damaged (Morton and Fontaine, 2000). Other causes include tamponade, mitral regurgitation, pulmonary embolism, cardiac dysrhythmias.

Compensatory mechanisms (as per hypovolaemic shock) can increase cardiac workload which is unable to meet the increased demand leading to further decrease in cardiac output (Woodrow, 2006). In addition to hypotension and tachycardia other clinical features include pulmonary oedema (dyspnoea, tachypnoea, productive cough (frothy, loose, white), ischaemic cardiac pain, hyperglycaemia, hypernatraemia, hypocalcaemia and dysrhythmias.

Cardiogenic shock can be a fatal condition (mortality 50–80 per cent (Bromet and Klein, 2004)) with the patient deteriorating very quickly. The goals of management are to correct reversible problems, prevent further ischaemia and improve tissue perfusion.

■ *Increase oxygen supply to the heart* – reperfusion of the coronary arteries through thrombolysis (Chapter 26) this may be counterproductive if the shock state occurs after the initial insult. Oxygen should be administered, titrated to arterial blood gas results.

■ *Maximise cardiac output* – treatment of dysrhythmias (Chapter 25); dobutamine may be used as it improves the contractility of uninjured myocardium and thus increases cardiac output. By stimulating the adrenergic receptor vasopressors (e.g. adrenaline) causes vasoconstriction, increasing blood pressure to an adequate mean level (but in doing so increases the workload of the heart)

■ *Decrease workload of the left ventricle* – if left ventricular failure is present diuretics are administered to decrease the pre-load and to improve stroke volume and cardiac output. Diamorphine may be indicated for pain control. Due to cardiovascular and respiratory symptoms, the patient may need to be positioned at a 45° angle

■ *Artificial aids may be required* – e.g. intra-aortic balloon pumps (IABP) and ventricular assist devices (VAD). It is beyond the remit of this book to discuss these interventions in detail.

Distributive shock

Neurogenic shock

Causes of neurogenic shock include traumatised or diseased brain stem, spinal cord injury and some anaesthetic drugs. Neurogenic shock occurs as the result of loss of sympathetic nerve activity from the brain's vasomotor centre (Collins, 2000). The vasoconstrictor tone is interrupted and as the autonomic nervous system controls systemic vascular resistance (SVR), there is massive vasodilatation and profound uncontrolled vagal (sympathetic impulse) stimulation as SVR is decreased. Here, blood volume has not decreased but the space containing the blood has increased, causing pooling of blood and a reduced venous return to the heart and consequently a reduced cardiac output. Bradycardia (due to parasympathetic activity) and hypotension occur. Excessive vasodilatation causes warm extremities.

The cause should be treated but failure of the autonomic response makes inotropic support ineffective (Woodrow, 2006). Poor circulating blood volume may be compensated with fluid replacement (colloids) and oxygen support. Prophylaxis against deep vein thrombosis should be instigated.

Anaphylactic shock

Anaphylactic shock results from an acute hypersensitive reaction to a substance to which the person has previously been sensitised; therefore, patients are more likely to have a reaction to a second dosage. Unrecorded previous exposure to the antigen may initiate a 'first dose' reaction (Woodrow, 2006). The hypersensitivity response occurs on the surface of the mast cell, which are located primarily in the lungs, small blood vessels and connective tissue. The antigen combines with sensitised antibodies from previous exposure (usually immunoglobulin E (IgE) type). The antigen also attaches to basophiles circulating in the blood. The immediate reaction is a release of histamine and other mediators (e.g. bradykinin causing vasodilatation and increased capillary permeability).

Clinical features usually manifest rapidly (within minutes) and include hypotension and tachycardia; visual changes are noted on the skin, e.g. urticaria; facial oedema (due to loss of protein-rich fluid in the tissues) possibly causing laryngeal obstruction ('stridor' breathing). This is a life-threatening situation (airway obstruction) and can be very frightening for both patient and nurse. Bronchospasm can also occur causing wheezing.

The goal is to stop the reaction, restore vascular tone, improve fluid volume and maintain an open airway. Therefore, it is imperative to remove the cause. The Resuscitation Council (UK) (2006) have produced an algorithm indicating the first line treatment for anaphylactic reactions. Adrenaline should be administered as a first line drug. It causes an increase in blood pressure through vaso-constriction and inhibits the mediators released by the immune response. The drug also causes smooth muscle relaxation and, therefore, bronchi dilation. Oxygen support is required. Antihistamines are used to stop the inflammatory reactions, usually piriton, but steroids (hydrocortisone) may be administered.

Fluid resuscitation should begin if drugs (antihistamine and hydrocortisone) do not reverse the shock status. Crystalloids remain the preferred fluid (Resuscitation Council (UK), 2006).

Signs and symptoms of infection (SSI)

This is formally known as systemic inflammatory response syndrome (SIRS). SSI describes the physiological response to severe infection and is the abnormal, generalised inflammatory response reaction occurring in organs remote from initial injury (Burdette and Parilo, 2007). There are no specific investigations for diagnosis, just routine observations and baseline blood tests.

The presence of two or more of the following is required for diagnosis:

■ temperature > 38°C or < 36°C;
■ heart rate > 90 bpm;
■ respiratory rate > 20/m, or $PaCO_2 < 4.3\,kPa$;

■ leucocyte count above 12,000 10^9/litre below 4,000 10^9/litre, or containing over 10 per cent mature neutrophils (ACCP/SCCM, 1992; Bone *et al.*, 1992).

Management

Oxygen therapy is administered to reverse hypoxaemia. Fluid replacement, usually colloids, is necessary to increase colloid osmotic and perfusion pressures. Inotropes will support myocardial contractility. If infection is present, antibiotics should be prescribed. Control of hyperglycaemia is crucial. Nutritional support should be started as soon as possible.

Septic shock

Septic shock is sepsis-induced hypotension (systolic B/P < 90 mmHg or MAP < 70 mmHg) in the absence of other causes of hypotension despite adequate fluid resuscitation (Dellinger *et al.*, 2008). Sepsis is the systemic response to severe infection in the body, commonly caused by gram negative bacteria (Oppert *et al.*, 2005). Its sequence is equal to the generalised inflammatory shock response seen in the progressive stage of illness (Bone *et al.*, 1992).

The inflammatory response is designed to protect the body from further injury and promote rapid healing. Vasodilatation, increased microvascular permeability, neutrophil activation and adhesion and enhanced coagulation occur. Histamine, prostaglandin and bradykinin initiate the vascular response. If regulatory mechanisms fail, uncontrolled systemic inflammation overwhelms the body's normal protective response. Excessive vasodilatation, hypotension and increases in vascular permeability occur (Kumar and Clark, 2006).

Sepsis remains life-threatening and mortality rate remains high (approximately 40–50 per cent) (Oppert *et al.*, 2005). Management must be initiated quickly. There are now international clinical guidelines available for the quick and comprehensive management of sepsis and septic shock (Dellinger *et al.*, 2008).

Management requires early detection and removal of cause. Clinical guidelines (Dellinger *et al.*, 2008) provide useful physiological parameters for goal-directed resuscitation. Principles of management include early diagnosis, resuscitation and antibiotic therapy. Fluid replacement via CVP with considered vasopressors (adrenaline and dopamine). Nutritional support and antipyretic agents should also be considered (Kumar and Clark, 2006).

Multi-organ dysfunction syndrome (multi-organ failure)

Shock can precipitate dysfunction in all organs.

■ Acute lung injury starts early. An increase in permeability of the lung microvasculature occurs, allowing pulmonary oedema to develop, even with low venous pressure. When severe, it can lead to adult respiratory distress syndrome (ARDS). Clinical features include severe hypoxaemia –

$PaO_2 < 8.0\,kPa$ on 40% inspired oxygen (Gunning and Rowan, 1988), radiological appearance of bilateral pulmonary infiltrates, reduced lung compliance.

- Volume-responsive acute kidney injury (Chapter 30) may occur as a result of hypoperfusion.
- Interference with glucose and oxygen supply to the brain may lead to agitation, confusion and coma.
- Liver cell necrosis occurs in shock lasting for more than 10 hours (Henrion *et al.*, 2003). Hepatic hypoperfusion produces intense angiotensin II release, precipitating vasoconstriction. Symptoms of liver impairment include encephalopathy, jaundice and bleeding problems.

Nursing implications

Nursing observations and monitoring of the patient's condition should be performed on a regular basis (initially 15–30 minutes until stable (Bench, 2004)). Ideally the same nurse should be monitoring the patient for the duration of the shift, placing them in a better position to notice subtle changes in the patient's condition.

Observations should be made of the patient's cardiovascular status, including heart rate/pulse, blood pressure, MAP, CVP, cardiac monitoring, temperature and urine output (Chapter 6). In addition, respiratory status (Chapter 15), including rate, depth, cough, degree of effort, and mental status (Chapter 9) should be noted.

Implications for practice

- Nurses are responsible for monitoring and interpreting patient data for the early detection of shock.
- Shock necessitates diligent monitoring of cardiovascular and respiratory function.
- Fluid replacement must be given with great caution, particularly in the older person.
- Gut ischaemia increases problems owing to the translocation of gut bacteria, enteral feeding should be encouraged/maintained whenever possible
- Some acutely/critically ill patients are immunosuppressed, so effective infection control is a must (Woodrow, 2006).
- Shock can cause prolonged complications, so management should focus on long-term effects; benefits may not be seen for a number of days.
- Administration of high flow oxygen limits hypoxaemia.

Summary

The nature of shock remains complex and controversial. Owing to the severity of the disorder, it is imperative that nurses are well informed in the different types of shock. Through close monitoring of the patient's cardiovascular and respiratory status, early identification and intervention can help to stop progression, thereby reducing morbidity and mortality.

Clinical scenario

Raymond Robinson, 52 years old, has just returned to England from a holiday in the Caribbean. Since his return five days ago he has suffered from acute diarrhoea and vomiting. He presents in A&E complaining of dizziness and excessive thirst.

Clinical examination reveals the following:

B/P	85/50 mmHg
Heart rate	144 bpm – sinus tachycardia
Pulse pressure	low
Respiratory rate	29 bpm
Temperature	37.2°C
Skin	pale, dry and warm to touch
Tongue	dry and furred
Mental status	anxious and lethargic but orientated to place and time

1 Identify the type of shock Raymond is suffering from. Give reasons for your answer.

2 With reference to physiological changes, discuss your assessment.

3 Formulate an evidence-based plan of care for Raymond.

Bibliography

Further reading

Bench (2004) offers a useful text in relation to nursing management.

Chapter 28

Heart failure

Philip Woodrow

Contents

Learning outcomes

After reading this chapter you will be able to:

- recognise signs of heart failure;
- develop a care plan for a patient with chronic heart failure;
- identify advice that should be offered to patients.

Fundamental knowledge

Cardiovascular anatomy and physiology.

Introduction

Heart failure is a major cause of chronic and often disabling disease in Western societies. In the UK, cardiovascular disease (including strokes) causes over one-third of deaths, more than any other disease. Heart failure may be

- acute
- chronic
- acute-on-chronic.

The type of heart failure may influence treatment, as chronic heart failure is ultimately a terminal disease.

Acute heart failure typically occurs from acute cardiac events, such as myocardial infarction or severe sepsis. It is sometimes called 'decompensated' heart failure, because the failing heart ejects small pulses, while compensatory mechanisms fail to sustain blood pressure. Hypotension usually causes hypoperfusion, progressing to cardiogenic shock (see Chapter 27), which usually necessitates transfer to coronary or intensive care units.

Chronic heart failure, sometimes called 'progressive' or 'compensated' heart failure, is more likely to cause, or co-exist with, acute ward admission, so is the focus of this chapter. With chronic heart failure, tachycardia often compensates for hypoperfusion, and chronic vascular disease either maintains normotension or causes hypertension. Heart failure may also be acute-on-chronic, but this often necessitates either transfer or (if end-stage) palliative care.

Heart failure is a syndrome causing patients to experience

- dyspnoea
- fatigue
- fluid retention.

(Mehta and Cowie, 2006; von Klemperer and Bunce, 2007)

It is mainly caused by coronary heart disease, usually following myocardial infarction (SIGN, 2007), but one-third of cases are caused by non-ischaemic cardiomyopathy – e.g. hypertension, thyroid disease, valvular disease, alcohol excess, myocarditis (SIGN, 2007). Heart disease is the most common cause of hospital admission in older people (Weir et al., 2005), and incidence is increasing. Even if heart failure does not cause admission, it may complicate other diseases, or precipitate crises.

This chapter outlines what heart failure is, the ways in which it can affect individuals, and so the nursing care in both acute crises and for health promotion during recovery/rehabilitation. Hypertension, an almost inevitable cause or effect of heart failure, is discussed. A brief overview of some commonly used drugs is included, with their main effects and side effects. However, this is not a pharmacology text; many more drugs are available, and each drug can have many other side effects.

Pathophysiology

Heart failure is caused by structural or functional cardiac dysfunction (von Klemperer and Bunce, 2007). It may be left- and/or right-sided – common causes are listed in Table 28.1.

Table 28.1 Common causes of heart failure

Left-sided	Right-sided
Coronary artery disease	Left ventricular failure
Hypertension	Tricuspid valve disease
Cardiomyopathy	
Congenital defects	

Left-sided failure is usually caused by coronary artery disease (Mehta and Cowie, 2006) and/or hypertension (Lakasing and Francis, 2006). Cardiovascular disease often affects both coronary and systemic arteries. While coronary heart disease affects heart structure, systemic vascular disease affects its function. Both contribute to the downward spiral of the syndrome.

The World Health Organisation and International Society and Federation of Cardiology (McKenna, 1996) classify cardiomyopathies as

- dilated
- hypertrophic
- arrhythrombogenic right ventricular cardiomyopathy or dysplasia
- restrictive;

the most common type being *dilated*. Cardiomyopathies are summarised in Table 28.2.

The heart uses more energy than any other organ (Neubauer, 2007), extracting nearly all oxygen delivered by the coronary arteries. This leaves little reserve if demand increases. Sustained increased demand causes compensatory responses – tachycardia (Mehta and Cowie, 2006) and muscle enlargement. But both of these further increase oxygen and energy demand, so structural changes accelerate. Structural changes in the heart, together with vascular resistance to output, cause progressive problems with cardiac output, and so tissue perfusion.

Left-sided heart failure causes pulmonary vascular congestion (von Klemperer and Bunce, 2007), causing

- breathlessness
- limited exercise tolerance.

Pulmonary vascular disease, often complicated by pulmonary oedema, impairs gas diffusion, often returning poorly oxygenated blood to the left side of the heart. In addition, breathlessness hinders normal activities of living, so patients

Table 28.2 Cardiomyopathies

	Effects	Main causes	Incidence
Dilated	Dilates (enlarges) both ventricles, so impaired systolic function; progressive	Usually alcohol; also street drugs such as cocaine (Hall and Henry, 2006), metabolic disorders, autoimmune disease, pregnancy	Most common type; usually older people
Hypertrophic	Ventricular (left and/or right) hypertrophy, usually asymptomatic	Genetic	Rare; usually young people
Arrhythromgenic right ventricular	Progressive replacement of (especially right) ventricular muscle with fat/fibre	Genetic	Rare
Restrictive	Heart normal size or slightly enlarged, but filling restricted	Endomyocardial fibrosis; primary disorder	Rarest type of cardiomyopathy

may be malnourished and dehydrated. Malnourishment may cause emaciation, but a significant factor contributing to many patients developing heart failure, and breathlessness, is obesity. Breathlessness is often especially bad at night, so patients often complain of difficulty sleeping.

Right-sided heart failure causes venous congestion and generalised oedema. Patients typically experience

■ lethargy
■ a feeling of 'fullness'.

Hepatic portal congestion can cause abdominal distension and ascites. Engorged jugular veins cause raised jugular venous pressure.

Because heart failure is a syndrome, diagnosis is made on the overall clinical picture, and not through any single test. Tests often used to contribute towards making diagnoses include:

■ echocardiography – checks heart size and function, including ejection fraction;
■ chest x-ray – views heart size and shape;
■ cardiac catheterisation – measures pressures in right heart chambers;
■ biopsy – views tissue cells.

Nurses should ensure their patients have given informed consent for procedures, and where significant risks are attached to procedures, that these have been explained to patients. Procedures may require other preparation (e.g. cardiac catheterisation is normally performed in a theatre-style suite), so nurses should check local requirements for planned procedures. Nurses should also check if there are any special post-procedure instructions.

Other information that contributes to diagnosis includes:

- vital signs (heart rate, blood pressure, respiratory rate)
- 12-lead ECG
- blood results (U+Es, FBC, LFTs)
- weight
- treatment aims are to improve both
  - life expectancy, and
  - quality of life.

(NICE, 2003b)

Incidence of chronic progressive heart failure

Up to 2 per cent (approximately 900,000 people) of the UK population have heart failure (von Klemperer and Bunce, 2007), most aged over 65 (Weir *et al.*, 2005). Incidence rises with age: by 70, one in ten people have heart failure (von Klemperer and Bunce, 2007) while by 85 it occurs in one in seven (Vassallo, 2008). The ageing population means numbers are likely to increase – by 2025 probably 60 per cent of the UK population will be hypertensive (Adrogué, 2007).

Hypertension

Hypertension is sustained blood pressure above 140/90 mmHg. In Western societies, over one-fifth of adults are hypertensive (Elliott, 2006). It usually develops in later years of life. Chronic hypertension increases resistance against which the left ventricle pumps, so chronic hypertension almost inevitably causes chronic left ventricular strain, and often left ventricular failure (LVF).

Primary hypertension is rare; hypertension is usually secondary to vascular disease (atherosclerosis, arteriosclerosis) – hardening of arteries and arterioles. Vascular disease increases resistance, and so systolic blood pressure. Therefore, pulse pressure (systolic minus diastolic) rises significantly, and is a quick indicator of the extent of vascular disease. Increased pulse pressure is visibly seen by increased gaps between systolic and diastolic marks on observation charts. Years of heart strain causes the heart to attempt compensation by enlarging (cardiomyopathy), especially of the left ventricle. This usually causes a left axis deviation on ECGs (see Chapter 25). But sustained strain eventually causes ischaemia and cardiac disease, which often manifests as chronic dysrhythmias, often symptomatic. Atrial fibrillation often develops (Mehta and Cowie, 2006), reducing cardiac output, causing venous congestion and chronic peripheral oedema. As cardiac output and perfusion decline, oxygenation of all tissues is impaired, and the person often develops problems with other organs/systems.

Normal ageing has a minimal effect on vascular health. Vascular disease is almost invariably a result of lifestyle. In isolated societies, incidence of hypertension is less than 1 per cent, but in industrialised countries about one-third of the population are hypertensive (Adrogué, 2007). The single most significant factor in development of vascular disease is smoking, but other significant modifiable factors include excessive alcohol intake (Adam *et al.*, 2008) and diet (saturated fats). Lack of exercise, stress and environmental pollutants also often contribute to disease.

Kidney disease

The renal artery is one of the largest in the body, taking one-quarter of cardiac output. But atherosclerotic changes often cause renal artery stenosis (Mehta and Cowie, 2006). Reduced renal bloodflow impairs urine output, but also causes intrarenal ischaemia. Glomerular filtration rate is often below 60 ml/minute (Mehta and Cowie, 2006). But other renal functions are also impaired. Reduced erythropoietin production often causes anaemia (Mehta and Cowie, 2006), while reduced renal bloodflow often stimulates renin production. These effects compound the problems of heart failure:

- oliguria accelerates oedema formation;
- anaemia further reduces oxygen delivery to body cells;
- increased renin release increases blood pressure.

Gender

The historical view that cardiovascular disease is largely a male disease is increasingly being challenged. Mehta and Cowie (2006) suggest chronic heart failure is more common in men, but Nicholson (2007) suggests that, on average, women have the same risk of developing the disease as men, only with a ten-year delay, and that cardiovascular disease is the leading cause of death among women in the developed world. It has long been known that pre-menopausal female hormones provide cardioprotection; what is currently unclear is whether post-menopausal hormone replacement therapy protects against cardiovascular disease (Nicholson, 2007).

Drugs

Blood pressure control is often poor. NICE (2006b) and the British Hypertension Society (Williams *et al.*, 2004) recommend drug therapy with sustained systolic pressures of 160 or diastolic pressures of 100 mmHg (Crichton, 2007), although Conen *et al.* (2007) suggest that even high normal BP (130–139/85–89) increases the ten-year risk of major cardiovascular event by 64 per cent, which suggests even tighter control may be beneficial. Williams *et al.* (2004) recommend making treatment decisions with systolic blood pressure over 140 or diastolic over

90 mmHg. Anti-hypertensives significantly reduce the incidence of heart failure, even in the over-80s (Beckett *et al.*, 2008). Heart failure causes a complex syndrome, and for each problem there are often many pharmacological options, with new drugs frequently being marketed. Key drug groups used to control heart failure are usually

- diuretics
- antihypertensives
- lipid-lowering.

But because of likely complications of heart failure, various other cardiac and non-cardiac drugs are also often needed for

- rate control
- anti-thrombotic.

Diuretics

Heart failure typically causes venous congestion and so oedema. Diuretic therapy reduces both oedema and preload, enabling the failing heart to function more effectively. Three main groups of diuretics are used:

- loop (e.g. furosemide, bumetanide)
- thiazide (e.g. bendroflumethiazide, metolazone)
- potassium-sparing (e.g. amiloride, spironolactone).

Loop diuretics inhibit reabsorption in the Loop of Helne, so not only reduce renal reabsorption of water, but also significantly reduce renal reabsorption of potassium. Loop diuretics can, therefore, cause hypokalaemia, which can impair cardiac conduction, so causing escape ectopics and dysrhythmias. Because urine is formed from arterial blood, but excess water is mainly either in the veins or tissues (oedema), diuretics often stimulate thirst. Oral fluids are absorbed into capillaries, which flow into veins. So oral (or intravenous) rehydration increases cardiac preload. Fluid restriction may, therefore, be necessary, which often increases patient's distress.

Antihypertensives

Blood pressure is the sum of cardiac output multiplied by resistance. Heart failure usually reduces cardiac output, but extensive vascular disease (arteriosclerosis, atherosclerosis, peripheral vascular disease), which significantly increases resistance, often exacerbated by tissue oedema. Increase in resistance is generally greater than fall in cardiac output, resulting in hypertension. Antihypertensives significantly reduce incidence of heart failure (Beckett *et al.*, 2008).

Hypertension is often divided between 'high renin' and 'low renin' (Williams *et al.*, 2004), the type affecting choice of drugs. With 'high renin', poor renal bloodflow, from both reduced cardiac output and renal artery stenosis, together with serum lipids (see below) stimulates release of the renal hormone renin, which initiates the renin–angiotensin–aldosterone cascade, which further increases blood pressure. Renin activates angiotensinogen (in the liver), to form angiotensin I. Angiotensin I, a mild vasoconstrictor, is converted by angiotensin-converting enzymes (in the lungs) to form angiotensin II, a very powerful vasoconstrictor. In addition, angiotensin II stimulates release of the hormone aldosterone (from the adrenal gland). Aldosterone increases renal reabsorption of sodium, which helps retain water. Thus, the renin–angiotensin–aldosterone cascade increases blood pressure by

- vasoconstriction (angiotensin, decreasing blood vessel volume)
- reabsorbing more saline into the bloodstream (aldosterone).

The main effect of this cascade occurs after angiotensin-concerting enzymes (ACE) form angiotensin II, so

- ACE inhibitors ('-pril's)

are one of the most widely used antihypertensives for heart failure. However, other antihypertensives may be used in addition or instead. ACE inhibitiors often cause a dry, tickly cough. As antihypertensive therapy for chronic heart failure should continue for the remainder of life, this irritating side effect sometimes causes non-compliance. So alternative therapy is

- angiotensin II type 1 receptor blockers (e.g. losarten)
- aldosterone antagonists.

The other widely used group of antihypertensives is

- beta-blockers ('-olol's, carvedilol).

Cardio-selective beta-blockers block stimulation of beta 2 receptors in the heart; in practice, all beta-blockers likely to be used now are cardio-selective, and a non-cardio-selective beta-blocker would also cause bronchoconstriction. Beta 2 receptors increase heart rate and stroke (pulse) volume, so increasing both factors that create cardiac output. Blocking beta receptors, therefore, reduces blood pressure by reducing cardiac output. Beta-blockers should be prescribed for all patients with heart failure (SIGN, 2007), yet, Vassallo (2008) suggests they are seldom used.

The electrical conduction and activity of both skeletal and (especially) cardiac muscle is created by movement of cations, of which calcium is the main one that affects both peak and duration of conduction. Therefore, blocking the calcium channel reduces cardiac excitability (heart rate) and vascular constriction. Another widely used group of antihypertensives is therefore

- the calcium channel blockers (e.g. nifedipine, amlopidine, diltiazem).

Lipid-lowering drugs

Atherosclerosis is a cyclical problem with a complex pathology. But one of the main causes of plaque forming in tunica media is intravascular chemicals, especially lipids such as cholesterol and low-density lipoproteins (LDLs). These chemicals also help trigger the renin cascade (above) (Singh and Mehta, 2003) and inhibit release of the endogenous vasodilator nitric oxide (Galley and Webster, 2004). Lipid-lowering drugs ('statins') not only inhibit plaque formation, but significantly reduce existing plaque (Jensen *et al.*, 2004). Joint British Societies' guidelines (Wood *et al.*, 2005) recommend

- TC < 4 mmol/litre
- LDL < 2 mmol/litre.

Statins cannot be used in liver failure, and liver function of all patients should be monitored. Other significant side effects of statins include:

- gastrointestinal (pain, nausea/vomiting, flatulence, diarrhoea, constipation)
- headache
- muscle damage.

Depending on symptoms experienced by patients, various other cardiac (and non-cardiac) drugs may be needed. Atrial fibrillation and angina frequently co-exist and need treating.

Rate control drugs

Rate, rather than rhythm, reduces mortality from atrial fibrillation (Roy *et al.*, 2008). Target rates with atrial fibrillation should be 60–80 bpm at rest and 90–115 with exercise (Fotherby, 2006). Digoxin should be omitted if heart rate is below 60 bpm. If a cardiac monitor is not being used, and peripheral pulse rate (brachial – measured by automated blood pressure monitors – or radial) is below 60 bpm, apex heart rate should be counted using a stethoscope over a full minute. Counting the apex-radial deficit, with one person counting using a stethoscope to count the apex rate over a full minute while another person counts the radial pulse over the same minute, is a useful way to monitor rate-control therapy – if there is a significant difference, rate is probably not being well controlled. Digoxin remains the most widely used rate-control drug, although its narrow therapeutic range necessitates frequent checking of serum levels.

Anti-thrombotic drugs

Atrial fibrillation causes loss of co-ordinated contraction of atrial muscle, and so with only passive emptying of atria, thrombi may develop, releasing emboli. Emboli from the left atrium are usually carried into the carotid artery, creating a six-fold increase of stroke-risk (Hart *et al.*, 2003). Therefore, people with permanent atrial fibrillation should be anti-coagulated. Warfarin is the most widely used anti-coagulant, and is superior to aspirin (Mant *et al.*, 2007; Waldo, 2008).

Angina drugs

Stable angina is usually treated with glyceryl trinitrate (GTN) inhalers. Unstable angina, an acute coronary syndrome, is described in Chapter 26.

Future drugs

The increasing burden of heart failure has encouraged research for new drugs. One current area of promise is the search for drugs that can improve adenosine triphosphate (ATP – cell energy) production/usage, prognosis may be improved (Neubauer, 2007).

Non-pharmacological treatment

In addition to drugs, helping people with chronic heart failure largely focuses on symptom relief. Although care will vary between patients, likely aspects of nursing care include:

- close monitoring of vital signs, fluid balance and daily weight
- oxygen therapy
- rest
- fluid management
- salt restriction (limiting hypervolaemia)
- health promotion.

British Thoracic Society (BTS, 2008) guidelines recommend oxygen therapy to achieve target saturations of 94–98 per cent provided hypercapnic respiratory failure is not also present; if the person also has COPD, target saturation should be 88–92 per cent until an arterial blood gas has been obtained. Changes in daily weight almost always indicates changes in body water, so weight gain over 1 day is likely to reflect accumulation of oedema, and the need for medical review of drug therapy. Fluid management often necessitates restriction to limit hypertension from hypervolaemia, but in acute wards could necessitate carefully monitored fluid challenges. Central venous cannulation may be necessary to titrate fluid therapy within specific targets for central venous pressure, remembering that heart failure increases central venous pressure, and a higher-than-normal target may be needed. Dieticians can advise about low-salt diets. With alcohol-related dilated cardiomyopathy, stopping drinking, nutritious diet and vitamin B supplements can enable the heart to its normal size, and prognosis is good compared with other forms of chronic heart failure, but if drinking continues, prognosis poor (Adam *et al.*, 2008).

Most acute hospitals offer management programmes for people with heart failure, although Clark and Thompson (2008) suggest supporting evidence for interventions is often weak. While heart failure limits lifestyle, rest should be carefully planned to include gently increasing activity and exercise, based on advice from physiotherapists and/or specialist cardiac nurses.

Metabolic syndrome

The term 'metabolic syndrome' has been coined within the last decade to describe a cluster of symptoms that frequently occur with heart failure. Criteria vary slightly, but the standard American criteria for metabolic syndrome are three or more of:

- fasting plasma glucose ≥ 6.1 mmol/litre;
- abdominal obesity (e.g. waist circumference >102 cm in men, >88 cm in women);
- triglyceride level ≥ 1.7 mmol/litre;
- high-density lipoprotein cholesterol (HDL-C) <1 mmol/litre in men, 1.3 mmol/litre in women;
- BP $\geq 130/85$ mmHg.

(Tonkin, 2004)

Insulin resistance (Tonkin, 2004) and pro-inflammatory responses (Eckel *et al.*, 2005) cause many of the problems of the syndrome, which may both cause and accelerate cardiovascular disease.

Prognosis

Because heart failure is a progressive, chronic disease, mortality is high. NICE (2003b) suggests nearly 40 per cent die within one year from diagnosis, although von Klemperer and Bunce (2007) suggest that five-year survival from the first hospital admission is about 50 per cent. What these two discrepant figures exclude is that progressive limitations to activities of living are physically, socially and mentally disabling. Although the precise future for each patient may not be fully predictable, nurses can offer useful advice to help people with heart failure limit their problems, and limit the progression of the disease. People admitted to acute hospitals with established chronic heart failure usually have an eventually terminal disease, so although acute problems can often be treated, the team (including the patient) should discuss appropriateness of interventions in the light of likely prognosis. Possible considerations include:

- What are the patient's wishes?
- Has the patient made a living will?
- What should be ceiling treatment?
- Should a 'do not attempt cardiopulmonary resuscitation' order be instigated, and if so how long it should remain in effect?

People with heart failure often have a poor understanding of their condition, and need both specialist information and psychosocial support (Aldred *et al.*, 2005), such as counselling. If palliative care is more appropriate than aggressive therapy, palliative care teams should be involved. If active treatment is appropriate, patients should be aware of their long-term prognosis so they can plan for their future – some patients may wish to make a 'living will' to limit potentially futile treatment in the future.

Health promotion

Patients discharged from acute hospitals with heart failure are likely to need long-term support within the community, so staff in acute hospitals may need to make referrals to community services. By the time of hospital admission, the person with heart failure has suffered much irreversible damage to their cardiovascular system. In most instances this has largely been caused by lifestyle choices. While the person should not be blamed for their chosen lifestyle, they should be offered advice about how they can modify their lifestyle to limit further damage (Peters *et al.*, 2007). Advice may vary with the causes of heart failure (see Table 28.1), but SIGN (2007) suggest advising about:

- avoiding excess alcohol;
- stopping smoking;
- taking regular low-intensity physical activity;
- limiting salt intake below 6 grams/day;
- monitoring weight.

(SIGN, 2007)

Cardiovascular disease is a major killer in Western societies, so widespread health promotion is needed. But because cardiac disease has traditionally been viewed as a male disease, some women may be especially unaware of the risks they face. Williams *et al.* (2004) offer detailed advice about healthier lifestyles.

Implications for practice

- Chronic heart failure is a progressive syndrome.
- Acute admission may be caused by acute or decompensated heart failure.
- Colloid fluids contain significant amounts of sodium, so may complicate heart failure.
- Vital signs and daily weight are important for monitoring acute episodes.
- Long-term follow-up and management in the community will be necessary after discharge.
- Heart failure needs pharmacological management (diuretics, antithrombotics, statins and often digoxin and aspirin).
- Lifestyle changes (exercise, diet) can significantly slow progression.

Summary

Chronic heart failure is a common, complex and progressive syndrome. It exerts a high human cost on its victims, but also a high financial cost on society – it is currently estimated to consume 2 per cent of the UK NHS budget (Neubauer, 2007), a figure that is likely to rise in the future. Not surprisingly, heart failure is, therefore, a major health target for politicians. However, the insidious nature of the disease means that most initiatives will take many years to show any benefits, and the effects of political changes on many unhealthy aspects of UK lifestyle are often questionable. Heart failure is, therefore, likely to remain a burden to individuals, healthcare and society for some years.

Clinical scenario

Alan Burnside, aged 78, is admitted via his GP for investigations for suspected heart failure. Increasing breathlessness has limited his mobility, and he now seldom leaves his house. His wife is his main carer.

Vital signs on arrival are:

- blood pressure 168/98 mmHg
- pulse 115 bpm
- respiratory rate 36 bpm
- temperature 37.6°C.

He has experienced difficulty in passing urine, and is currently unable to supply a sample for testing. His ECG reveals atrial fibrillation.

1   Using the early warning score used in your workplace, calculate Alan's score. Identify what actions the score requires you to make. Is there any additional information you need before proceeding?

2   List further investigations which you, as Alan's nurse, are likely to initiate within the first 24 hours of his admission to an acute hospital.

3   Completing his admission paperwork, you also begin preparing his discharge planning. From what you know so far, what aspects are likely to need attention for discharge? Identify relevant care.

Bibliography

Key reading

Various national guidelines have been produced by NICE (e.g. 2003b; 2006b), the British Hypertension Society (Williams *et al.*, 2004) and SIGN (2007). The NICE 2003 guidelines should currently be being updated, while the British Hypertension Society usually produce new guidelines approximately every 5 years, so although the ones cited are current at time of writing, readers should check for updates.

Further reading

Over the last decade a number of useful books on heart failure have been published, including Stewart and Blue (2004). Nicholas (2004) provides a useful review of nursing care.

Chapter 29

Fluid and electrolyte disturbances

Tina Moore

Contents

Learning outcomes

After reading this chapter you will be able to:

- outline the homeostatic mechanisms of water and electrolyte balance;
- conduct an appropriate assessment of patient's fluid and electrolyte status;
- identify appropriate intervention for the prevention and treatment of actual/potential disturbances;
- understand the aetiology of electrolyte disturbances;
- monitor fluid balance appropriately.

Fundamental knowledge

Basic knowledge of the functions and homeostatic mechanisms of water and electrolyte balance; sources of water intake and losses; sources of various electrolyte intake and areas of loss; nephron physiology.

Introduction

Clear guidelines and knowledge need to be available which clarifies and challenges why and if patients require a fluid balance chart, what needs recording, and what impact does it have upon the overall care. Despite this, there appears to be little value placed on the assessment of patient's fluid status and the overall use of fluid balance charts in clinical practice. Loss or gain of relatively small amounts of fluid and electrolytes can tip a very delicate balance in an unstable patient.

All nurses have a fundamental role in the prevention, early detection and treatment of fluid and electrolyte imbalances. Yet it is a role that appears to be given the least priority. Failure to properly recognise and treat fluid and electrolyte disturbances in the acutely/critically ill patient may have fatal consequences. Successful management is dependent upon accurate assessment of the patient.

Fluid balance

Water is an essential element for all body processes. It is involved in

- the transportation of substances to and from the cells;
- the promotion and maintenance of necessary chemical activity;
- the regulation of sodium balance, aiding the control of blood pressure.

Water and electrolyte disturbances generally occur simultaneously. However, to enable clarity of information within this particular chapter fluid and electrolytes will be discussed separately.

In the 'average' adult male approximately 60–65 per cent of total body weight is water (i.e. 40–45 litres). In the 'average' female, due to higher body fat content this figure is reduced to 50 per cent (Marieb, 2008). Consequently obesity also incurs a lower total body weight (water) percentage.

With age, the body increases its fat content and loses a significant amount of muscle mass (muscle holds 40 per cent of total body water). Therefore, the older person is more at risk of becoming dehydrated.

There are two main body fluid compartments:

1 Intracellular fluid (ICF) is contained within the cells and accounts for approximately 40 per cent of total body weight.
2 Extracellular fluid (ECF) surrounds the cells and is subdivided into two types:

2.1 *Interstitial fluid* (water between the cells and outside the blood vessel). The transcellular compartment (also considered part of the interstitial fluid) consists of a collection of biochemically distinct fluids, including cerebrospinal, synovial, pleural, pericardial, peritoneal fluids and digestive secretions, which are separated from the interstitial compartments by a layer of epithelium (Flanning, 2000).

This space (known as the third space) increases in illness, taking place as a consequence of increased capillary hydrostatic pressure, decreased plasma colloid osmotic pressure or both. It enables movement of fluid (transcellular fluid) into body cavities, e.g. in paralytic ileus (pooling of fluid in the bowel), oedema and effusion.

2.2 *Plasma fluid volumes* (20 per cent of total body weight). Plasma (intravascular) is contained within the blood vessels and plasma volume.

Normally, the composition and concentration of ECF is altered and modified as the body reacts with its surrounding environment, ICF remains relatively stable. During acute/critical illness there is an alteration in the normal distribution of fluids, namely a depletion of ICF and an increase in ECF.

Maintaining fluid balance

Initially, fluid volume and osmolality are maintained within normal limits by the hypothalamic thirst mechanism and by several hormones, notably aldosterone, antidiuretic hormone (ADH) and atrial natuiretic peptide, which act on the kidney to regulate urine volume and osmolality. A reduction in plasma osmolality inhibits ADH release and thus increases the excretion of water. An increase in osmolality stimulates ADH (via osmoreceptors) production and increases kidney tubular reabsorption of water. A reduction in circulating blood volume stimulates baroreceptors to trigger ADH.

In normal ageing, the release of ADH appears to be increased in response to a variety of stimuli that can result in the retention of fluid. Aldosterone is an important regulator of fluid volume that is released by the adrenal cortex. The release of aldosterone is stimulated by an increase in potassium levels and decrease in sodium levels. It promotes reabsorption of sodium in the distal tubules in the kidney and from the colon. Water, sodium and potassium need to be in constant motion between the intracellular and extracellular body compartments (Edwards, 2001).

Fluid and electrolyte homeostasis is maintained by the cardiovascular, renal, respiratory and gastrointestinal systems, the skin and brain. In illness where cardiac volume is insufficient (resulting in renal impairment), selective reabsorption takes place. Sodium is retained and potassium is excreted, maintaining normal osmolality and blood volume. The lungs influence loss of fluid through ventilation.

There are two principal forces that govern movement of water:

1   *Osmotic pressure* – pressure that must be applied to a solution on one side of a membrane. Sodium and protein are important for the maintenance of osmotic pressure and volume in the ECF compartment. Any changes in

sodium concentration will lead to fluid volume changes (water follows sodium). Potassium is the main intracellular cation and maintains the ICF osmotic pressure. Electrolytes do not move between the cell walls and capillaries as easily as water.

Sodium and potassium concentrations are maintained inside and outside the cells through active transport in the ECF; sodium is pumped out of the cell (keeping intracellular sodium low) and potassium is pumped into the cell (maintaining high intracellular potassium level). Renal mechanisms aid this distribution, regulating sodium excretion. Despite variations in potassium, levels are kept constant. Constancy is achieved by the renal tubular absorption of potassium and the secretion of variable amounts of potassium. When potassium is lost from the body (e.g. in urine) potassium moves out of the cells into the ECF to maintain potassium equilibrium between the ICF and ECF.

In the ECF compartment there is an exchange of water and electrolytes between the interstitial fluid compartment and the intravascular compartment. The principal difference in composition between these compartments is the presence of proteins in the plasma. Proteins cannot pass through the capillary membrane and therefore function as osmotically active substances holding fluid in the blood vessels. The osmotic pressure exerted by plasma proteins is referred to as oncotic pressure, at approximately 20–30 mmHg. With sodium, the plasma proteins control intravascular volume.

2 *Hydrostatic pressure of blood* is the pressure exerted by fluid against the vascular wall. When the osmotic pressure changes in one fluid compartment water moves across the semi-permeable membrane from an area of lesser osmotic pressure to that of greater osmotic pressure until equilibrium is achieved. The volume of blood flowing through the vessels creates hydrostatic pressure and this driving force causes filtration of fluid through the semi-permeable membranes of the capillaries. Water and small electrolyte molecules pass easily; larger colloid substances and protein are held back.

Disturbances to fluid balance

Water balance disorders are manifested by alterations in plasma osmolality (which measures the ability of a fluid to hold water and to draw it through semipermeable membrane). Normal osmolality is 280–290 mOsm/kg of water and this provides an environment that is favourable for cellular activity. In disturbances such as dehydration, hyperosmolality occurs.

Time out 29.1

1 Reflect upon patients you nursed who had developed fluid and/or electrolyte disturbances. How were these disturbances detected (i.e. symptoms manifested)?
2 What caused the imbalances and how were they corrected?
3 Think about why monitoring fluid balance is important.

The osmolality of the ICF compartment must balance that of the ECF compartment in order to maintain a correct and orderly distribution of fluid between the cell and its environment.

Monitoring fluid balance

Loss or gain of relatively small amounts of fluid and electrolytes can influence a delicate balance in an unstable patient. Fluid imbalance is present when regular mechanisms are insufficient to compensate for abnormal intake or output of fluid.

Movement of water, electrolytes and albumin occurs into the interstitial spaces. This third space fluid shift leads to localised swelling and lymph blockage causing localised interstitial oedema. A patient might appear hypovolaemic or dehydrated. Fluid has moved into the interstitial spaces, so the total amount of body water may not have changed but just become unequally distributed. These patients can easily become overloaded with fluid replacement, even though the central venous pressure (CVP) is low. Minimum urine output for acutely/critically ill patients should be at least 1 ml/kg per hour or about 1,700 ml per 24 hours (Perkins and Kisiel, 2005). Hourly monitoring of input, output and calculation of the overall balance is essential.

Fluid loss: hypovolaemia

Depletion of ECF volume occurs when water loss exceeds water intake over a period of time and the body is in negative fluid balance. Irrespective of the cause of fluid loss, cardiac output will be impaired (diminished pre-load). Presenting problems will reflect the effects of reduced cardiac output, disruption of normal cellular metabolism and the resulting activation of homeostatic mechanism to compensate.

Sometimes patients will develop hypovolaemia with fluid overload, e.g. oedema due to increased capillary permeability. Despite clinical signs of shock, positive fluid balance is present. While interstitial overload is present the aim is to expand the vascular space with fluids that will not leak into the interstitial spaces and risk worsening the oedema. Reducing water and sodium intake together with diuretic therapy (optional) should result in a negative balance.

Fluid loss may be:

- *Hypertonic* – body water losses. Losses may occur because of food and water deprivation. An increased body or environmental temperature, hyperglycaemia, diuresis (diabetes insipidus) or hyperalimination.
- *Hypotonic* – loss of fluids and electrolytes. May occur because of loss of body fluids containing salt, haemorrhage, burns, peritonitis or surgical intervention.
- *Isotonic* loss in excess of water excretion (hypernatraemic dehydration). Commonly seen in the critically ill patient. Occurs when a disproportionate amount of free water is retained in the intracellular compartment. Often associated with diabetic ketoacidosis, disorders causing excessive gastrointestinal loss and excessive use of diuretics.

Clinical features

Clinical signs of hypovolaemic shock include increased heart rate, thready pulse, reduced blood pressure and CVP, increased systemic vascular resistance (SVR), tachypnoea and decreased urine output (increased in diabetes insipidus).

Fluid balance results indicate a negative gross balance. Skin is of a dehydrated appearance (although older patients' skin elasticity is lost, therefore this sign alone will not truly reflect a fluid deficit). The patient's oral cavity, mucous membranes and tongue are dry, while the skin is often cold and clammy. Skin colour changes suggest under-perfusion of tissues and a reduction in capillary refill is noted. Excessive perspiration accompanies increased body temperature. Patients may appear apprehensive and restless and there may be acute weight loss (except when a third space occurs).

Owing to the compensatory mechanisms, the severity of the illness may be misjudged. The older person is particularly vulnerable to hypernatraemic dehydration. This may be present; initially there may be little change in the B/P (compensatory responses). In severe cases, mental confusion, hallucinations and a dangerous reduction in renal blood flow may occur.

Diagnostic tests include elevated blood urea nitrogen (BUN) levels, electrolyte disturbances (variable depending upon the type of fluid lost); increased urine specific gravity (kidney's attempt to conserve water) and increased urine osmolality.

Management

Management dependent upon treating the known cause. The overall fluid balance should be monitored initially on an hourly basis. Insensible loss (i.e. fluid loss through respiration, skin and faeces) need to be estimated; this accounts for approximately 500 ml of water per day. Fluid replacement will be given to induce a positive balance. Any infused intravenous fluids will directly enter the ECF compartment, primarily the vascular space, and will then be distributed into the respective fluid compartments, according to their composition.

The type of fluid replacement will depend upon the type of fluid loss and the severity of the deficit:

- Oral fluids may be encouraged, if tolerated.
- Isotonic saline (0.9%) is appropriate for rapid volume replacement; it expands ECF only and does not enter ICF.
- Hypotonic saline (0.45%) solution is used in the management of patients who have both volume depletion and hypernatraemia or hyperglycaemia (e.g. diabetic ketoacidosis).
- Glucose and water is used to treat water deficit; it is useful in replacing fluid volume without altering electrolytes (both in ECF and ICF).
- Mixed saline/electrolyte solutions provide additional electrolytes.
- Blood and albumin expands the intravascular portion of the ECF only (acute haemorrhage).

■ Dextran, a colloid solution that expands the intravascular portion of the ECF.

■ If there is no response in stroke volume to a fluid challenge then positive inotropic support and vasodilators or vasoconstrictors will be necessary.

■ Low sodium fluid replacement is used in hypernatraemia dehydration (fluid intake of at least 2,500 ml/day unless contraindicated).

If the patient has periodic fluid challenges, then vital signs need to be monitored and evaluated. There should also be daily measurements of serum electrolytes.

For further information on hypovolaemic shock, see Chapter 27.

Fluid gain: hypervolaemia

Expansion of the ECF is termed *hypervolaemia*. Iatrogenic fluid overload is preventable with appropriate monitoring of treatment.

Fluid gain may be:

■ *Hypertonic* (more water than sodium is lost or ECF concentration of sodium increases). This can result from increased solutes in the ECF compartment, leading to water being drawn out of the cells.

■ *Isotonic* (sodium and water are lost in equal proportion). This results from increased fluid and electrolyte gains. Expansion of both ICF and ECF compartments occur. Excessive infusion of isotonic solutions, congestive heart failure, acute renal failure, liver cirrhosis can be classified as causes.

■ *Hypotonic* (water intoxication). Here, water moves from the ECF, causing overhydration and swelling of cells. Possible causes include: excessive fluid intake, renal impairment, and retention of irrigation fluid, physiological stress (ADH production is affected and increases rapidly, overriding normal regulation). It can result in reduced urine output and osmolality, leading to water retention and hyponatraemia.

Clinical features

Clinical features of overload result in an increased heart rate and BP (unless left-sided heart failure is present); increased CVP (neck vein distention may be evident); delayed capillary filling time; tachypnoea; dyspnoea and pulmonary oedema may be evident. Lung auscultation reveals crackling rhonchi and wheezes. Urinary output may be increased or decreased depending on the underlying cause and renal function. Urine osmolality increases in fluid volume deficit (this test reflects the concentrating ability of the kidneys, normal range = 300–1,200 mOsml/litre). Diagnostic findings are related to haemodilution.

Fluid balance is gross positive. Signs of systemic overload are apparent; generalised, and/or pitting oedema, weight gain is noticeable (rapid gains are generally associated with changes in fluid volume). Skin may be warm, moist and swollen with the appearance of being tight and shiny. The patient's general behaviour may include irritability and a deteriorating level of consciousness.

Management

The goal is to treat the precipitation problem and return ECF to normal. Patient may require fluid and sodium restrictions, monitoring of patient's fluid balance aids evaluation of treatment and indicates deterioration or improvement in the patient's condition. Caution should be taken when administering fluid with sizeable amounts of sodium (e.g. 0.9% normal saline), a change in the solution or a slow infusion rate may need to be prescribed. Diuretics may be indicated; loop diuretics (e.g. furosemide) in severe hypervolaemia. Patients receiving intravenous medication need to have it diluted in the minimum amount of solution. Careful monitoring of vital signs (BP, CVP, MAP, respiratory status) should be performed, initially on an hourly basis. In life-threatening hypervolaemia, haemodialysis is indicated.

Time out 29.2

1 Make a list of the electrolytes you can remember.
2 How does a disorder in each affect the patient's physiological status?

Table 29.1 provides information about electrolyte disturbances.

Implications for practice

- Nurses should have in-depth knowledge in this aspect of care.
- Prevention, early detection and early treatment should occur.
- The older person and critically ill patients are particularly vulnerable to developing fluid and electrolyte disturbance.
- Close monitoring is required including serum electrolytes.

Summary

Fluid and electrolyte disturbances are common features within clinical practice. All nurses have a fundamental role in the prevention, early detection and treatment of fluid and electrolyte imbalances, yet this is a role that appears to be given a low priority. Failure to recognise and treat fluid and electrolyte disturbances properly may have fatal consequences. Successful management is dependent upon accurate assessment of the patient. Nurses must have knowledge and understanding of the normal physiological processes of fluid balance in order to deliver safe care. Risks of imbalance must be predicted, detected and evaluated through accurate monitoring and recording of fluid intake and output.

Table 29.1 Electrolyte disturbances

Electrolyte	Causes	Clinical features	Treatment
Potassium • Closely related to reabsorption of sodium and hydrogen ions • Major cation in the ICF compartment, maintains osmotic pressure and volume within ICF • Essential for transmission and conduction of nerve impulses (contraction of skeletal, cardiac and smooth muscles) • Necessary for movement of glucose into cells • Required for carbohydrate metabolism and is essential for the conversion of glucose to glycogen and its storage • Normal range = 3.5–4.5 mmol/l	**Hypokalaemia** (<3.5 mmol/l) • Reduced potassium intake (anorexia malabsorption and alcoholism) • Excessive loss – diarrhoea and vomiting • Diuretic phase of acute kidney injury • Iatrogenic, e.g. excessive use of diuretics, prolonged and excessive aspiration of GI tract, IV alkali, e.g. sodium bicarbonate, nephrotoxic drugs, e.g. aminoglycoside antibiotics	• Usually become apparent when levels are below 3.0 mmol/l (Wheeler and Marini, 2006) • Reduces contractility of smooth skeletal and cardiac muscle. May cause cardiac arrhythmias • Weakness of respiratory muscles, leg and generalised body cramps • Confusion, disorientation • Anorexia decreased gastric motion, paralytic ileus	• Hypokalaemia can produce serious effects that demand prompt recognition and intervention • Potassium replacement oral or slow IV infusion. May act as irritant, therefore, frequent inspection of the infusion site and monitoring of the infusion rate is required (Chapter 30)

Table 29.1 continued

Electrolyte	Causes	Clinical features	Treatment
Hyperkalaemia	• Increased potassium intake • Iatrogenic – excessive use of potassium supplements • Increased supply – hypercatabolic states (e.g. ACS, cardiac arrest, massive injury, infection), resulting in wide release of potassium ions from the cells into the ECF • Acidosis – hydrogen ions cross cell membranes into ECF in exchange for potassium ions, cells become potassium depleted but plasma ECF levels increase • Poor excretion due to renal failure, diabetes • Haemolysis (e.g. vaso-occlusive crisis)	• ECG changes – peaked T waves, widening of QRS complex • Bradycardia, atrial and ventricular tachycardia • Risk of cardiac arrest (levels <7.0 mmol/l) • Respiratory failure • Tingling in extremities • Hypotension	• Depends on underlying condition, level and cause • Emergency treatment is aimed at counteracting the cardiac effects and shifting extra cellular potassium into the cells – 10 ml 10% calcium gluconate or calcium chloride protects the heart, raises the threshold and prolongs repolarisation; rapidly, but temporarily reverses adverse effects on the heart • Calcium salts potentiate the effects of digitalis, so should be given with caution to patients already receiving cardiac glycosides. If potassium remains persistently high (dangerous levels) haemodialysis or haemofiltration will need to be considered • Sometimes insulin and glucose, 50 units in 50 ml glucose IV slow bolus or 10 units in 500 ml over 1 hour • Continuous ECG monitoring

Sodium
- Sodium is widely distributed in the body, although most of it is in the ECF
- Essential for nerve impulses and muscle contractions
- Influences acid base balance; chloride and potassium levels; maintains osmotic pressure and volume in ECF compartment
- Normal values: 135–145 mmol/l

Hyponatraemia
- Diarrhoea and vomiting, GI suction, surgery/inappropriate replacement of GI losses, e.g. water without sufficient amounts of sodium
- Skin – perspiration in fever; burns
- Nephritis (renal tubules do not respond to ADH)
- Abuse or overuse of diuretics
- Water gain in CCF, liver cirrhosis, nephrotic syndrome and dilutional hyponatraemia results even though total body sodium may be in excess
- Hyperglycaemia (increases tubular flow rates and may promote renal sodium loss in excess of water). Can occur in hypervolaemia (dilution of sodium)

- Most common imbalance in the acutely ill
- Can lead to serious neurological disturbances, e.g. coma, convulsions, confusion
- Can cause headaches
- Causes a reduction in the osmotic pressure within the ECF (water then moves into the ICF leading to overhydration of the cells) and disturbance of fluid volume
- Initiates the movement of potassium out of the ICF leading to the addition of potassium imbalance
- Muscle cramps, nausea and vomiting

- Calcium resonium (mild hyperkalaemia) (Chapter 25)

- Treatment is dependent on cause and severity of symptoms; if cause is fluid volume deficit 5% glucose may be administered
- 0.9% sodium chloride will also be administered

Table 29.1 continued

Electrolyte	Causes	Clinical features	Treatment
Hypernatraemia	• Develops when in response to increased ECF osmolality (water moves out of the cells, leading to cellular dehydration) • Dietary – increased intake or overinfusion of sodium containing fluids • GI tract – severe diarrhoea and vomiting • Excessive perspiration • Renal and congestive cardiac failure both involves sodium retention • Reduced water intake/inability to respond to fluid deficit	• Clinical features associated with fluid volume disturbances – excess or deficit • In severe hypernatraemia convulsions, drowsiness, lethargy, confusion, coma may occur	• Dehydration is treated with IV, e.g. 5% glucose • Overhydration is treated through the correction of sodium (restricted intake of sodium) and with the use of diuretics (e.g. thiazide which blocks sodium absorption and water reabsorption)

Magnesium

- A major ICF cation closely related to potassium
- Essential in the function of many enzyme activities
- Has a depressant effect at the neural synapsis. Also affects neuromuscular transmission and cardiovascular tone
- Renal function is central to magnesium homeostasis
- Normal values some controversy but most suggest 1.25–2.5 mmol/l

Hypermagnesaemia

- Renal failure
- Excessive magnesium administration, e.g. some antacids

- These mainly include cardiac problems, for example:
  - bradycardia
  - complete heart block
  - hypotension
- In severe cases cardiac arrest and coma

- Directed towards promoting urinary output
- IV fluid replacement and diuretics are used to 'flush out' excessive magnesium
- Calcium chloride via IV infusion (should counteract effects of cardiovascular system)

Hypomagnesaemia

- Common in the critically ill, usually due to malnourishment, diarrhoea/vomiting and alcohol abuse
- Increased renal excretion
- Reduced intestinal absorption

- Muscular weakness/cramps, twitching and tremors
- Cardiac arrhythmia – SVT, VT
- Carpopedal spasm (tetany)
- Convulsions and coma in severe cases

- IV replacement which necessitates ICU admission (for continuous cardiac monitoring)
- Kidney function should be assessed prior to treatment
- Nutritional replacement

Table 29.1 continued

Electrolyte	Causes	Clinical features	Treatment
Chloride • A major anion in the ECF helps maintain ECF osmotic pressure and water balance • Digestion – essential for production of hydrochloric acid • Normal values 95–108 mmol/l	**Hyperchloraemia** • Increased retention or intake • Excessive IV sodium chloride • Renal failure	• Weakness, lethargy • Deep and rapid respirations (if caused by metabolic acidosis)	• Treat the cause
	Hypochloraemia • Increased loss from GI tract • Excessive diuretic use • Excessive perspiration • Generally associated with disorders of sodium loss	• Those of fluid loss	• Treat the cause

Part 5

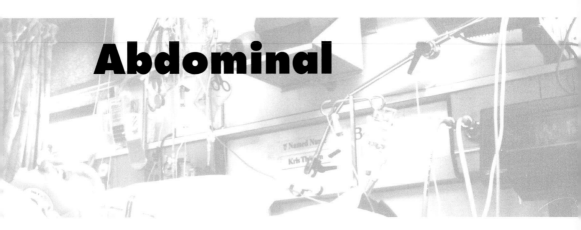

Abdominal

Chapter 30

Acute kidney injury

Philip Woodrow

Contents

Learning outcomes

After reading this chapter you will be able to:

- define the three stages of acute kidney injury;
- identify signs of kidney failure;
- explain the importance of maintaining renal perfusion.

Fundamental knowledge

Renal anatomy and physiology – nephron (filtration), renal tubule (selective reabsorption and secretion); renal functions (including acid/base and electrolyte balance).

Introduction

Acute kidney injury is a clinical syndrome characterised by rapidly reduced excretory function (Davenport and Stevens, 2008). Few patients are admitted to hospital with kidney disease, but acute kidney injury (AKI, previously called 'acute renal failure') is a common, and often avoidable, complication of acute illness. Up to one-quarter of surgical patients develop AKI (Sykes and Cosgrove, 2007). With kidney injury complicating underlying disease, mortality is high – about half will die (Ympa *et al.*, 2005).

Chronic, and acute-on-chronic, kidney injury can also cause problems for patients, but usually either existing treatments will be continued or specialist nephrology input will be sought. This chapter, therefore, focuses on acute failure, which can often be prevented, or treated, on general wards. It includes an overview of ward urinalysis.

Identifying acute failure

The British Renal Association (Davenport and Stevens, 2008) define AKI as any one of:

- serum creatinine rising ≥26.4 micromol/litre within 48 hours;
- a rise in serum creatinine ≥150–200 per cent (1.5–2-fold) within 48 hours
- urine output <0.5 ml/kg/hour for more than 6 hours.

Urea is noticeably not included; urea levels may be raised for non-renal reasons. Creatinine (normal 60–120 micromol/litre) remains a useful marker, as creatinine is produced by muscle metabolism, so rises fairly steadily by 50–100 micromols for each day of failure. The kidney's ability to compensate for impaired glomerular filtration delays detection of failure. Most laboratories now, therefore, routinely measure glomerular filtration rate (GFR), normal healthy adult GFR being 90–130 ml/minute (Murphy and Robinson, 2006).

The kidney has many functions, most of which are affected by failure. Urine is obviously the main function. Healthy kidneys adjust urine volume to maintain fluid balance, but failing kidneys produce insufficient urine to clear toxins. Traditionally, often accepted minimum urine volume of 30 ml/hour would be adequate if patients weighed 60 kg or less, but this is increasingly uncommon.

Reasons for oliguria

Oliguria may be

- volume-responsive (previously called 'pre-renal')
- intrinsic/intra-renal or
- post-renal.

Volume-responsive AKI is the most common cause of oliguria in acute hospitals. The kidneys produce urine from blood, so inadequate renal bloodflow (perfusion) causes oliguria. Inadequate bloodflow is usually caused by systemic hypotension (hypovolaemia and/or cardiac failure), but may also be caused by renal artery stenosis. If the kidney can be adequately perfused, volume-responsive AKI is quickly reversed. Hence, giving adequate fluid prevents volume-responsive AKI. Volume-responsive AKI caused by cardiac failure can be reversed if cardiac function can be improved. Renal artery stenosis is unlikely to be reversed during acute illness.

Box 30.1 Signs of volume-responsive AKI

- Oliguria (<0.5 ml/kg/hour)
- History of hypovolaemia
- Concentrated urine – SG >1.018 (Rahman and Treacher, 2002)
- (Usually) hypotension
- Responds to fluid challenge

Intrinsic failure is caused by damage to kidney tissue. This can be from nephrotoxic drugs, but more often occurs from inadequate, or delayed, treatment of volume-responsive AKI. Inadequate renal perfusion (volume-responsive AKI) not only causes oliguria, but also deprives renal cells of oxygen and nutrients, resulting in cell necrosis. Renal tubules are especially susceptible to necrosis, and when sufficient tubule cells necrose, acute tubular necrosis (ATN) occurs. Volume-responsive and ischaemic ATN cause three-quarters of hospital cases of AKI (Stevens, 2007). One night of unresolved volume-responsive AKI can cause ATN. Fortunately, renal cells normally recover well, but recovery often takes a couple of weeks, during which kidney injury complicates the patient's underlying disease. Provided the patient does not die beforehand, full renal function is usually regained.

Post-renal failure is caused by obstruction to urinary flow after the kidney. This is usually caused by prostrate enlargement or cancers or stone in the urinary tract, although less frequently can be caused by other problems, such as strictures. These are insidious problems, common in the community, and often necessitating urological intervention. But they are unlikely to occur in acute hospitals, unless patients already have them on admission.

Polyuric renal failure

Recovery from intrinsic failure begins once new cells grow. Initially, these cells are immature. Immature cells do not usually function efficiently. The purpose of renal tubular cells is to selectively reabsorb and secrete substances, so that water and electrolyte losses in urine are minimised, while waste product removal is maximised. Immature cells fail to optimise transfer, resulting is polyuria. Despite the large volumes of urine, toxin clearance is poor – serum creatinine remain high. Although the polyuric phase is a sign of recovery, hypovolaemia is frequently a problem.

Serum potassium

Various electrolyte imbalances can occur with renal dysfunction, but potassium is usually the most significant. Nine-tenths of potassium loss normally occurs in urine (Burger, 2004). Therefore, oliguria often causes hyperkalaemia, while polyuria often causes hypokalaemia. Cardiac function relies on maintaining serum potassium within relatively narrow limits (normal physiological range 3.5–4.5 mmol/litre). Serum potassium below 3.5 or above 5.0 can cause cardiac dysfunction (ectopics, dysrhythmias), and more extreme abnormalities are likely to cause cardiac arrest. Therefore, serum potassium should be monitored with kidney injury, and abnormalities treated. Mild hypokalaemia should be treated with oral potassium supplements (e.g. Sando-K, Kay-Cee-L), while more severe hypokalaemia should be treated with intravenous supplements (limited to a 40 mmol/litre bag unless patient has a central line, and are nursed where they can be suitably monitored (NPSA, 2002)) – this usually means in a high dependency unit. Mild hyperkalaemia (5–6 mmol/litre) is usually treated with calcium resonium. Severe hyperkalaemia (>6 mmol/litre) is usually treated with glucose and insulin (see Chapter 25). As insulin and glucose remove potassium from the blood, but not the body, rebound hyperkalaemia can occur later, so often calcium resonium will also be given.

Urinalysis

Ward urinalysis is probably the most frequent urological investigation in hospitals. It can provide useful screening, but is also useful for monitoring renal function. Except for specific gravity, pH and urobilinogen, normal levels for tests below are zero/negative. Tests available vary slightly between test-strip manufacturers, but usual tests include:

Appearance

Visual appearance can indicate likely causes, although there can also be less likely causes for many aspects:

- dark ('golden syrup') – concentrated (dehydration);
- rusty – rhabdomyolosis;
- cloudy – infection;
- frothy – protein.

Drugs can also affect urine colour; for example, rifampicin creates an orange tint.

Blood/leucocytes

Like plasma proteins, blood cells are not normally filtered by the glomerulus. Inflammatory disease may allow cells to pass into urine, or trauma to the urinary tract (e.g. stones, cancers, catheterisation) may cause bleeding. If blood is present, protein will inevitably be detected also. Leucocytes (white blood cells) are part of the immune system, and are usually only found in urine if infection is present (urinary tract infection – UTI).

Nitrite

Bacteria convert nitrate, which is normally in urine, to nitrite (Steggall, 2007), so nitrite will only be found if urine is infected. However, absence of nitrite cannot exclude urinary tract infection, as some bacteria do not convert nitrate (Steggall, 2007).

Urobilinogen/bilirubin

Bilirubinuria is only likely to occur if blood bilirubin levels are significantly raised. This usually indicates gall-bladder and/or liver disease. Bilirubinuria usually causes urine to look dark.

Protein

Protein is not normally filtered by the glomerulus, so proteinuria usually indicates an inflammatory response (disease, such as infection) in the kidney that has enabled it to pass through the glomerulus (Steggall, 2007). Proteinuria is the single most important indicator of kidney injury (Barratt, 2007).

pH (normal: 5–6)

Urine is made from blood. Blood pH is normally 7.4. A major factor in maintaining normal blood pH is excretion of excess hydrogen ions (an essential chemical for acids) into the renal tubule. Thus, urinary pH varies according to physiological needs, but is almost always acidic. Provided renal function is reasonable, high pH may reflect alkalaemia, while low pH may reflect acidaemia.

Specific gravity (SG) (normal: 1.002–1.035)

Urine is mainly water. The SG of pure water is 1.0 (= low SG), so urine normally is just slightly more concentrated. High SG suggests more water is being reabsorbed by the kidneys, usually in response to dehydration – i.e. volume-responsive AKI. SG is often lower in older people as age-related decline in function reduces their ability to concentrate urine (Wilson, 2005). Low SG (watery urine) often means excessive water in urine. With poorly controlled diabetes, this is caused by glycosuria. Intrinsic and post-renal failure often causes low SG, as damaged renal tubules lose their ability to concentrate urine (Barratt, 2007). Polyuria can cause various electrolyte imbalances, especially excessive loss of potassium, magnesium and phosphate.

Ketones

Ketones are a waste product of fat metabolism. Blood sugar, not fat, is normally the main source of cell energy, so ketones in blood (and urine) indicate lack of availability of blood sugar. The two main reasons for this are

■   lack of insulin (diabetic ketoacidois – see Chapter 33)
■   starvation.

As well as indicating problems, ketones may form acids, hence the metabolic acidosis found with diabetic ketoacidosis.

Bilirubin

Bilirubin is a waste product of erythrocyte metabolism. Normally converted by the liver into bile which flows to the gall bladder, bilirubin may be detected in urine with gall-bladder disease (Wilson, 2005).

Glucose

The kidneys filter blood sugar, but normally reabsorbs it all provided blood sugar is below 10 mmol/litre. Glycosuria, therefore, usually indicates hyperglycaemia. Glucose has a high osmotic pressure, reducing water reabsorption, causing polyuria and dilute urine (low SG). Diabetes is often initially detected from routine urinalysis. Acute illness and many drugs (especially cardiac) can cause transient hyperglycaemia.

Treating kidney failure

Urine is the most obvious renal function, but kidneys have many functions. Some, such as erythropoiesis, are not significantly affected by acute injury, but AKI is likely to cause

■   metabolic acidosis
■   electrolyte imbalance (especially hyperkalaemia)
■   neurotoxicity (confusion)
■   drug toxicity.

Treating AKI should, therefore, focus on causes of problems and needs of individual patients (symptom support).

Historically, many patients with AKI were managed by either fluid restriction or loop diuretics (e.g. furosemide). Both approaches were more likely to increase mortality. Replacing the term 'pre-renal failure' with volume-responsive AKI focuses on the most common problem: hypovolaemia. With intrinsic AKI, kidneys will not respond to fluid, so hypervolaemia and oedema can develop. But restricting fluid in fluid-responsive AKI almost invariably causes acute tubular necrosis (intrinsic AKI). The best way of finding whether kidneys will respond to fluid is to try a fluid challenge: rapid infusion of intravenous fluid. Because fluid challenges are important both for diagnosis and treatment, they should be adequate to achieve a clear answer. Generally, this means giving 500 ml as quickly as possible ('stat', over no more than 30 minutes). Where there are significant concerns of heart failure, more caution may be necessary, although monitoring central venous pressure, and titrating fluid input to this, may be preferable to risking acute tubular necrosis. Choice of fluid for challenges varies: some clinicians prefer crystalloids (usually 0.9% sodium chloride; sometimes Hartmann's) while others use gelatins. Choice of fluid is probably less important than volume and rate.

Most potassium loss occurs through the kidneys, so oliguria usually causes hyperkalaemia, while polyuria usually causes hypokalaemia (see p. 310).

The historical practice of giving loop diuretics, such as furosemide, to treat AKI is dangerous. If the patient has volume-responsive AKD, diuretics worsen hypovolaemia, and hasten acute tubular necrosis, and increase mortality (Mehta *et al.*, 2002). If they do result in more urine being produced, it is likely to be poor quality (not removing adequate waste products), and to induce a false belief among staff that the problem has been resolved. Diuretics, generally, merely convert oliguric kidney failure in polyuric kidney failure, and so should not be routinely used (Ho and Sheridan, 2006; Davenport and Stevens, 2008). Pharmacological therapy, and especially the once-popular drug dopamine, has no role in treating AKI (Davenport and Stevens, 2008).

Malnutrition may cause AKI by causing hypovolaemia, but it can also exacerbate disease (Druml, 2005). Appropriate nutrition is an important treatment, but because kidney injury impairs waste removal, nutritional guidance should be sought from dieticians. If there is any significant delay in dieticians being able to offer advice, the UK Renal Association guidelines (Davenport and Stevens, 2008) offer useful advice.

Preventing kidney injury

Maintaining renal perfusion prevents volume-responsive AKI – Sarnak *et al.* (2005) suggest aiming to maintain blood pressure at 130/80. The Surviving Sepsis target of mean arterial pressure of 65 mmHg (see Chapter 27) is probably a better target to use, as mean arterial pressure is a better indicator of perfusion. Preventing malnourishment and dehydration are also important.

Many drugs are nephrotoxic – some of the worst offenders being ace-inhibitors, non-steroidal anti-inflammatories (NSAIDs) and metformin. Where kidney function causes concern, advice should be sought from pharmacists.

Vigilance is often the key to prevention. The first visible sign of kidney injury is often oliguria, although compensation can often cause significant delays before this becomes apparent. Where there is cause for concern, accurate fluid balance charts should be maintained and a urinary catheter inserted. Daily weight is a useful indicator of significant fluid loss or gain, but this does cause a 24-hour delay in obtaining information, which is long enough to cause acute tubular necrosis. No laboratory markers are ideal for detecting renal failure, although raised creatinine is probably the most reliable. Reduced glomerular filtration rate is also a significant cause for concern. But nurses may be the first to detect renal problems by taking routine urinalysis; proteinuria indicates kidney injury.

Implications for practice

- Renal function should be measured by the ability of the kidneys to achieve and maintain homeostasis, not simply by the amount of urine produced.
- The most common cause of AKI in hospitalised patients is volume responsive.
- Volume-responsive AKI can often be prevented if patients receive adequate support to maintain perfusion.
- Diuretics may increase urine volumes, but have no place in treating volume-responsive AKI.
- If volume-responsive AKI is not treated promptly and effectively, ATN almost invariably occurs, often within a relatively few hours.
- Kidney injury prevents excretion of hydrogen ions from the body, so causes metabolic acidosis.
- The many other metabolic functions of the kidney mean that kidney injury causes complications for all other major systems.
- Recovery from AKI is usually complete, provided the patient does not die first.
- About half of patients who develop AKI will die.

Summary

AKI is rarely the cause of acute hospital admission, but it is a common complication for many patients and, together with the underlying disease, too often causes preventable morbidity and mortality. AKI in hospitalised patients is usually volume responsive, so adequate rehydration should be given. Without adequate rehydration, volume-responsive AKD usually progresses into intrinsic AKD, which takes longer to resolve, and is more likely to end in avoidable mortality. Recent UK guidelines will hopefully improve treatments and outcomes for this sizeable group of hospitalised patients.

Clinical scenario

Norma Dray, an inpatient, develops profuse diarrhoea which is suspected to be caused by *C. difficile*. When giving her 6 p.m. antibiotics you notice that she has only passed 120 ml of urine over the last four hours (she weighs 80 kg). You bleep the doctor-on-call, but the team is busy in A&E, and as the patient has passed 30 ml an hour, you are asked to continue monitoring it and call again if volumes fall.

1   List your concerns about Norma's kidney function. Identify why these aspects cause concern.

2   List possible means available within your hospital to pursue your concerns.

3   Discuss with your medical colleagues what fluids, volume and time they would initially prescribe for treating AKI. Ask reasons for their preferences.

Bibliography

Key reading

UK guidelines (Davenport and Stevens, 2008) provide excellent advice for all staff, and can be accessed online (www.renal.org/guidelines). All staff should also be familiar with NPSA advice about intravenous potassium (NPSA, 2002). Useful overviews, such as Stevens (2007), often appear in various medical journals.

Further reading

Considering its frequency, there is relatively little recent nursing literature on AKI. Reviews of urinalysis appear periodically (e.g. Wilson, 2005; Steggall, 2007).

Chapter 31

Gastrointestinal disorders

Philip Woodrow

Contents

Learning outcomes

After reading this chapter you will be able to:

- understand why patients with upper gastrointestinal bleeds and acute pancreatitis may need urgent treatment;
- recognise and understand priorities of care, including assessment and observation, involved with gastrointestinal emergencies;

■ devise a plan of nursing care for patients admitted with these conditions.

Fundamental knowledge

Gut anatomy and physiology (including pancreas).

Introduction

The two most frequent and life-threatening gastrointestinal emergencies are:

■ upper gastrointestinal bleeds
■ pancreatitis.

Pathophysiology is briefly described, but discussion focuses on nursing interventions. Underlying causes of these conditions may be chronic, possibly necessitating later medical or surgical treatments, but this chapter focuses on acute care. Once immediate dangers to life have been removed, care and treatment increasingly focuses on causes, underlying problems and needs.

The gut is highly vascular, so susceptible to major bleeds. Upper gastrointestinal bleeds from

■ oesophageal varices or
■ ulcers (gastric or duodenal)

may develop rapidly, prove fatal, and are the most common gastrointestinal emergency (British Society of Gastroenterology Endoscopy Committee, 2000). Shock and other signs are often present (see Box 31.1). Priority should therefore be given to restoring circulating volume, and stopping haemorrhage.

Bleeds in the lower gut are usually from chronic conditions. They can be life-threatening, requiring major surgery or aggressive medical treatment, but are less likely to necessitate emergency admission. Lower GI bleeds are briefly discussed, together with bowel care.

Box 31.1 Signs of upper GI bleeds

■ Haematemesis (often massive)
■ 'Coffee-ground' vomit
■ Hypotension
■ Tachycardia
■ Other signs of shock (pale, often clammy)
■ Pain relieved by eating (gastric ulcers)
■ Pain after eating (duodenal ulcers)
■ Melaena

Note: These may not all appear.

Acute pancreatitis usually resolves spontaneously, but one-fifth of mild cases progress into severe acute disease (Uhl *et al.*, 1999). Progression of acute pancreatitis is unpredictable and often rapid, with mortality of 2–10 per cent (Mitchell *et al.*, 2003). Severe pancreatitis can cause

■ infected necrosis
■ shock from systemic inflammatory response syndrome (SIRS)
■ inflammation (De Waele *et al.*, 2007).

Mortality rates significantly increase with severe disease – more than 50 per cent with infection (Pickworth, 2003). Survival has not significantly improved since the 1970s (Goldacre and Roberts, 2004).

Potential dangers and urgency surrounding upper gastrointestinal bleeds and acute pancreatitis means that nurses looking after these patients need to be able to detect early signs of deterioration and know what treatments to initiate.

Oesophageal varices

The gut has a rich blood supply, to facilitate absorption of nutrients. Most blood from the gut flows to the liver, where most nutrient metabolism occurs. Cirrhosis of the liver, usually (but not always) from alcoholic liver disease, obstructs bloodflow, causing congestion (hypertension) in veins draining into the liver, the largest being the hepatic portal vein. Ninety per cent of people with portal hypertension develop oesophageal varices within a decade. Half of cirrhotic patients develop varices (Fallah *et al.*, 2000). Hypertension from congestion causes about one-third of these to rupture and bleed (Ghost *et al.*, 2002; Koti and Davidson, 2003), of which 30–50 per cent prove fatal (Fallah *et al.*, 2000). Most (70 per cent) survivors rebleed (Sharara, 2001).

Sudden and major haemorrhage usually necessitates:

■ intervention to stop haemorrhage – drugs, urgent endoscopy, balloon tamponade;
■ fluid resuscitation;
■ system support (especially oxygen);
■ replacing clotting factors.

Reducing portal hypertension can stop or prevent bleeds. In acute bleeds, drugs such as somatostatin (or analogues) and terlipressin are usually used.

Endoscopy

Urgent endoscopy may be needed to stop bleeding. This enables direct visualisation and treatment of bleeding points by:

■ injecting sclerosants

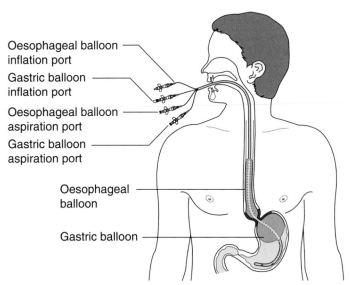

Oesophageal balloon
inflation port

Gastric balloon
inflation port

Oesophageal balloon
aspiration port

Gastric balloon
aspiration port

Oesophageal
balloon

Gastric balloon

Figure 31.1 **Balloon tamponade ('Minnesota') tube**

- laser treatment
- ligation ('banding').

Sclerosants such as adrenaline or ethanolamine are injected directly into bleeding points to cause atrophy. Endoscopic sclerotherapy stops 71–95 per cent of variceal bleeds (Kokozides, 2006). Ligation, which draws varices into the endoscope then places ligatures (bands) around them, is more effective than sclerotherapy, so remains the treatment of choice (Stanley and Hayes, 1997). Laser treatment has largely replaced diathermy.

Shunts

Transjugular intrahepatic portosystemic shunt (TIPPS) uses a catheter to create a fistula between the portal vein and hepatic artery. TIPPS is the best treatment for recurrent bleeds (Vargas *et al.*, 1999) and the treatment of choice if endoscopy fails (Therapondos and Hayes, 2002). Surgery is rarely performed for variceal bleeding.

Balloon tamponade

Direct pressure (*tamponade*) can be placed on bleeding varices with 'Minnesota' or 'Sengstarken' tubes. Placed orally through the oesophagus and into the stomach, these usually have two balloons (oesophagus, stomach) and two aspiration ports (oesophagus, stomach). Like nasogastric tubes, these are easier to insert if cold (Smith, 2000), so are best stored refrigerated.

Balloon tamponade stops most (70–80 per cent) oesophageal bleeds (Fallah *et al.*, 2000), but half rebleed on removal (Stanley and Hayes, 1997), so tamponade is an emergency measure until more effective treatments are available (Vargas *et al.*, 1999).

Prolonged pressure may cause ulceration, so tamponade is usually limited to 12 hours (Therapondos and Hayes, 2002). Periodic deflation to prevent ulceration is controversial, as deflation may restart bleeding. There is little consensus about optimum pressure. Traction is sometimes used but this is also controversial.

Blood loss and impaired consciousness normally necessitates nursing these patients in the recovery position. Blood and other fluids in the oesophagus could be aspirated into the lungs, so should be removed either with continuous low suction, or through periodic removal.

Vasoactive drugs, such as

- terlipressin, to constrict smooth muscle (Vargas *et al.*, 1999);
- nitrates, to vasodilate (Sharara, 2001);
- beta-blockers, to reduce hypertension (Bosch and Abraldes, 2005)

may be used to prevent rebleeding, but require close cardiovascular (ECG, BP) monitoring.

Ulcers

Ulceration may develop anywhere in the gut, but most upper gastrointestinal bleeds are caused by peptic ulcers (British Society of Gastroenterology Endoscopy Committee, 2000; Kokozides, 2006). Hydrochloric acid, secreted by the stomach, is very strong, making resting stomach pH about 2. Mucus protects the stomach from acid erosion, but failure of this mucosal barrier exposes the stomach wall to acid. Until acid chyle from the stomach is neutralised by pancreatic juice (pH 8), failure of protective mucus in the duodenum can cause duodenal ulcers. One-quarter of people with duodenal ulcers develop haemorrhage or other major complications (Shiotani and Graham, 2002).

Eating typically relieves pain from gastric ulcers, but aggravates pain from duodenal ulcers. Gastric ulcers frequently cause vomiting (Cole *et al.*, 2006). Early endoscopy is usually performed to stop bleeding (Kokozides, 2006), using similar techniques to those described above.

Mucosal barrier failure is particularly associated with

- non-steroidal anti-inflammatory drugs (NSAIDs);
- the gram-negative bacterium *Helicobacter pylori*.

For people needing long-term anti-inflammatory drugs, such as for arthritis, cox-2 inhibitors cause less gastric ulceration than NSAIDs (Sikes *et al.*, 2002; Lisse *et al.*, 2003). *Helicobacter pylori*, one of the most common human infections, is a major cause of gastrointestinal disease (Fuccio *et al.*, 2008). Eradication is problematic, but should be considered in people with, or at risk of, developing gastric cancer (Fuccio *et al.*, 2008).

Acute illness stimulates a stress response, which increases gastric acid secretion. If patients are eating little, or are nil-by-mouth, absence of food to reduce gastric acidity and excessive hydrochloric acid production increases risk of ulceration. Debate about the best prophylaxis for stress ulcers remains inconclusive. Some studies, such as Cook *et al.* (1998), recommend ranitidine or other H$_2$-blockers, while other studies, such as Messori *et al.* (2000) indicate these are ineffective, or may cause other problems such as obstruction or albumin toxicity (Bradley, 2001). With gastric ulcers, proton pump inhibitors are normally prescribed to reduce future bleeds (Kokozides, 2006). Nutrition should be given early and enterally, whenever possible (Marik and Zaloga, 2004; UK Working Party, 2005; Kingsnorth and O'Reilly, 2006; Meier *et al.*, 2006), including following gastric surgery (Lewis *et al.*, 2001).

Complications

Severe haemorrhage usually causes hypovolaemic shock. Even if shock does not prove fatal, perfusion failure to other main organs often causes

- acute kidney injury (acute tubular necrosis);
- increased myocardial work, possibly resulting in infarction;
- liver failure, resulting in many complications (see Chapter 34);
- hypoxaemia (from anaemia).

Complications may progress into multi-organ dysfunction syndrome (MODS), which makes survival unlikely.

Blood contains protein, so blood in the gut may be digested like any other protein. Protein metabolism produces ammonia, which with impaired liver function may not be metabolised, resulting in neurotoxicity. Toxic ammonia levels increase blood–brain barrier permeability, leading to encephalopathy, confusion and possible coma.

Therefore, once bleeding has been stabilised, blood should be removed from the gut, usually with oral laxatives, aiming for more than one stool each day.

Lower gastrointestinal bleeds

About one-fifth of acute gastrointestinal bleeds are from the lower tract, mostly in older patients (Fearnhead, 2007). Although diverticulitis can cause massive bleeds (Hoedema and Luchtefeld, 2005), lower GI bleeds tend to be less acute. However, prolonged bleeding, problems often not being so immediately obvious, and embarrassment preventing some people from seeking help even when signs do appear, can cause anaemia, morbidity and preventable mortality. Many patients are reluctant to discuss abnormal stools, but if asked whether they have noticed any blood, darkness or other abnormality may report symptoms. Normal bowel transit time is about 24 hours, with individual variations sometimes extending to several days. Constipation may reduce gut motility further, resulting in signs not appearing in stools until several days after bleeds begin.

Lower GI bleeds may resolve with conservative treatment or endoscopy, but persistent bleeds may necessitate early surgery (e.g. hemicolectomy).

Nursing care

Major gastrointestinal bleeds often need urgent resuscitation:

- oxygen;
- fluids (preferably colloids, with probable need for blood and platelet transfusion);

together with close monitoring, including vital signs. Medical help should be summoned urgently. Lying the patient flat and raising the foot of the bed may sustain cerebral circulation until fluids are prescribed. As far as possible, privacy and dignity should be maintained. Anything that may provoke bleeding, such as passing nasogastric tubes, should be avoided unless benefits outweigh risks.

Blood may distress patients and families, so soiled linen should be removed, the patient offered a wash, and the environment cleaned as necessary. The taste of blood can be removed with a drink or mouth-wash (including brushing teeth). The patient should be reassured, with information being honest and realistic. Visitors should be informed about what has occurred, warned that their loved one may look and often feel very ill, and that they may see some blood. As distressed visitors might faint, staff should accompany them to the bedside and encourage them to sit down.

GI bleeds are often caused by preventable factors, so health promotion before discharge should explore ways to help patients prevent future problems. GI bleeds, especially varices, are often alcohol-related, so staff should explore whether help should be offered to those willing to change their lifestyle. If damage is caused by medicines, such as aspirin or NSAIDs, alternative prescriptions should be explored. *Helicobacter pylori* can be eradicated, although this requires a prolonged course.

Bowel care

Healthy bowel function is important for eliminating solid waste from the body, yet bowel care is frequently overlooked (RCN, 2008a). Nurses should assess and monitor bowel function. Initially, this usually means asking patients, or their families, about bowel function and habit. Any recent changes in bowel function, difficulty passing stool, or blood, should be investigated further. If bleeding is suspected, a stool sample should be obtained. Social stigma may prevent some patients from reporting bowel problems, and healthcare professionals from asking/assessing. Restlessness, agitation and confusion are often caused by constipation, so nurses should assess restless patients by asking when they last opened their bowels. Reluctance to eat may be caused by constipation.

All bowel motions should be recorded; many observation charts include a place for recording bowel movements, although this is often not completed. It is also valuable to record the type of motion (e.g. colour, consistency, amount). The Bristol Stool Chart (discussed in *Intensive Care Nursing*) is increasingly used to monitor bowel function. Contrary to widespread belief, not everyone normally opens their bowels daily, so asking what is normal for the person should be part of routine nursing assessment on admission. Nurses should also ask whether people have noticed any change in regularity or abnormalities in their stool. Abnormalities include:

- constipation
- diarrhoea
- blood
- fat (streatorrhoea).

Constipation may have various causes, including reduced mobility and dehydration. So mobilising patients is usually an important part of bowel care. But initially, constipation often necessitates laxatives:

- *stimulant laxatives* (e.g. senna) increase gut peristalsis, so are often the first choice of laxative for new constipation;
- *osmotic laxatives* (e.g. lactulose) lubricate the stool, so may be useful with severe constipation, often in combination with stimulant laxatives;
- *bulk-forming laxatives* (e.g. bran) increase faecal volume, so are generally the best choice where chronic constipation is likely, such as from severely reduced mobility.

If laxatives are ineffective after a few days, suppositories, and later enemas, may be needed to evacuate bowels.

Bowel assessment may need digital rectal examination, and occasionally manual evacuation may be needed, but both procedures should only be performed if necessary, following individual assessment, and with patient's consent (RCN, 2008a).

Diarrhoea may be reduced by drugs which slow gut motility (e.g. codeine phosphate), although if diarrhoea caused by bacteria, stopping diarrhoea may reduce elimination of the problem. Severe diarrhoea can cause fluid and electrolyte imbalances, necessitating replacements. Diarrhoea is discussed further in Chapter 7.

Long-term use of laxatives should be discouraged. Where patients have persistent problems with constipation, dieticians can provide advice about high-fibre diets.

Pancreatitis

Pancreatitis may be acute or chronic. Acute pancreatitis can rapidly, and unpredictably, progress to life-threatening disease, so should be closely monitored and promptly treated. This chapter focuses on acute, rather than chronic, pancreatitis.

Pancreatitis is a relatively common, and increasing prevalent, disease (Kingsnorth and O'Reilly, 2006; Siva and Pereira, 2007), which may be so mild it causes only vague abdominal pain. People with very mild pancreatitis may not seek medical help or be admitted to hospital, but more severe cases require urgent admission with provision of high dependency (level 2) and sometimes intensive (level 3) care. A minority of people with pancreatitis progress, often rapidly, from appearing relatively well (other than abdominal pain) to severe acute pancreatitis. Progression is unpredictable, and can occur within a few hours. Therefore, when

> **Box 31.2 Signs of acute pancreatitis**
>
> - Abdominal pain – often severe, radiating to back
> - Tachypnoea
> - Tachycardia
> - Pyrexia

pancreatitis is suspected or confirmed, nurses should observe and monitor patients closely and frequently, providing physical and psychological care. Signs of pancreatitis are listed in Box 31.2.

The pancreas has both endocrine and exocrine functions. Endocrine functions include hormone production:

- glucagon (alpha cells)
- insulin (beta cells)
- somatostatin (delta cells).

Although endocrine activities may be affected, pancreatitis primarily affects exocrine function. As an exocrine organ, the pancreas secretes digestive enzymes, including amalyse, into the duodenum. These powerful pancreatic enzymes are alkaline (pH 8), to neutralise gastric acid. With pancreatitis, the pancreatic or common bile duct is blocked. Unneutralised acid in the duodenum continues to stimulate enzyme production, which eventually ruptures the pancreatic duct and begins autodigesting surrounding tissue – mainly the pancreas itself and peripancreatic fat. Fistulae may form into surrounding tissues, including the colon. Bacteria entering necrotic tissue usually suppurate.

Serum amylase is probably the most widely used biochemical marker (normal = <100 mmol/litre), but serum lipase is the recommended test (UK Working Party, 2005), pancreatitis causing levels >110 units/litre. C-reactive protein (CRP) is a useful marker of severity (UK Working Party, 2005).

Pancreatitis is typically associated with either

- gallstones/biliary disease; or
- alcoholism;

although only a minority of people with gallstones or chronic alcoholism develop pancreatitis. There are many other rarer causes of pancreatitis. Biliary causes often occur in women in their fifties (Hale *et al.*, 2000), while alcohol-related pancreatitis typically occurs in men in their forties (Hale *et al.*, 2000). Chronic pancreatitis is usually caused by alcohol (Hughes, 2004).

Classification

The Atlanta consensus classification is the only widely accepted classification (Bollen *et al.*, 2008), and should be followed in the UK (UK Working Party, 2005):

- acute

- ■ mild acute
- ■ severe acute
- ■ acute fluid collection
- ■ pancreatic necrosis
- ■ acute pseudocyst
- ■ pancreatic abscess.

People with mild pancreatitis often recover with minimal or no intervention, but should be observed and monitored in case they develop severe pancreatitis. Later complications, such as fluid collection, pseudocysts and abscesses, should also be observed and monitored for, but may occur following discharge.

Pancreatitis may be sterile or become infected, usually from gut bacteria (Uhl *et al.*, 1998). About half of people with severe pancreatitis develop bacterial infections (Steinberg and Tenner, 1994), so preventing infection is the most promising treatment for pancreatitis (Uhl *et al.*, 1999). Infected pancreatic necrosis necessitates early surgical debridement (Nathens *et al.*, 2004; Malangoni and Martin, 2005). Severe pancreatitis stimulates gross hypermetabolism, so pyrexia (often 38–39°C) may occur without infection.

Complications

Severe pancreatitis can rapidly affect most major organs and systems in the body. The main problems are usually:

- ■ pain
- ■ cardiovascular
- ■ respiratory
- ■ metabolic.

Pain

Most patients with severe pancreatitis experience severe, rapidly progressing, abdominal pain. Attempting to relieve this pain, they often sit forward, with knees bent (Banks, 1998). Pain usually causes nausea and (often) vomiting. Opioids, usually morphine, and anti-emetics are usually needed.

Cardiovascular

Inflammation and stress cause large shifts of fluid from the bloodstream into tissues, causing

- ■ hypovolaemia and shock;
- ■ ascites and oedema;
- ■ pericardial effusions, often causing dysrhythmias and raised ST segments;
- ■ electrolyte imbalances.

Autodigestion can also cause aneurysms.

Aggressive fluid therapy should be given to prevent organ failure (UK Working Party, 2005). Close monitoring, including urine output (target >0.5 ml/kg/hour), continuous ECG, fluid balance and central venous pressure, are usually needed.

Respiratory

Severe attacks often cause acute lung injury and pulmonary oedema. Breathing may also be compromised by

- pain
- diaphragmatic splinting from ascites
- pleural effusions
- pulmonary oedema.

Supplementary oxygen is often needed (Tham and Collins, 2000). Close and frequent respiratory monitoring should include rate, depth and oxygen saturation. Further support, such as non-invasive ventilation, may be needed.

Metabolic

Impaired insulin release, insulin antagonism and excessive glucagon release often cause hyperglycaemia. Aggressive insulin therapy and frequent (1–2 hourly) blood glucose monitoring may be needed. Survival is improved if blood sugar is kept at 4.4–6.1 mmol/litre (van den Berghe, 2001), although application of this to severe pancreatitis remains presumptive. Many electrolyte imbalances occur, partly from fluid shifts and partly from poor diet or impaired intake. Blood calcium, needed for cardiac conduction, clotting and cell repair, is often low (Hale *et al.*, 2000). Biochemistry (U+Es) should be checked and stabilised.

Medical treatment

Treating pancreatitis remains problematic. Gallstones may be removed using endoscopic retrograde colangio-pancreatography (ERCP) or lithotripsy. Cholecystectomy may be performed to prevent recurrence (Mitchell *et al.*, 2003). Various drugs have been trialled, and most abandoned, so treatment is largely limited to supporting failing systems and preventing/limiting further complications.

Nursing management

With severe pancreatitis, extensive medical treatments necessitate nursing care being focused largely on administering prescribed drugs and fluids, preventing complications and monitoring patient's progress, and relieving pain. Nurses' knowledge of their patient's social history, together with close rapport often built up with families, can valuably contribute to diagnosis and treatment. Patients with severe pancreatitis are often able to do little for themselves, so maintaining, as far as possible, normal activities of living (such as hygiene and mouth-care) valuably contributes to quality of care.

With severe pancreatitis, hypodynamic circulation and prolonged immobility predispose to pressure sores and deep vein thrombosis (DVT). DVT prophylaxis (thromboembolic stockings and low molecular weight heparin) are usually needed and active/passive exercises should be encouraged (Turner, 2003).

Less severe cases may progress rapidly, so patients should be closely observed, and early indications of progression, such as symptoms of shock or deteriorating blood results, should be reported quickly to medical staff and Critical Care Outreach.

Nutrition is needed for recovery. Patients with pancreatitis should be fed early and enterally if their gut is able to absorb – 80 per cent can be fed enterally (UK Working Party, 2005; Meier *et al.*, 2006). People with alcohol-related pancreatitis should be encouraged to moderate or discontinue alcohol. People with biliary-related pancreatitis usually benefit from low-fat diets.

Implications for practice

- Large bleeds and severe pancreatitis need urgent fluid resuscitation and close haemodynamic monitoring.
- Balloon tamponade can quickly stop many variceal bleeds, but is only a temporary measure until endoscopic treatment is available.
- When balloon tamponade is removed, many patients rebleed.
- Following gastric bleeds, patients should be offered drinks or mouth-care to remove the taste of blood.
- Severe pancreatitis causes acute pain, usually needing opioid analgesia and often anti-emetics.
- Hyperglycaemia may occur with pancreatitis, while people with gastric bleeding may be malnourished, so blood sugar should be assessed. With pancreatitis, blood sugar may need to be monitored regularly; insulin infusions may be needed.
- Nurses should ensure nutrition is optimised; if possible, orally or enterally (gastric or jejunal tubes).

Summary

Upper gastrointestinal bleeds and pancreatitis often require urgent intervention. Most cases of pancreatitis remain mild, but an unpredictable minority progress rapidly to acute severe pancreatitis, with significant mortality. Medical treatment of severe acute pancreatitis is difficult and remains largely limited to supporting failing systems. Nursing care focuses around providing relief from pain and nausea, providing other care that patient needs, and close observation and monitoring or that any deterioration can be reported and treated promptly.

Clinical scenario

Charles Hill, aged 49, is admitted with acute pancreatitis. On arrival, he is in obvious pain, despite having been given 10 mg oromorphine an hour previously. The medical team have prescribed an aggressive fluid regime of Gelofusine® 500 ml over one hour, which has been commenced immediately before transfer. They will review him further within that hour, by when results from the serum amylase test should be available. He is separated from his wife, and gives his next-of-kin as his daughter, whom he describes as 'close', and who manages a care home 'about 50 miles away'.

1   List the immediate priorities of nursing care you would give Charles. Identify rationales for care.

2   Charles' vital signs are: HR 115 regular, BP 90/60 mmHg, RR 35 bpm, temperature 38.5°C. His blood sugar is 24 mmol/litre. He is oliguric, passing 15 ml during the last hour. The medical team have just arrived and are now reviewing Charles. What treatments do you anticipate they will offer him? Include rationales for interventions.

3   The medical team's decisions coincide with your expectations. Devise a plan of care for Charles for the next 12 hours, remembering possible complications that may occur. His daughter is expected shortly; include information and support that you will offer her.

Bibliography

Key reading

UK medical guidelines include the UK Working Party (2005). Kingsnorth and O'Reilly (2006) and Kokozides (2006) provide useful medical reviews. RCN (2008a) offers comprehensive guidance on bowel care.

Further reading

Many studies and reviews support early enteral nutrition with pancreatitis, key articles being cited in this chapter. Fewer nursing articles on these topics have been published in recent years, compared with the 1990s, probably reflecting limited change, but Hughes (2004) and Fawcett and Smith (2005) provide a useful nursing review, while Cole *et al.* (2006) provide review initial assessment. Meier *et al.* (2006) provide European (ESPEN) guidelines for nutrition with pancreatitis.

Chapter 32

Haematological disorders

Tina Moore

Contents

Learning outcomes

After reading this chapter you will be able to:

- identify the trigger factors for sickle cell anaemia/causes of DIC/thalassaemia;
- to demonstrate knowledge of the associated symptoms of all disorders;
- understand the related pathophysiological dangers;
- Devise a plan of care (with rationale) for a patient during a vaso-occlusive crisis/DIC/thalassaemia.

Fundamental knowledge

Normal physiology of the erythrocyte; complications of blood transfusion; normal physiology of coagulation.

Introduction

Haematology is concerned with circulating blood and blood-forming products. The three major functions of the haematopoietic system are: the distribution of oxygen and nutrients to all cells of the body; protection of organism from invading microbes and regulation homeostasis. Many disorders manifested by abnormalities of the haematopoietic system are secondary to abnormalities of other organ system failure. Three haematological disorders will be discussed in this chapter: sickle cell anaemia, disseminated intravascular coagulation (DIC) and thalassaemia.

Sickle cell anaemia

Sickle cell anaemia is an inherited blood disorder mostly affecting Afro-Caribbean people but can be found in Eastern Mediterranean and Middle Eastern people (WHO, 2006). This disease is one of the most common genetic blood disorders in the world (Westerdale, 2004). Sickle cell anaemia occurs when a person inherits two genes from Haemoglobin S (HbS; one gene from each parent). HbS forms long polymers upon deoxygenation. These rod-like polymers change the normally round and pliable red blood cells into rigid cells with a crescent or sickle shape that has a life span of only 10 days. Bundles of these deformed cells act as plugs within the capillaries. This results in a reduction of bloodflow, causing localised tissue hypoxia and promoting further sickling. If uncorrected, tissue necrosis and infarction follow, causing severe pain, multisystem organ damage and possibly early death (Gladwin *et al.*, 2004; Taher, 2007).

A sickle cell (vaso-occlusive) crisis occurs when the inflexible sickled cells become lodged in the arterial and micro-circulation causing stasis, obstruction of bloodflow and damage to surrounding tissues and organs, resulting in infarction. A crisis can last for a matter of minutes or several months (De, 2005). Triggers for sickling of the blood include infection (especially viral), stress (both emotional and physiological), dehydration or sources of external temperature, hypoxia, hypothermia, smoking and alcohol (Firth, 2005).

Time out 32.1

Consider a patient with acute sickle cell anaemia.

1 Identify main clinical features the patient will exhibit.
2 Explain how these occur.
3 What are the patient's main needs?

Clinical features

The most common clinical picture during adult life is a vaso-occlusive crisis. Pain is considered a major symptom of sickle cell, and is thought to be due to the site and degree of vaso-occlusion. This pain is variable and can be localised or diffused, constant or intermittent. Patients' symptoms will vary from mild–moderate–severe. Some patients suffer from fever and swelling in the joints of the hands or feet. Long bones can also be affected. Occasionally, abdominal pain is the major symptom and this may be associated with distension and rigidity (a picture very similar to an acute abdomen requiring surgery). This is usually due to splenic involvement. The spleen is a site in which recurrent sickling typically occurs (Berliner, 2004). Splenic sequestration is a pooling of red blood cells within the spleen causing an enlargement of the spleen causing acute abdominal pain.

The degree of pain can be so severe that it is comparable to that experienced in myocardial infarction (Pasero, 1996), yet, in patients with sickle cell this complaint is still not taken seriously or treated with the same degree of urgency. It is a symptom that continues to be doubted by a significant number of nursing and medical staff (Yale *et al.*, 2000). Patients' commentaries throughout the literature also support this. Studies show a relationship between the frequency of painful crisis and early death (Pasero, 1996). However, with extensive patient and healthcare professional education this can change (Larsen *et al.*, 2001).

Secondary symptoms predominantly result from the pain experienced and include disablement and fright. Hostility and anger may result if nurses are perceived to be slow to respond or are openly sceptical of the pain reports from the patient.

Sickle cells have a short life span in comparison with 120 days of the normal red blood cell causing chronic haemolysis and haemolytic anaemia (Adjei, 2004). Due to the increased levels of bilirubin, patients may also look jaundiced (mainly seen in the conjunctivae). Tachypnoea, hypertension, nausea, vomiting and fever may also accompany symptoms.

Patients are highly susceptible to infection, this is thought to be related to the spleen becoming scarred from the sickling process and, therefore, losing its immunological function (Wendell *et al.*, 2000). Patient's temperature should be closely monitored. Vigilance is required as regular paracetamol for pain control masks symptoms of a raised temperature.

There may be multiple organ involvement, with micro-infarcts affecting the heart, lung, central nervous system and spleen. Urinalysis may indicate haematuria, infection or elevated bilirubin levels (increased as sickle cells are destroyed).

Management

Most practices indicate that accurate pain assessment, administration of analgesics, humidified oxygen and intravenous hydration are the first steps in managing a vaso-occlusive crisis. Where an underlying infection is present, IV antibiotics are administered.

Controlling the patient's pain can be challenging for nurses. Continuous intravenous infusion of an appropriate analgesia is usually required and this may be in the form of morphine. Satisfactory doses are necessary to ensure that the patient remains mobile, and maintaining deep breathing exercises helps to avoid atelectasis. Prescriptions should be written on an individual basis.

Over-prescribing of opioids may lead to respiratory depression. When appropriate, patient-controlled analgesia (PCA) should be started. Many healthcare professionals remain apprehensive about patients becoming addicted to the analgesia. At present there is no conclusive evidence to demonstrate the link between sickle cell pain and drug addition. Indeed, under-treating the pain actually encourages such behaviour and predisposes the patient to pseudoaddiction syndrome (Marlowe and Chicella, 2002) and causes unnecessary suffering (Firth, 2005). Epidural may be considered if the patient is unresponsive to intravenous analgesia.

The treatment sometimes can be detrimental to the patient, e.g. patients receiving high doses of narcotics need to be monitored for side effects, such as constipation, urinary retention, nausea and vomiting. In addition to pharmacological treatment, alternative methods to pain control could be considered/implemented, e.g. aromatherapy, distraction, heat and cold application.

Patient's familiarity with opioids and specific requests for a particular drug or dosage can be misinterpreted. There is a high level of analgesic tolerance in patients with recurrent episodes of severe pain (Firth, 2005). Many patients with sickle cell pain receive covert or sometimes overt messages from healthcare professionals (including nurses) who believe that the pain is exaggerated and that medication is wanted for non-medical reasons (Yale *et al.*, 2000). From the patient's perspective, this accusation becomes both humiliating and unprofessional.

Dehydration not only precipitates a crisis but can also occur during one. Intravenous hydration 0.9% saline and or 5% glucose in saline should be administered aiming for 3–4 litres a day (Mak and Davies, 2003). If patients are able to drink, this should be encouraged. Replacement of insensible loss (particularly due to fever) is required. Hydration decreases blood viscosity and maintains renal perfusion. Careful monitoring for signs of fluid overload (e.g. tachycardia, hypertension, jugular vein distension and crackles) should be performed.

The use of oxygen therapy has been controversial. One view is that the sickling process is caused by hypoxia, so preventing hypoxia helps prevent sickling (Hoffbrand *et al.*, 2006). Another view is that the effect of suppressing erythropoietin is not immediate, therefore, oxygen therapy is only beneficial during the early stages of a crisis (Taher, 2007). Patients can become acidotic, so regular monitoring of arterial blood gas should be carried out as pulse oximetry readings provide a falsely high SpO_2 during sickle cell crises (Chapter 16).

In the early stages of the crisis blood transfusions are of a low priority. At this point many patients have developed chronic haemolytic anaemia and, therefore, have lower haemoglobin and haematocrit levels. Patients with sickle cell can manage relatively well with low haemoglobin and haematocrit levels (Hoffbrand *et al.*, 2006). During more acute situations an exchange transfusion of packed red blood cells may be performed. This involves removing one unit of blood and transfusing one unit, then repeating the process. Alternatively, this can be achieved via a plasmapheresis machine (Distenfield and Woermann, 2002). This approach may cause blood to become more viscous and increase the chances of sickling. This procedure may compromise both cardiac and respiratory functions.

Folate stores are often depleted and will require supplementation. Problems associated with multiple transfusions, including iron overload, should be considered. Limb tourniquets and blood pressure cuffs should be used with caution, as they may cause local hypoxia and so may precipitate sickling. Any major procedures are best carried out after an exchange transfusion.

Patients vary in their coping abilities. Many describe feelings of helplessness against the disease and express concerns about premature death (Gorman, 1999). This may lead to depression. Treatment can be enhanced by approaches that incorporate psychological, social and behavioural components. Empowering the patient to reduce stress through appropriate strategies (Chapter 13) should help reduce anxiety and allow time to regain some control over the situation.

Complications

Acute lung infarction (acute lung syndrome) is one of the most common causes of death from sickle cell (Gladwin *et al.*, 2004) and accounts for a large proportion of admissions of these patients. It is caused by infection, fat embolism (from necrotic bone marrow) or pulmonary infarction due to sequestration of sickle cells (Kumar and Clark, 2002). This is illustrated by deteriorating radiological appearances of the chest and blood gas analysis (showing increasing hypoxia). Regular arterial blood gas analysis should be monitored for signs of respiratory failure and not to rely on pulse oximetry results alone.

Respiratory status including colour needs to be monitored – cyanosis will be difficult to observe due to dark skin. This complication is managed by analgesics. However, some patients require very high doses which could have a counteractive response. Management includes respiratory support (oxygen in the first instance), antibiotics and transfusion (Firth, 2005).

Damage to the kidney, promotes an inability to concentrate urine, resulting in polyuria and nocturnal enuresis. In older patients there is chronic glomerular damage that may lead to chronic renal failure. Sickling in the liver can lead to liver failure. A combination of the pooling of blood and a drop in haemoglobin can be life-threatening. There may be periods of transient bone marrow aplasia (aplastic crisis), resulting in a low white cell count and an increased risk of infection.

Cerebrovascular accidents causing permanent disability and retinopathy may also occur. Repeated crises may cause permanent damage to the vital organs, precipitating multi-organ failure.

DIC

DIC is not a disease or a symptom, but a syndrome. Its presence always indicates an underlying disease, it is rarely of idiopathic origin. DIC is characterised by systemic intravascular activation of coagulation, leading to widespread deposition of fibrin in the circulation (Becker and Wira, 2008). This means that DIC is a thrombohaemorrhagic disorder that manifests in bleeding or thrombosis. DIC can be a disastrous complication for the critically ill patient.

DIC involves an extremely complex pathophysiological process (Levi, 2008). Normally, coagulation is a dynamic action with the balance between clot or thrombus formation and lysis being carefully regulated to provide competent homeostasis.

DIC syndrome results from an inappropriate, excessive and uncontrolled activation of the haemostatic process in which excessive procoagulant is released by the vascular endothelium (Box 32.1), i.e. the loss of balance between the clot-forming activity of thrombin and the clot-lysing activity of plasmin (Schmaier, 2004).

Box 32.1 Clotting cascade

Platelets and coagulation factors are activated by a disease stimulus and are rapidly consumed

↓

Thrombin is formed very rapidly and inherent inhibitors cannot stop the formation of the vast amounts of thrombin generated

↓

The fibrinolytic system lyses fibrin and impairs thrombin formation
↓

Fibrin degradation product (FDP) result from fibrinolysis, changing platelet aggregation and inhibiting fibrin polymerisation

---

Endothelial or tissue injury acts as a trigger for the excessive release of procoagulant material. This is usually in the form of cytokines (interleukin 6) and tissue factors. As a result the intravascular formation of fibrin causes thrombotic occlusion of small and mid-size vessels, possibly precipitating organ failure. Severe bleeding complications may result from the consumption and subsequent exhaustion of platelets and coagulation proteins initiated by the ongoing activation of the coagulation process (fibrinolysis). Two proteolytic enzymes, thrombin and plasmin, are activated and circulate systemically. Their balance determines a thrombotic or bleeding tendency.

Acute DIC is more serious, profound and unexpected and usually manifests as a haemorrhagic disorder. This involves excessive plasmin formation and thrombolysis. Massive blood loss may lead to further coagulation factor and platelet depletion, thus aggravating the situation.

In chronic DIC (compensated) subacute tendency towards diffuse thrombosis, confined to a specific anatomic location has been associated with aortic aneurysm and giant haemangionomas. Here, the activation of coagulation and fibrinolysis does not occur rapidly enough to exceed the rate of production of clotting factors and inhibitors (Levi, 2008). Microcirculation and microcirculatory thrombosis leads to hypoperfusion, infarction and end-organ damage with the possibility of shock.

Causes

These include any factors that result in damage to the endothelium or tissue thus triggering the accelerated clotting response. Common causes include:

- Gram negative bacterial sepsis. A common pathogenic feature resulting from severe infection is the generalised inflammatory response, characterised by systemic release of cytokines (Levi, 2008).
- Viruses, especially varicella, hepatitis.
- Obstetric damage during delivery/abortion (placenta and brain are especially rich in thromboplastin). Obstetric complications associated with activation of blood coagulation are eclampsia and haemolysis elevated liver enzymes and low platelets syndrome (HELLP).
- Trauma, particularly head trauma (due to the relatively large amount of tissue factor in the cerebral compartment (Levi, 2008)). A combination of mechanisms including release of tissue material in the circulation (fat, phospholipids), haemolysis and endothelial damage may also be a contributing factor to DIC (Levi, 2008).
- Disorders that produce necrosis, e.g. severe burns and trauma, brain tissue destruction.
- Neoplastic disease, e.g. acute leukaemia, metastatic carcinoma (Becker and Wira, 2008).
- Other disorders including incompatible blood transfusion, drug reaction, shock, diabetic ketoacidosis, pulmonary embolism, sickle cell anaemia, cardiac arrest surgery.

Clinical features

These can be quite challenging to diagnose as the primary disorder may initially mask symptoms. Symptoms may include:

- microvascular thrombosis, including dyspnoea, haemoptysis (pulmonary infarct may lead to ARDS), confusion/disorientation, renal failure;
- haemorrhagic (more commonly, epistaxis), generalised bleeding/bruising, persistent bleeding from invasive sites, e.g. venepuncture sites, urethral catheters;
- a mixture of thrombosis and haemorrhaging in various systems.

The major problem and presenting feature of acute DIC is bleeding. When DIC occurs in acutely ill patients with multi-organ dysfunction the prognosis is poor.

Time out 32.1

1 Assess the patients within your own clinical practice setting.
2 Identify those patients who you think are susceptible to developing DIC.
3 Give reasons why you think this is so.

Diagnostic tests

Early recognition and prompt intervention is essential if the patient is to have a chance of survival. In addition to the clinical examination, diagnosis is made on the basis of laboratory findings. The main tests are listed in Box 32.2

There is no single test to accurately diagnose DIC. As haemostasis is complex, test results may be variable and difficult to interpret. Significant DIC can be present despite normal standard coagulation tests and also some patients may show laboratory features of DIC without any clinical sequence (Becker and Wira, 2008). A combination of a clinical condition that may be complicated by DIC with a number of laboratory results will establish the presence of DIC with an acceptable level of certainty (Levi, 2008).

Box 32.2 Diagnostic tests: DIC

- Platelet count (decreased)
- Fibrinogen levels (decreased)
- Prothrombin time (likely to be prolonged)
- Partial thromboplastin time (prolonged)
- Fibrinopeptide (elevated)
- Fibrin degradation product (FDP) (detectable in the plasma)
- D-dimer test (specific fibrinogen breakdown test for DIC) (raised)

The D-dimer and FDP tests offer the best assessment for the diagnosis of DIC (Yu *et al.*, 2000).

Management

The management of DIC is controversial and complex. However, the principles of management appear to be threefold:

1 identifying and treating the cause;
2 optimising the patient's condition;
3 replacing clotting factors as appropriate.

In some cases, the DIC will completely resolve within hours after resolution of the underlying condition. Throughout, measures should be undertaken to support organ function, thus maintaining adequate tissue perfusion and preventing further clinical deterioration.

Thrombic

These patients are prone to developing deep vein thrombosis (DVT), calves should be regularly checked for signs of inflammation, redness, heat and pain. Blockage to the lower extremities may manifest in cold, mottled-looking limb(s). When the patient is stationary, elevating the legs 15–30° together with limb exercises may help prevent venous stasis. The patient's respiratory status should be monitored very closely for signs of distress resulting from pulmonary emboli.

Drugs may include antifibrinolytic agents (e.g. aminocaproic acid and transexamic acid) to inhibit fibrinolysis; vitamin K (phytonadione) and folate. Anti-platelet drugs may also be used. Thrombolytic agents, e.g. streptokinase, tissue plasminogen activator (TPA), are not indicated in patients with thrombosis as they may facilitate excessive bleeding. The use of heparin is controversial, as it potentiates the naturally occurring plasma protease inhibitor, anti-thrombin, that keeps in check any accelerated coagulation reaction. Hence, too much heparin can accelerate the bleeding. In some cases (thromboembolic disorders) low molecular weight heparin used with caution can prove useful (Becker and Wira, 2008).

Haemorrhagic

Assessment of the patient would include signs of bleeding (internally and externally). Puncture sites (IV sites, etc.) should be inspected regularly for visual signs of blood. Urinalysis should be used to check daily for blood. Invasive blood pressure monitoring may be an alternative for these patients as it reduces the risk of bleeding under the skin caused by external cuff pressures. Changing the patient's position must also be done with caution. Vigorous brushing of the teeth should be avoided and the gums must be inspected regularly. If the patient has limited mobility then two-hourly inspection/turning should occur.

Blood component replacement, i.e. fresh frozen plasma, cryoprecipitate (for patients with markedly decreased fibrinogen levels) may be prescribed. If indicated, red blood replacement and vitamin K and folate should be given. Platelet transfusion may be considered for patients with severe thrombocytopenia or those who are bleeding/at risk of bleeding from invasive procedures (Levi, 2008).

Complications

These can be either haemorrhagic or thrombotic:

- lungs: especially ARDS, pulmonary emboli and pulmonary hypertension;
- kidneys (intrinsic renal failure);
- liver failure;
- cerebral: microthrombi may cause confusion or cerebrovascular accidents;
- hypoxia and anoxia may lead to severe striated muscle pain;
- shock and coma;
- after fibrinolysis, severe to fatal haemorrhaging of vital organs can occur without warning.

Thalassaemia

Beta thalassaemia (thalassaemia major) is an inhered blood disorder that begins in early childhood. It affects both male and female. Thalassaemia occurs more frequently in Mediterranean countries, North Africa, the Middle East and England. Haemoglobin (Hb) contains a large amount of iron. When red blood cells are broken down, more of the iron from the Hb is used again to make new Hb. In thalassaemia the Hb is fragile and suffers premature breakdown and, therefore, there is not enough Hb in the body.

Symptoms include paleness, headaches, fatigue, short of breath, jaundice (from hyperbilirubinaemia) and splenic enlargement. The skull and the bones may be deformed, and there may be cortical bone thinning. Cardiac failure, arrthymias and iron overload may occur. Severe anaemia if untreated can result in cardiac failure, increased iron deposition resulting from multiple life-long transfusions.

Diagnosis is from microscopic examination of the blood revealing small red blood cells. Primary treatment involves regular blood transfusions (usually every week). Multiple transfusions lead to haemolysis resulting in iron overload. This may initiate liver failure. Injections of desferal (an iron-chelating agent) are administered, allowing excess iron to be easily removed from the body. The dosage and length of therapy is dependent upon the severity of the condition.

Implications for practice

- Nurses should be open and alert to the needs of the patient with sickle cell anaemia, particularly pain control.
- Through clinical supervision and reflective practice, the care of patients during sickle cell crisis and those patients with DIC should improve.
- Any acutely ill patient has a potential to develop DIC, therefore, nurses must carefully monitor the patient for unexplained haemorrhaging or interference with normal tissue perfusion.
- Early recognition of DIC is essential if the patient is to have a chance of survival.
- Strategies need to be adopted to try and prevent further injury to the patient particularly during invasive procedures.

Summary

Sickle cell anaemia, DIC and thalassaemia are disorders of the blood which can pose a challenge for nurses. Each are potentially life-threatening. Early detection and administration of treatment is required to enable a reasonably favourable outcome for the patient.

Clinical scenario

Philip Anthony is 35 years old, and has suffered from sickle cell anaemia since his childhood. He is usually admitted to hospital twice a year for treatment of vaso-occlusive crises. This time, on admission he is complaining of severe abdominal pain. The pain ruler score is ten.

Pulse – 135 (sinus tachycardia)
Blood pressure – 100/150 mmHg
Temperature – 38.2°C
Hb 8g/dl
Sickle cell test is positive.

Philip is very anxious and very vocal in his expression of pain.

1　Identify the priorities for the nursing management during his sickle cell crisis.

2　Discuss the specific care required by Philip during an exchange transfusion. Include the identification of potential problems and evidence with your answer.

3　Evaluate Philip's condition and suggest health promotion strategies to help reduce the occurrence of another sickle cell crisis.

Chapter 33

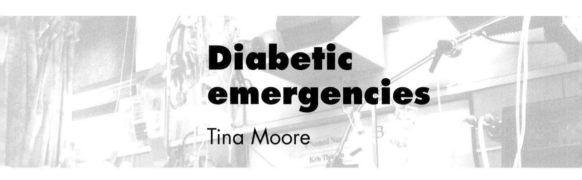

Diabetic emergencies

Tina Moore

Contents

Learning outcomes

After reading this chapter you will be able to:

- identify the causes of diabetic ketoacidosis (DKA), hyperglycaemic hyperosmolar state (HHS) and hypoglycaemia;
- prioritise nursing assessment and intervention for each emergency;
- understand the underlying principles of fluid resuscitation and management in DKA and HHS;
- recognise and initiate emergency treatment for hypoglycaemia;
- consider health promotion strategies to minimise/prevent such emergencies occurring.

Fundamental knowledge

Control of blood glucose; acid base balance; aetiology of diabetes mellitus.

Introduction

Although diabetic emergencies do not occur too often, they can provoke life-threatening situations with fatal consequences (particularly if they are not identified quickly and treated appropriately). Hence, a thorough assessment of the patient is required, exercising caution in the assessment of the older person (as some symptoms may mimic other less acute conditions).

Many of these emergencies are preventable (mainly through patient education), thus the role of the nurse as a health educator/promoter is essential. This chapter will discuss the three main diabetic emergencies that nurses may be exposed to within clinical practice.

Time out 33.1

1 Using physiology outline normal blood glucose control.
2 When normal control fails, identify and explain symptoms of high and low blood glucose.

Control of blood glucose is dependent upon effective metabolic processes. Glucose is essential to maintain brain, renal and erythrocyte energy sources. Insulin and glucagons are hormones responsible for carbohydrate metabolism and glucose control. Interference will upset homeostasis. Disorders include diabetes mellitus, gestational diabetes and stress responses.

Diabetic ketoacidosis (DKA)

This can be a life-threatening disorder (even if the patient is not comatosed). The onset usually occurs over the course of hours or sometimes days. DKA is a complication of diabetes mellitus (mainly Type 1) but can also feature in Type 2 (results from severe insulin deficiency leading to the disordered metabolism of proteins, carbohydrates and fats).

The outcomes of such pathological events are hyperglycaemia, hyperosmolality, ketoacidosis and volume depletion. Observing for symptoms (such as glycosuria, ketonuria and hypotension) is required in order to confirm diagnosis and enable prompt intervention. The ability of the healthcare professional to recognise the clinical features of DKA profoundly affects outcome and survival rates.

Precipitating factors

Precipitating factors include anything that would initiate a physiological or psychological stress response (e.g. sepsis). Patients may have a history of uncontrolled insulin-dependent diabetes mellitus (Type 1), mainly due to accidental or deliberate omission of insulin (e.g. patients undergoing surgery, illness and acute/critical illness) can precipitate DKA through an exaggerated stress response.

The stress response relates to a cascade of metabolic and neurohormonal changes. Stress-induced hyperglycaemia is attributed to hypersecretion of the counter-regulatory hormones: catecholamines (adrenaline (epinephrine) and noradrenaline (norepinephrine)), glucagons, cortisol and growth hormone. Release of catecholamines results in decreased insulin and increased glucagon secretion by the pancreas (Ganong, 2005). The effect is a surge in circulating glucose derived from glycogenolysis and impaired utilisation of glucose (hyperglycaemia itself impairs glucose utilisation and residual insulin secretion).

Patients who have an inadequate secretion of insulin and taking fixed doses of insulin are unable to increase insulin production to counteract these intense catabolic effects. The sympathetic branch of the autonomic nervous system plays a key role in the stress-mediated glycaemic response, causing increased heart and respiratory rates and blood pressure. The patient's physiological response to stress can cause considerable added strain on failing organs.

Clinical features

In the older patient symptoms can be less overt, these symptoms may be associated with disorders of ageing; other diseases may mask symptoms, e.g. urinary frequency may be associated with prostatism in men or infection in women. Kussmaul breathing may be mistaken for respiratory problems associated with heart failure or chest infection.

The severity of the condition is determined by the degree of acidosis: mild (pH 7.2–7.3); moderate (pH 7.1–7.2); severe (pH < 7.1) (Wolfsdorf et al., 2006). Metabolic acidosis (Chapter 17) is due to excessive acid production, commonly, lactic and keto acids occurring with a significant fall in plasma bicarbonate concentration. Clinical presentations of metabolic acidosis include headache and lethargy. Severe acidosis can cause deep, rapid respirations (respiratory system is stimulated to increase the excretion of carbon dioxide in an attempt to restore acid base balance), cardiac dysrhythmias and eventually coma.

Hyperglycaemia

Osmotic diuresis causes large volumes of water and electrolytes to be lost. Dehydration depletes the intracellular compartment (largest of the body's fluid spaces); an increased serum osmolality causes movement of water out of the cells, resulting in a reduction in the level of consciousness. Counter-regulatory hormones are released and their catabolic action further exacerbates hyperglycaemia.

> **Box 33.1 Summary of problems associated with hyperglycaemia**
>
> Glucose concentrations should not be too high for the following reasons:
>
> - Cellular dehydration can be caused by glucose exerting a large amount of osmotic pressure in the extracellular space.
> - Glycosuria (caused by excessive high levels of glucose concentration) causes fluid and electrolyte depletion.
> - Glucose is the main source of cell energy, without glucose cells die, and organs start to fail.

Dehydration

Generally, the renal threshold varies and can be as low as 6 mmol/litre, but is usually 10 to 12 mmol/litre (Higgins, 2007). Glucose exerts a high osmotic pressure in the extracellular fluid and if the glucose concentration rises to excessive values this can cause considerable dehydration. Fluid is also lost via hyperventilation, nausea, vomiting, increased perspiration and decreased oral fluid intake. Some 6–8 litres of free water can be lost (Kitabachi *et al.*, 2006). Clinical signs are a dry mouth and skin and acute weight loss. Compensatory mechanisms include polydipsia (increased thirst). Compensation stimulated by hypovolaemia helps maintain blood pressure. Intracellular dehydration occurs and the intravascular volume falls leading to hypotension and shock. Vomiting will also worsen electrolyte loss and imbalances, especially potassium, precipitating hypokalaemia and possible cardiac complications.

Electrolyte imbalances

These are caused by polyuria and vomiting (ketonaemia, dehydration and electrolyte imbalances) (Marini and Wheeler, 2006). Low serum concentrations of potassium, phosphate and magnesium can cause cardiac dysrhythmias including asystole (Chapter 29). Hypokalaemia can result from haemodilution following fluid resuscitation and inadequate potassium replacement. Initially plasma potassium is decreased. However, as the vascular volumes fall, renal function will be affected. If the kidneys fail to conserve sodium, this will decrease and the exchange (sodium/potassium) will not occur, producing high serum potassium levels despite the total body reduction (and cellular level), increasing sometimes to dangerously high levels (Rucker, 2008).

Sodium plasma concentrations are usually normal or slightly low (130–140 mmol/litre). Hyponatraemia is caused by the osmotic gradient moving water from the intracellular compartment and diluting extracellular sodium. Hypophosphataemia can cause muscle weakness, malaise, confusion, respiratory failure, decreased oxygen delivery.

Glycosuria

Glycosuria is also responsible for the loss of water through osmotic diuresis. This and hyperglycaemia create a favourable medium for the growth of yeast organisms, consequently the patient may complain of pruritis (itching), particularly around the genitalia.

Ketonaemia and ketonuria

Insulin deficiency prevents normal utilisation of serum glucose leading to cellular starvation. The unmet energy requirements of the cells stimulate gluconeogenesis and glycogen conversion in the liver through the release of counter-regulatory hormones. In the absence of glucose availability, the body is then forced to break down fat and protein stores to meet energy requirements. Ketone bodies (waste product of fat metabolism) accumulate in the blood, lowering the blood pH level.

Kussmaul respirations

Kussmaul respirations represent an increased rate and depth of breathing (Hipp and Sinert, 2008), resulting from a low pH that stimulates the respiratory centre producing hyperventilation (bodies attempt to 'blow off' carbon dioxide and compensate for acidosis). The odour of the breath smells fruity (acetone).

Management

Patients who present severe DKA are usually semi-conscious with marked hypotension, severe acidosis and/or electrolyte disturbance. The first 24 hours are the most critical and require very close monitoring by nurses and medical staff. Managing the patient with severe DKA may present a challenging situation.

Box 33.2 The aims of treatment

- Reduce serum glucose
- Correct dehydration
- Correct metabolic acidosis
- Find and treat cause (if possible)

Guidelines (NICE, 2004c, 2008) adopt a proactive approach and advocate for health education prior to the development of DKA (thus avoiding this situation). They are, however, unhelpful in their guidance when such an emergency occurs. Local protocols exist within Trusts, so nurses are encouraged to be familiar with these.

Fluid replacement

Detailed clinical guidelines exist, e.g. De Beer *et al.* (2008), but readers are advised to be conversant with their own Trust guidelines. Fluid replacement is determined by hydration status (should be via a central line). By rehydrating the patient hyperglycaemia should be reduced (improved glomerular filtration). Replacement of fluid should take account of the patient's age, degree of dehydration and issues such as history of cardiac disease.

Extracellular volume is expanded to restore renal function. Some patients may develop hypovolaemic shock. The choice of fluid is isotonic saline (0.9% saline) treated via rapid infusion in order to restore renal blood flow. One to two litres over the first 1–2 hours is given, and half the fluid deficit over the first 6–8 hours, and the remainder over the next 16 hours (Brenner, 2006).

In severe dehydration, fluid is lost initially from the largest spaces (intracellular space), rehydration using a similar sodium concentration may be used, e.g. hypotonic saline 0.45%. The aim is to correct water and electrolyte deficits over the first 24–48 hours to replete extracellular fluid volume and restore intravascular volume.

Hypotonic saline may be used if sodium levels are greater than 160 mmol/litre and then only 1 litre over 8 hours. Isotonic saline (half strength) is used in hypernatraemia. Colloids may be indicated in some cases if systolic pressure is <100 mmHg (English and Williams, 2004). Colloids aid fluid retention in the intravascular space (only one-quarter to one-third of crystalloid will remain in the intravascular space, the remainder enters the interstitial space – depending upon the fluid as well as capillary permeability). However, resuscitating the severely hypovolaemic patient (requiring ICU transfer) with crystalloid fluids may only cause a massive expansion in the intracellular spaces and can result in peripheral, pulmonary or cerebral oedema. When blood glucose levels are <13 mmol infusion fluid should be changed to 5% glucose (Kitabachi *et al.*, 2006).

Vital signs such as blood pressure, pulse pressure, mean arterial pressure, central venous pressure (CVP) should be closely monitored. ECG rhythm should also be observed for dysrhythmias associated with initial hyperkalaemia (peaked T waves, widening QRS complex, prolonged PR interval, flattened to absent P wave). Hypokalaemia may show depressed ST segments, flat or inverted T waves or increased ventricular dysrhythmias.

Insulin replacement

Repletion of potassium should begin before insulin infusion if the serum potassium is too low. The use of insulin will further decrease extracellular potassium levels (Morton *et al.*, 2006). Insulin shifts potassium from the extracellular to the intracellular space as glucose enters the cell and restarts the sodium–potassium pump

An intravenous infusion using a sliding scale insulin regime helps lower serum glucose and inhibits ketogenesis (production of ketones) and so begins the reversal process for metabolic acidosis. Serum glucose needs to be analysed (initially 1–2 hourly) via laboratory rather than a portable glucometer to enable accuracy of results.

Hypoglycaemia is one complication that should be avoided through careful monitoring. The infusion should continue until the patient is eating and drinking, and then substituted with the subcutaneous route.

Insulin resistance may occur because of the effects of counter-regulatory hormones and acidosis; this may be significant when weaning a patient from the IV route to subcutaneous. Intravenous infusions of insulin should not be stopped abruptly as the patient can become totally insulin deficient within 10 minutes. The infusion dosage should be reduced on an hourly basis. NICE guidelines exist on the management of insulin pumps (NICE, 2008).

Once the urine is clear of ketones and blood glucose is maintained within the normal limits, subcutaneous insulin can be commenced. IV infusion regime must only be discontinued at the same time as the first dose of subcutaneous insulin is given. Premature discontinuation of insulin is the most common cause of lapsing in DKA (Marini and Wheeler, 2006).

Correcting metabolic acidosis

The role of bicarbonate in treating DKA acidosis remains controversial. Sodium bicarbonate (8.4%) can cause alkalosis, hypokalaemia, hypocalcaemia and hypernatraemia. Excessive sodium load causes pulmonary oedema, thrombosis of the peripheral veins, tissue necrosis and extravasation. Other treatments should be considered only using bicarbonate as a last resort, i.e. except in extreme cases of acidosis when the pH is <7.1–7.2 (Hipp and Sinert, 2008). Close monitoring of the patient, particularly cardiovascular status is required. Baird *et al.* (2005) suggest that acidosis is best corrected by insulin therapy. Arterial blood gas monitoring is also required to establish the degree of metabolic acidosis and to evaluate acid base balance.

Effective treatment of DKA should instigate a reduction or curing of abdominal pain within 6–12 hours. If pain persists, another cause is likely. Infection is treated with intravenous antibiotics. Patients are at risk of developing deep vein thrombosis, therefore, low doses of heparin should be administered.

Complications

- Gastric stasis can lead to acute abdominal distension with copious vomiting and a high risk of aspiration pneumonia. A nasogastric tube should be inserted in order to aspirate stomach contents.
- Sodium and water depletion can cause shock and renal insufficiency.
- Over-rapid correction of the biochemical abnormalities can cause hypoglycaemia, hypocalcaemia and hyperkalaemia.
- Respiratory complications/failure presenting with rapidly progressive shortness of breath and hypoxaemia. The pathophysiology is unclear but possible links have been made to decreasing osmotic pressures and increased left atrial pressure from excessively rapid fluid replacement (Page and Hall, 1999).

- Mediastinal surgical emphysema (usually affects the chest and neck) can occur in patients with severe acidosis. Symptoms include prolonged hyperventilation and vomiting. Increased alveolar pressure can damage the alveolar walls and allows air to escape into the interstitial lung tissue.
- Cerebral oedema – due to fluid shift.

Hyperglycaemic hyperosmolar state (HHS)

HHS is less common than DKA and relates predominately to patients over 60 years old presenting with Type 2 diabetes mellitus (indicating some insulin production). Mortality is high – up to 40 per cent (DOH, 2001). This condition can lead to ketosis.

HHS is characterised by insulin deficiency (a raised plasma glucose, dehydration, plasma hyperosmolarity and renal impairment). Generally potassium is unaffected. This condition is the second major clinical presentation of uncontrolled diabetes mellitus. In comparison to DKA the onset is more insidious with clinical features developing gradually, sometimes up to two weeks. Acidaemia is not pronounced.

Precipitating factors

- Drugs that reduce insulin secretion such as beta-blockers, thiazide/loop diuretics.
- Drugs that increase insulin resistance such as corticosteroids.
- Excessive IV glucose administration.
- A preceding illness resulting in several days of increasing dehydration, e.g. vomiting.

Clinical features

Frequently, older patients do not manifest acute clinical symptoms of illness and can become critically ill before symptoms are recognised. Patients may present with non-specific symptoms, e.g. anorexia, malaise, weakness. Hyperglycaemia is more severe than in DKA, resulting in a significant serum hyperosmolality and pronounced osmotic diuresis. Severe dehydration can occur, patients can loose up to 25 per cent of body weight resulting in intracellular dehydration. The blood becomes more viscous and flow is impeded, increasing the risk of thromboemboli. Increased cardiac workload and decreased renal and cerebral blood flow may result in myocardial infarction, renal failure and stroke.

Other features include polydipsia and polyuria, tachycardia, hypotension, tachypnoea with shallow respirations, profound weakness, focal seizures and hypokalaemia. Neurological deficits may be mistaken for senility in the older patient. Some patients may be unconscious or suffer impairment of conscious levels, this is proportional to the severity of hyperosmolarity.

Although the body's available insulin is insufficient to control blood glucose, it usually is adequate to prevent the formation of ketone bodies, avoiding metabolic acidosis. However, some patients may present with ketonuria (hence the replacement of the term hyperosmolar non-ketotic state (HONK) with HHS).

Management

Though pathophysiologically different, treatment is very similar to DKA but patients have a much greater sensitivity to insulin. Insulin is usually administered in low doses via the intravenous route (because of poor tissue perfusion). Fluid replacement and electrolyte replacement via central line of 0.9% saline may be prescribed, sometimes requiring up to 9 litres in 48 hours (Stoner, 2005). Potassium, sodium, phosphate and magnesium supplements are given on the basis of laboratory values. Fluid replacement requires flexibility in relation to patient's level of dehydration/electrolyte imbalances and blood glucose levels, and general cardiovascular status.

Initially, a large volume of fluid may be given rapidly, e.g. 1–2 litres over the first two hours. The aim is to replenish intravascular volume and correct hyperosmolarity. Many patients respond to fluid resuscitation alone, but IV insulin can correct hyperglycaemia (Sagarin and McAfee, 2001). The aim is usually to replace the fluid deficit (average 8–10 litres) over 48 hours approximately. Close monitoring for signs of fluid overload is crucial.

For patients who are comatosed safety is the priority and airway management is required and prompt transfer to ICU. Prophylactic anti-coagulation should be given to prevent venous thromboembolism (DOH, 2001). Correction of HHS must be cautious as abrupt reversal of serum hyperosmolarity may produce intracellular water intoxication leading to diaphoresis and seizures.

Time out 33.2

Outline the major differences between DKA and HHS (consider the aetiology, precipitating factors, clinical features and management).

Hypoglycaemia

Hypoglycaemia is the commonest cause of a diabetic emergency and is usually sudden in onset, but correctable. Serum glucose levels fall below 1 mmol/l. Causative factors include: missed meal, overdose of insulin, changing insulin therapy/preparations, liver and adrenal insufficiency and beta-blockers.

If the patient is unconscious, procedures to maintain patient safety should be taken. During prolonged hypoglycaemia growth hormone and cortisol are secreted. Both reduce the rate of glucose utilisation by most cells of the body, converting instead to greater amounts of fat utilisation. This helps the blood to return the level of glucose towards normal. During severe hypoglycaemia the hypothalamus stimulates the sympathetic nervous system. Adrenaline is secreted by the adrenal glands, so furthering release of glucose from the liver.

If hypoglycaemia is not promptly corrected, irreversible brain damage and acute myocardial infarction can occur. Prompt reversal of hypoglycaemia should be a priority (administration of concentrated glucose). Still, there is the danger of precipitating hyperglycaemia with the administration of too much glucose.

Clinical features

Clinical features include altered behaviour (including 'inappropriate' behaviour); withdrawal; irritability; sometimes difficulties in motor function (e.g. walking) and slurred speech (gives the impression of drunkenness). Physiological symptoms include increased heart rate, sweating and tremor. It may even present with epilepsy, in severe cases stupor, seizure and comas are present.

Patient education

Once the priorities of management and care have been addressed consideration needs to be given to health promotion. The focus here is on prevention. Some patients require a revision of diabetes mellitus (aetiology, clinical features and the control of blood glucose). Educational guidance is available (NICE, 2004c, 2008).

The importance of preventing diseases as far as possible, e.g. common cold, infection should be emphasised. Tips should be given on how to manage stress. Food nutrition management and the importance of continuing insulin therapy and medication (even when experiencing nausea and vomiting from other illness) when ill should be explained. Patients should be re-educated regarding the need to monitor their blood glucose and urine regularly.

The symptoms of hypoglycaemia should be revisited. In some circumstances it may be possible to induce hypoglycaemia under a controlled situation. In the event of conscious hypoglycaemia, oral glucose should be ingested.

Some patients find it extremely difficult to implement the recommendations by healthcare professionals in relation to modifying diet; complying with self-monitoring; taking of medication; adapting personal lifestyle habits and returning for follow-up. Healthcare professionals should work with patients to identify and agree a plan of action. Recommended techniques for patient education and counselling, providing factual information and motivational encouragement (needed for meaningful change) should be employed.

Implications for practice

- Prompt recognition of diabetic emergencies and appropriate intervention is required.
- Nurses must conduct a thorough assessment of the patient to aid confirmation of diagnosis.
- Maintenance of effective fluid balance is an essential aspect of care.
- Caution must be adopted when assessing the older person, as some symptoms may mimic other less acute conditions.

Summary

There are three main diabetic emergencies, all requiring prompt recognition and appropriate intervention. The selected intervention requires the maintenance of fluid and electrolyte balance, as well as controlling hyperglycaemia. Once the patient's condition improves, health promotion should begin.

Clinical scenario

Ceylan is 23 years old and has Type 1 diabetes mellitus. She has found it difficult to manage her diabetes with several subsequent admissions with DKA. Normally her diabetes is controlled with Novorapid (short-acting insulin taken with meals) and Glargine (long-acting insulin daily). Recently she has complained of feeling unwell and has a two-day history of fever and sore throat. Her visual appearance indicates dehydration, her skin is thin and dry, and her tongue is furred. She also has lower right quadrant abdominal pain. On admission she is semi-conscious.

GCS – 11
Pulse – 136 beats/minute
B/P – 94/67 mmHg
Temperature – 39.2°C
Respirations – 35/minute (Kussmaul respirations)
Blood values:
pH – 7.12
pO_2 – 10.1 kPa
HCO_3 – 8.9 mmol/litre
pCO_2 – 2.6 kPa
Glucose – 34 mmol/litre

Urinalysis indicates ketones and glucose. Her clinical symptoms and laboratory results confirm a diagnosis of DKA.

1 From the assessment data, offer a rationale for Ceylan's symptoms.

2 Devise a plan of care for the first six hours of admission together with criteria for evaluation.

3 Consider the possible causes of Ceylan's admission. What health promotion is required to reduce the chances of recurrence?

Chapter 34

Acute liver dysfunction

Philip Woodrow

Contents

Learning outcomes

After reading this chapter you will be able to:

- understand the main causes of liver failure;
- recognise usual symptoms of acute liver failure;
- be able to plan nursing care for patients with acute liver failure.

Fundamental knowledge

Hepatic anatomy and physiology.

Introduction

Liver failure may be acute, chronic or acute-on-chronic. Acute failure, often caused by paracetamol (or other drugs), or viruses, is fairly rare, although can be devastating when it happens. Chronic liver failure, often caused by alcohol, implies an end-stage disease, fatal unless a liver transplant or artificial support are provided, although exacerbations may necessitate admission to acute wards. Acute liver failure is potentially reversible, but it can rapidly progress to multiorgan failure, necessitating urgent transplantation. While acute liver failure is relatively rare, many acutely ill patients may experience liver dysfunction as a complication of other disease. As with any other organ dysfunction, early detection and prompt and appropriate treatment make significant differences to outcome. But more so than other major organs, signs of liver failure may take a relatively long time to appear, and even longer to cause concern to the individual.

The liver is a complex organ, so dysfunction can cause many problems. Yet treatment options are limited, compared with other organ failure. Acute care largely focuses on symptom relief and system support.

After briefly summarising the main liver functions, this chapter identifies likely causes of liver failure and the main symptoms and effects of liver failure that may cause or complicate illness. However, the liver has many more functions, and liver disease can cause many more complications than can be described here, so care should be individualised to meet the needs of each patient.

Liver functions

The liver has many functions, but these can be grouped into four main areas:

- detoxification (drugs, alcohol, hormones);
- digestive (bile formation, nutrient metabolism), including protein synthesis (albumin, clotting factors);
- infection control (Kuppfer cells, complements);
- storage (glycogen, vitamins).

Pathophysiology

Hepatitis (inflammation of liver) may be caused by many toxins, including:

- viruses
- drugs (especially paracetamol)
- chemicals (especially alcohol)
- idiopathic (unidentified causes).

Although hepatocytes regenerate well, connective tissue between hepatocytes may generate more rapidly, especially with prolonged inflammation, causing cirrhosis. Cirrhosis (a chronic condition) is the end-stage of fibrosis in the liver. Obstructed blood flow increases pressure in the hepatic portal vein (portal hypertension). Cirrhosis usually progresses to chronic liver failure and cancer.

Classification

O'Grady's (1999) classification for acute liver failure is widely used:

- *hyperacute*: encephalopathy develops within 7 days of jaundice appearing;
- *acute*: encephalopathy develops between 8–28 days of jaundice appearing;
- *subacute*: encephalopathy develops between 4–12 weeks of jaundice appearing.

Symptoms

The key signs of liver failure are usually

- jaundice
- encephalopathy (confusion, drowsiness or other neurological changes)
- coagulopathy (e.g. bruising, bleeding).

Severe/chronic liver failure often causes ascites, but this is often a late complication. Liver failure may also cause

- abdominal pain
- sweet, sickly-smelling breath
- respiratory failure
- hypotension
- infections
- malnourishment, especially vitamin deficiency.

Patients' medical and social history may suggest liver disease, although they may also deny or moderate risk factors such as alcoholism or sexually transmitted diseases. Recent foreign travel may have exposed them to viral hepatitis.

Death from liver failure is usually caused by either

- cerebral oedema progressing to herniation of the brainstem into the spiral column (*coning*);
- overwhelming sepsis (Krumberger, 2002).

So liver dysfunction should be identified before it causes fatal complications.

Liver function tests (LFTs)

When the liver fails, anything it produces (such as plasma proteins) is likely to be deficient, while anything it metabolises (e.g. serum bilirubin) is likely to be raised. Because the liver has so many functions, there are many possible tests for liver failure, but the main markers are listed in Table 34.1. Jaundice, a visible sign of

Table 34.1 Main liver function tests (LFTs)

Liver function tests (including clotting)	Normal range
Main LFTs	
Bilirubin	1–20 μmol/litre
Alanine Aminotransferase (ALT)	<40 iu/litre
Gamma Glutamyl Transpeptidase (GGT)	10–48 iu/litre
Alkaline Phosphatase (Alk Phos; ALP)	<100 iu/litre
Albumin	35–50 g/litre
Total Protein	60–80 g/litre
Other LFTs	
Aspartate Aminotransferase (AST)	<40 iu/litre
(Activated) Partial Thromboplastin Time (PTT/APTT)	26–39 seconds or 6 seconds above control
Thrombin Time (TT)	15 second or 2 seconds above control
Prothrombin time	9.6–12.5 seconds
International Normalised Ratio (INR)	0.9–1.1

failure, typically occurs once serum bilirubin reaches 0.3 mg/dl (Krumberger, 2002).

Plasma proteins have many functions, including maintaining blood volume – holding the water part of blood in the bloodstream. Low plasma proteins therefore contribute to oedema formation and hypovolaemia. Plasma proteins are produced by the liver from protein in the diet. Although total protein levels are often measured, albumin is by far the main plasma protein, and is a useful marker of disease – albumin is lower in sicker patients. Albumin, and other plasma proteins, will be low if diet and/or liver function are poor. Nutrition, especially protein foods, is usually the best way to reverse low levels (hypoalbuminaemia, hypoproteinaemia). However, just as plasma proteins take time to noticeably fall, so improved levels take time to appear – significant improvement often does until a week after normal(ish) diet commences.

Cell damage releases intracellular enzymes. With damage to liver cells, blood tests will show raised levels of hepatic enzymes, such as:

- alanine aminotransferase (ALT)
- gamma glutmyl transferase (GGT).

Clotting factors are produced in the liver, so liver failure causes prolonged

- (activated) partial thromboplastin time (PTT or APTT)
- prothrombin time (PT)
- international normalised ratio (INR)
- alkaline phosphatase (Alk Phos; ALP)

Time out 1.1

Using Table 34.1, examine liver function test results of patients in your workplace. Where LFTs appear raised, what aspects (if any) of the patient's social or medical history might have caused liver dysfunction? How far has any liver dysfunction contributed to diseases for which they are currently being treated.

Paracetamol

Unlike most other countries, paracetamol overdose has long been the main cause of liver failure in the UK. Metabolism of paracetamol is individual, so small overdoses may prove fatal to some people, while others may survive significantly larger overdoses. As little as 4–6 g can cause liver damage (Mokhlesi *et al.*, 2003). Paracetamol is rapidly absorbed. Plasma levels usually peak within 1–2 hours after ingestion (Smith, 2007), but may take up to 4 hours to be interpretable (Bateman, 2007). Levels exceeding 200 mg/litre after 4 hours or 50 mg/litre after 12 hours usually cause hepatocyte damage (Wyncoll, 2003) and can cause renal tubular necrosis (Bateman, 2007).

Initial symptoms may be limited to nausea, but damage is slow and progressive, peaking 72–96 hours after ingestion. Intravenous acetylcysteine (Parvolex®) or oral methionine given within 10–12 hours of overdose can prevent hepatic failure, and may prevent damage if given within 24 hours.

Alcohol

Alcohol causes chronic, rather than acute, liver failure, but alcoholics may be admitted with acute complications, such as gastrointestinal bleeding. Current UK recommendations for daily maximum alcohol intake are 3–4 units/day for men and 2–3 for women. Deaths in the UK from alcohol are increasing (Day, 2002). Drugs may be needed to minimise withdrawal symptoms from alcohol.

Viruses

Many viruses can cause hepatic failure, including varicella, Epstein-Barr and cytomegovirus. Some hepatitis viruses, such as hepatitis A and hepatitis E, are transmitted through ingestion, so tend to be prevalent where sanitation is poor. Hepatitis B is blood-borne, causes a small but significant number of infections in the UK, with limited treatment options and high mortality if it causes acute liver failure. Hepatitis C is also a blood-borne infection, mainly associated with intravenous drug abuse (Fahey, 2007). It may cause early jaundice, but usually causes chronic failure and cancer after two or more decades (Fahey, 2007). Incidence of hepatitis C is increasing. Hepatitis D is a defective virus, only able to survive in the presence of hepatitis B. Infection is rare and usually self-limiting (Thomas, 1999), but it may accelerate hepatic failure or cause chronic hepatitis. Other hepatitis viruses have been identified, but infection is very rare.

Complications

Neurological

The liver normally metabolises many neurotoxins. For example, serum ammonia, normally no more than 800–1,000 mcg/ml, can rise to 5,000 mcg/ml. Other toxins, such as gamma aminobutyric acid (GABA), increase blood–brain permeability, resulting in encephalopathy (Jackson and Wendon, 2000). Hepatic encephalopathy occurs in up to four-fifths of cirrhotics (Sargent, 2007).

Symptoms of neurotoxicity often include:

■ acute confusion
■ drowsiness/coma.

Nursing care should include skilful psychological support of both patient and relatives, as well as maintaining safety (e.g. preventing aspiration) and providing fundamental aspects of care. Nursing staff may also need to involve other professionals for specialist support (e.g. social workers).

Most people with acute liver failure develop cerebral oedema, with related symptoms:

■ tachypnoea;
■ dysconjugate eye movement, dilated pupils and slow pupil reaction to light;
■ reversed sleep patterns;
■ increased muscle tone, sometimes causing decerebrate posture.

Fitting is, however, rare.

Respiratory

Metabolic acidosis and cerebral oedema may stimulate tachypnoea, drowsiness may compromise the airway, ascites or other abdominal distension may limit diaphragmatic expansion, and hypoalbuminaemia may cause pulmonary oedema. So patients are at risk of

■ hypoxia
■ ventilatory failure
■ aspiration.

Patients may also have co-existing respiratory disease.

Cardiovascular

Visible signs of liver failure often include bruising and bleeding. Portal hypertension, and often other factors such as extensive vascular disease, cause central (and jugular) venous pressure to be raised. Cirrhosis causes systemic vasodilatation, reducing blood pressure and perfusion This causes a compensatory increase in cardiac output, resulting in warm peripheries, tachycardia and a bounding pulse (McKinnell and Holt, 2007). Vascular disease, frequently occurring in alcoholics, may mask hypotension, causing an apparent normalisation of their normally high blood pressure.

Renal

Severe liver failure can cause intrinsic renal damage, but progressive cardiac failure causing acute tubular necrosis (ATN) is the main cause of renal complications. More than half of patients with acute liver failure develop acute kidney injury (McKinnell and Holt, 2007). Up to two-fifths of cirrhotics develop hepatorenal syndrome from renal vasoconstriction (McKinnell and Holt, 2007). Failure to clear neurotoxins exacerbates acute confusion. People with hepatorenal syndrome can be supported with MARS (molecular adsorbents reticulation system – an extracorporeal circuit) (McKinnell and Holt, 2007), renal failure usually resolving with liver transplantation. Both treatments are usually only available in tertiary centres, to which the patient should be referred.

Metabolic

The liver is the main metabolic organ, so liver failure causes extensive complications. These can vary greatly, but often include:

■ hypothermia or pyrexia
■ hypoglycaemia
■ (metabolic) acidosis.

With severe failure, hypoglycaemia can occur rapidly, so may necessitate monitoring blood sugar every 2–4 hours. Although not immediately life-threatening, malnourishment and vitamin deficiency complicate recovery, so vitamin supplements are usually commenced quickly, and dieticians should be involved.

Infection

The liver produces complements, part of the body's infection control mechanism. It also contains Kuppfer cells, specialised macrophages, to destroy bacteria which transfer across from the gut into the blood. With liver failure, both these defences fail. Most patients with liver failure develop infections, many of which are fungal. Minimising infection risks is, therefore, important.

Ascites is the most common complication of cirrhosis (Gines and Cardenas, 2008). Pathology is debated, and probably multi-factorial, likely factors including:

■ hypernatraemia
■ capillary leak from congestion
■ hypoalbuminaemia.

Ascites is protein-rich, drawing further fluid into the abdominal compartment, causing hypovolaemia. Abdominal distension places pressure on all surrounding organs. The most obvious effect is likely to be respiratory compromise (breathlessness, basal atelectasis); mechanical compression causes further liver damage.

Sodium is restricted, and diuretic therapy commenced (Gines and Cardenas, 2008), but large collections of ascites compromise function of major organs, including lungs and kidneys, so are usually drained. Intravenous albumin is then given to draw further fluid back into the bloodstream.

Prognosis

Outcome depends partly on the extent of liver damage, and partly on complications and co-existing diseases. Liver dysfunction from systemic hypotension and poor perfusion causes additional complications to the underlying disease. Severe acute liver failure can be fatal within a few days (Stocklmann *et al.*, 2000). Once ascites develops, prognosis becomes significantly worse (Gines and Cardenas, 2008), so patients are likely to be referred to regional centres.

Implications for practice

- Although signs of liver dysfunction are often less apparent than signs from other dysfunctioning organs, key signs of liver failure are jaundice (usually occurring when blood bilirubin exceeds 100 micromol/litre).
- Nurses may detect other signs (such as increasing drowsiness) or receive laboratory results which suggest liver failure. Identifying concerns to medical colleagues may result in earlier and more effective treatment.
- Monitor for hypoglycaemia, which may develop rapidly.
- Liver dysfunction exposes patients to greater risks of opportunistic infections, so infection control becomes especially important.
- If clotting is prolonged, minimise traumatic aspects of nursing care (e.g. wet shaving).
- As patients become more drowsy they may need information to be repeated and stated simply.
- Causes of liver failure, such as alcoholism or paracetamol overdose, may cause guilt and/or anger among relatives, creating psychological needs for both them and the patient.

Summary

Liver failure may be the cause of admission, but liver dysfunction may develop from other diseases. Symptoms of liver failure are often less immediately obvious than symptoms from other main organs failing. But the liver's many functions means that dysfunction or failure causes many and diverse effects. Early detection of hepatic dysfunction can, therefore, significantly improve outcome. Treatments for the failing liver are largely supportive, but if end-stage liver disease is suspected, patients should be referred early to regional centres. Personality changes can make supporting the patient with liver failure stressful for both staff and family, so skilful nursing care, and involvement of other professions in care can make significant differences to quality of life.

Clinical scenario

John Sanders, aged 28 years old, was staying in a hotel. This morning he was found in a drowsy state. In the ambulance he admitted having taken a paracetamol overdose the previous evening, but would not admit to how many he had taken. There were two empty packs of 32 tablets nearby. He stated that he wished to die, having recently been left by his long-term partner. A stomach washout in A&E produced only a few remains of tablets. He has been transferred to a medical assessment ward, with a parvolex infusion already in progress. He is now less drowsy with a Glasgow Coma Score of 11.

John is self-employed. His next of kin is his widowed mother, who lives 250 miles away; she has been contacted and is travelling to the hospital by train.

1   From this chapter, and any other sources available, list the nursing priorities immediately following John's arrival in Medical Assessment.

2   Using this list of priorities, devise a plan for John's immediate nursing care.

3   Paracetamol levels, which were taken in A&E after the washout, are reported as being 200 mg/litre. John has been referred to the regional liver centre, who will review his case in one week. Meanwhile, he is to be transferred to a general medical ward once a bed is available. What aspects of physical and psychological care should be highlighted to the ward nurses?

Bibliography

Further reading

Specialist medical journals *Gut* and *Gastroenterology* are generally useful sources for material on this topic. Articles also often appear in general medical and nursing journals. Sargent is a leading nurse specialist in liver failure, and has published widely; her 2007 article on hepatic encephalopathy is especially useful.

Chapter 35

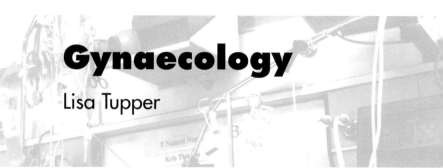

Gynaecology

Lisa Tupper

Contents

Learning outcomes

After reading this chapter you will be able to:

- understand the causes, pathophysiology and clinical characteristics of acute gynaecological disorders;
- provide effective management of emergency gynaecological problems;
- devise a care plan for a patient with an acute gynaecology

emergency based on nursing, medical, social and psychological needs;

■ identify and manage post-operative adverse events.

Fundamental knowledge

Gynaecological anatomy and normal physiology; human reproduction; vital signs; fluid balance.

Introduction

The female reproductive organs are essential to a woman's health and fertility. Gynaecological emergencies require prompt diagnosis and treatment to preserve organ function. Elective or emergency surgery may be necessary, resulting in loss of part or all of the reproductive system. Nurses should be aware of the impact this has on emotional and sexual well-being, as well as physical health.

This chapter outlines common acute gynaecological events and how to provide effective nursing care to women experiencing:

■ haemorrhage in early pregnancy – ectopic pregnancy rupture and miscarriage;
■ haemorrhage due to non-pregnant conditions – menorrhagia (heavy periods) and gynaecological malignancies;
■ pelvic infections;
■ post-operative complications.

Early identification and treatment of acute disorders can significantly reduce morbidity and mortality. It is vital nurses are aware of current practice, and significance and outcome of diagnostic investigations so they can alert medical staff. Monitoring vital signs and blood loss, fluid and dietary management, personal care, pain and nausea control and elimination are all fundamental in the care of gynaecology patients. Good psychological support can also reduce distress. Knowledge of surgical and medical practices enables nurses to empower women with explanations and advice, and to offer reassurance.

This chapter also highlights some rarer acute gynaecology complications:

■ ovarian cysts – acute events (rupture, haemorrhage and torsion);
■ ovarian hyperstimulation syndrome (OHSS).

Awareness of OHSS can minimise potential risks. National guidelines (RCN, 2006; RCOG, 2006) state women presenting with the condition should be treated in specialist gynaecological units.

Chronic gynaecological illnesses may also progress to acute emergencies. Complications from advanced gynaecological cancers result from large pelvic tumours impairing bowel or kidney function. Management options are identified.

Delivering efficient and effective point-of-care treatment, and achieving diagnosis in a timely manner, enables safe resolution of acute conditions.

Haemorrhage in early pregnancy

Ectopic pregnancy rupture

Ectopic pregnancy occurs where embryos implant outside the uterine cavity, usually presenting at 6–8 weeks' gestation. UK incidence, reported at 1 in 60–100 pregnancies (Impey, 2004), is increasing, due to increased prevalence of sexually transmitted infections that can cause pelvic inflammatory disease (PID) and acute salpingitis (inflammation of fallopian tubes) – predominantly chlamydia. If women of child-bearing age and capability present with abdominal discomfort, a urine pregnancy test should be performed. If this is positive or borderline, a blood sample for the pregnancy hormone beta-human chorionic gonadotrophin levels (β-hCG) is required. Urine pregnancy tests detect levels >50 iu/ml – reached at about four weeks' gestation. Only competent practitioners should be performing and interpreting pregnancy testing devices, as errors can be subject to litigation. RCOG (2004) recommend diagnosis is made through assessing:

- Symptoms – presence of unilateral iliac fossa pain or general lower abdominal tenderness, shoulder pain, unscheduled vaginal spotting (brownish in colour, continuous).
- Previous obstetric/gynaecological history (PID, endometriosis, previous pelvic surgery).
- Pelvic ultrasound – may reveal adnexal masses consistent with an ectopic (tubal) pregnancy.
- Serial β-hCG serum levels – levels should increase by 60 per cent or more every 48 hours, indicating viable intrauterine pregnancy. With ectopic pregnancies, levels can rise suboptimally, stay static or even decrease slightly. Increased levels can make diagnosis difficult.

Nurses caring for women with a possible ectopic pregnancy should be able to interpret diagnostic data and alert medical staff. Regular observations of pulse, blood pressure and respirations are required to monitor for hypovolaemia. A group and save serum and full blood count is required, in addition to establishing venous access. The woman should remain nil-by-mouth as a possible pre-operative measure, and intravenous fluids commenced.

Two clinical patterns occur, depending on the extent of tubal wall damage by the invading trophoblast – subacute or acute (Oats and Abraham, 2005).

Subacute presentations may be characterised by some pelvic discomfort interspersed with occasional attacks of sharp pain and faintness due to episodes of intraperitoneal bleeding. Resolution occurs as symptoms cease (indicating complete tubal abortion), or patients experience acute attacks (Oats and Abraham, 2005).

In acute presentations, the tube ruptures and internally haemorrhages into the pelvic cavity, causing severe pain and collapse. This occurs in one-third of cases, especially where implantation occurs in the isthmus (Oats and Abraham, 2005). Subdiaphragmatic irritation by blood causes referred shoulder tip pain (Symonds and Symonds, 2004). This acute presentation is potentially life-threatening, requiring emergency laparoscopy. Women with ruptured ectopic pregnancies show signs of hypovolaemia and distributive shock (see Chapter 27):

- tachycardia, weak rapid pulse
- hypotension
- abdominal distension
- pallor.

Remember – young otherwise healthy women may appear well despite internal haemorrhaging. Tachycardia may not be evident until 30 per cent of circulating blood volume is lost (Marieb, 2004).

Classical management of ectopic pregnancies is laparoscopic removal of the affected tube and pregnancy (salpingectomy) or removal of the pregnancy from the tube (salpingostomy). If the tube has ruptured, laparotomy may be required. Assessment of the tubes can be made during surgery; if bilateral tube damage is seen, the woman must be counselled that risk of subsequent ectopic pregnancies is significantly increased. Removing a tube reduces fertility, increasing anxiety for women hoping for future natural conception. Seven out of ten women have successful consecutive pregnancies, but one in ten have a further ectopic (Impey, 2004). Subsequent pregnancies are deemed to be higher risk so need monitoring by the local hospital-based Early Pregnancy Assessment Unit (EPAU) on discovery of a positive urine pregnancy test.

Following surgery, anti-D immunoglobulin is given to rhesus negative patients. This prevents antibody formation where surgical instrumentation may allow potentially rhesus positive embryo blood to cross the placenta into the mother's bloodstream. Anti-D serum is a blood product and should be administered intramuscularly once the correct checks have been made.

Medical management of ectopic pregnancy using methotrexate can be considered if β-hCG level is low – in practice levels <1,000 IU/ml – and there is no evidence of tubal rupture, and the patient is clinically stable. There are strict guidelines for use (RCOG, 2004) and patients should be made fully aware of risks. Methotrexate is a systemic chemotherapy drug, administered in a single dose in a chemotherapy unit to terminate the pregnancy. Follow-up of β-hCG results is required to ensure that the pregnancy is failing. The drug restricts the woman falling pregnant again for three to six months. Methotrexate is not always effective, so a second dose or surgery may be required. Risk of subsequent ectopic pregnancy is increased if the tube is damaged. This treatment remains controversial.

Miscarriage

Miscarriage is expulsion of a foetus before it reaches viability. Most miscarriages occur between the sixth and tenth weeks of pregnancy. Around one in eight pregnancies result in miscarriage, risk increasing with age. The Miscarriage Association (2008) identify the main causes of miscarriage:

- Genetic – chromosomal abnormalities account for over half of all early miscarriages. Incidence of genetic abnormalities increases with maternal age (Campbell and Monga, 2006).
- Endocrine – falling plasma progesterone levels from a failing corpus luteum; polycystic ovarian syndrome, poorly controlled diabetes and thyroid disease are also major risk factors (Symonds and Symonds, 2004).
- Infection – severe maternal febrile illnesses associated with bacterial or viral infections such as influenza, malaria and syphilis (Symonds and Symonds, 2004).
- Anatomical abnormalities – uterine congenital abnormalities and cervical incompetence (Impey, 2004).
- Immunological – antiphospholipid syndrome and thrombophilia may be discovered following recurrent miscarriages (Campbell and Monga, 2006).

Smoking and harmful chemical agents present risks during early pregnancy.

Natural miscarriage is an option offered to women with first trimester pregnancy loss. This is safe practice providing they have follow-up through EPAU, and are advised to seek medical help if experiencing excessive symptoms. Abdominal pain with heavy vaginal bleeding during miscarriage is an indication for hospital admission. A side-room is preferable so that her partner or alternative support person can stay. Bleeding and uterine cramps may continue if incomplete miscarriage causes products of conception to be retained within the uterus. This necessitates surgical evacuation of retained products of conception (ERPC). Anti-D is required for rhesus negative patients following ERPC.

If surgical intervention is delayed due to non-availability of an operating theatre, nurses may have to manage active miscarriage on the ward. Intramuscular opioid analgesia may be needed to reduce pain from uterine cramping, and a prophylactic anti-emetic. Fluid replacement with crystalloids is advisable, and excessive bleeding can be reduced using a synthetic oxytocin/ergometrine infusion or injection to contract the uterus. Pooling of clots and blood occurs when lying down, so bed rest is advised to prevent sudden heavy bleeding and fainting. Heavy bleeding necessitates one-to-one care, with regular pad changes for patient comfort. Taking time to explain interventions in an empathetic manner, answering questions and allowing couples to verbalise their feelings helps provide emotional support at this distressing time. Patient and partner are grieving and may harbour feelings of guilt. Reassurance that miscarriage is a natural process and not a result of their actions can be comforting. Encouragement is helpful where bleeding is slight or stops, but offering false hope should be avoided (Johnson, 2005). Clots and products should be assessed, to ensure retention of the embryo or placenta for histology to check for abnormalities. The products are sent for sensitive disposal by cremation unless the bereaved wish to make alternative arrangements. Each hospital will have individual protocols for disposal, so readers should check local guidelines. The hospital chaplain is usually available for advice and support, regardless of faith or culture.

Products of conception can distend the cervical canal, causing lower abdominal pain, hypotension, bradycardia and shock. Once removed, the uterus is able to contract (Symonds and Symonds, 2004). Secondary endometritis (infection of endometrial lining of womb) and haemorrhage can occur from tissue retained following caesarean section, elective termination of pregnancy or ERPC. Clinical signs are:

- heavy, often offensive smelling vaginal bleeding;
- pelvic pain or tenderness;
- pyrexia and tachycardia – if infection has spread beyond the uterus.

Endotoxic shock occurs in 5 per cent of septic miscarriages, requiring transfer to intensive care units (Oats and Abraham, 2005; Impey, 2004). Signs of endotoxic shock include:

- pyrexia
- rigors
- hypotension
- tachycardia
- renal failure
- acute respiratory distress syndrome
- disseminated intravascular coagulation.

If ultrasound reveals products retained in the uterus, further ERPC is indicated once infection has subsided, following intravenous antibiotic administration. Management of pelvic infections is discussed later. With heavy blood loss, a full blood count should be taken before discharge, to assess need for iron tablets or blood transfusion to correct anaemia.

In the absence of pain or bleeding, miscarriages may not be detected until the 12-week scan. Some women find it very distressing to continue carrying failed pregnancies, and opt for ERPC to guarantee a finite resolution, so they can grieve. Loss of a pregnancy can be very traumatic for a woman and her partner, especially under circumstances requiring emergency treatment. Grief intensity is more closely related to psychological attachment to the baby than length of gestation (Covington, 2000). Emotional support and sensitivity is required from nurses. Information about the Miscarriage Association, support groups and counselling should be offered on discharge. Advising couples to allow time to grieve and recover physically before trying to conceive again is paramount in preventing recurrent miscarriages. Future pregnancies should be referred to the EPAU for monitoring.

Menorrhagia

Menorrhagia is excessive blood loss during menstruation which interferes with the woman's physical, emotional, social and material quality of life (NICE, 2007c). It is the commonest reason for non-pregnant gynaecological referral.

Heavy bleeding in the absence of any abnormal pathology is referred to as dysfunctional uterine bleeding.

Underlying organic causes for menorrhagia include:

■ Uterine fibroids (myomata) – benign smooth muscle tumours arising from myometrium can increase endometrial surface area and vascularity, increasing blood flow, particularly submucous fibroids (Campbell and Monga, 2006).
■ Endometrial polyps – necrosis of surface of benign fine fibrous tissue core polyps can interfere with normal menstruation, causing heavy irregular bleeding (Symonds and Symonds, 2004).
■ Adenomyosis – infiltration of basal endometrial cells into myometrium stimulates myometrial proliferation and enlargement of the tumour (Oats and Abraham, 2005).
■ Endometriosis – endometrial lining displaced outside the uterus.
■ Inert or copper-containing intrauterine contraceptive devices (IUD) – a common iatrogenic cause of increased blood loss at menstruation (Symonds and Symonds, 2004).

Admission to hospital is necessary if:

■ serum haemoglobin level falls significantly to <8 g/litre, necessitating blood transfusion; or
■ bleeding is excessive, with clots.

Heavy bleeding is alarming for patients, who may experience shortness of breath and associated anxiety, so reassurance should be provided, pads changed and observed regularly, and treatment commenced as soon as possible. Good communication is essential, supported by evidence-based information to allow women to make informed decisions about their care and treatment (NICE, 2007c).

Diagnosis is made through pelvic examination, pelvic ultrasound and hysteroscopic inspection with endometrial biopsy. Management options depend on diagnosis and whether a woman wants to preserve reproductive function, requires contraception or has associated dysmenorrhoea (painful periods). NICE (2007c) recommend pharmaceutical management of symptoms:

First-line
■ Levonorgestrel intrauterine system (Mirena® coil) – can remain in utero for up to five years, reducing blood loss by more than 90 per cent, in addition to providing contraception (Impey, 2004).

Second-line
■ Antifibrinolytic agent – Tranexamic acid can reduce menstrual loss by half (Wellington and Wagstaff, 2003).
■ Non-steroidal anti-inflammatory drugs (NSAIDs) – prostaglandin synthetase inhibitor, e.g. mefenamic acid.
■ Combined oral contraceptive pill – blood loss reduced by half (Campbell and Monga, 2006).

Third line

■ Synthetic progestogens (norethisterone and medroxyprogesterone) – control heavy bleeding by preventing proliferation of endometrium.

Surgical treatments offer complete resolution of symptoms if pharmaceutical management fails, or is deemed necessary by the gynaecologist. These include endometrial ablation, hysterectomy, myomectomy or uterine artery embolisation, depending on the pathology, age, anatomy, surgical history and future fertility aspirations of the woman. All surgical procedures present a small risk of organ perforation, infection or haemorrhage. Laparoscopic surgical interventions are increasingly performed to reduce post-operative recovery time. Vaginal and laparoscopic hysterectomies present greater risks of complications than abdominal hysterectomy, but can significantly reduce post-operative recovery time and length of hospital stay when performed without incident. Severe perioperative complications occur in 3 per cent of hysterectomies (McPherson *et al.*, 2004). Risks decrease with age and increase with parity and history of serious illness.

Gynaecological malignancies

Irregular intermenstrual or postmenopausal bleeding in non-pregnant conditions should always be investigated, due to possible underlying malignancy. Advanced cervical and endometrial cancers may present with symptoms of heavy vaginal blood loss.

Bleeding points on cervical lesions can be embolised. Palliative radiotherapy may ease symptoms. In an emergency, vaginal packing can be used as a short-term measure. Anaemia should be rectified by blood transfusion provided kidney function is not impaired.

Total abdominal hysterectomy and removal of tubes and ovaries is the preferred surgical management for endometrial carcinomas. Pelvic nodes are also removed if there is suspicion of spread beyond endometrium.

Pelvic infections

Upper genital tract infections encompassing the uterus, ovaries and fallopian tubes are diagnosed under the blanket term pelvic inflammatory disease (PID). Many infections are asymptomatic. Pathogens enter via the vagina and cervix. In extreme cases, infection spreads via the lymphatic system causing sepsis and pelvic peritonitis. Most cases are triggered by untreated sexually transmitted bacterial infections such as chlamydia or gonorrhoea (Campbell and Monga, 2006).

The Royal College of Obstetricians and Gynaecologists (RCOG, 2003) have produced guidelines for management of acute PID. Clinical features for definitive diagnosis include:

■ lower abdominal pain and tenderness (bilateral adnexal tenderness);
■ deep dyspareunia (pain on intercourse);
■ abnormal vaginal or cervical discharge;

- cervical excitation (pain on moving the cervix);
- fever (>38°C).

Pyrexia may also generate a tachycardia >120 bpm. Raised white cell count (WCC) and C-reactive protein (CRP) support diagnosis. High vaginal swabs, routinely taken on admission, take 3 days to culture. Negative swab results do not exclude PID, as poor collection technique or delay in transport to laboratories may give false negative results (RCOG, 2003). Negative high vaginal swabs do not necessarily exclude infection if other clinical indicators suggest otherwise, so full antibiotic treatment should be given.

Ultrasound scanning can exclude other abnormalities as the source of pain. Detection of pyosalpinx, hydrosalpinx – pus or fluid in the tubes respectively, or pelvic abscesses – enhances suspicion of PID.

Acute episodes require in-patient admission for intravenous antibiotics and strong analgesia. If septicaemia is suspected, blood cultures should be taken. Samples take 48 hours to culture so broad-spectrum antibiotics are commenced on admission to cover *Neisseria gonorrhoeae, Chlamydia trachomatis* and anaerobic infections. RCOG (2003) recommend that in-patient treatment should continue until acute symptoms subside and the patient remains apyrexial for 24 hours.

IUDs can cause endometritis. Actinomycosis is a fungal infection seen almost exclusively in women with IUDs. Symptoms may mirror PID. Actinomycosis can be detected by cervical cytology. Undetected infection can cause widespread pelvic involvement, inflammatory masses fixing pelvic organs in 'frozen pelvis syndrome' (Campbell and Monga, 2006). Removal of the IUD by a doctor is necessary, followed by a course of intravenous and oral antibiotics. This syndrome significantly impacts on future fertility. Uterine infection in postmenopausal women is commonly linked with malignancy. Pyometrium occurs where pus accumulates in the uterus and cannot escape.

Pelvic infections can disastrously affect fertility. Scarring of tubes increases risks of ectopic pregnancy and subfertility. STIs readily spread through unprotected sexual intercourse so on diagnosis nurses should emphasise the need for women to contact ex-partners to be investigated. Advice on contraception and sexual health promotion can be discussed informally on discharge. Good communication skills and tact are required to tackle these sensitive and often embarrassing issues. Information on self-referral to a sexual health clinic should be offered, with assurance that confidentiality is absolute. Referral to the HIV clinical specialist nurse is recommended for any patient concerned about risk of HIV transmission or requiring counselling prior to testing.

Post-operative complications

Post-operative haemorrhage

Observation of post-operative vaginal bleeding is of paramount importance when nursing gynaecology patients. In combination with physiological assessments, early signs of haemorrhage and/or hypovolaemia can be detected. The uterus is highly vascular, especially a fibroid uterus or ante/post-partum.

Following vaginal hysterectomy or vaginal prolapse repair, the vagina is packed with proflavine-soaked gauze for 24 hours to reduce bleeding. On removal, patients remain on bed rest for one hour until blood loss is reassessed, to ensure it is minimal before mobilisation. If observed vaginal loss is moderate or clots appear, medical assistance should be summoned. While patients remain on bed rest, vital signs are monitored and pads changed regularly for patient comfort. Low molecular-weight heparin is given to prevent thromboembolism, but it can exacerbate post-operative haemorrhaging. Group and save serum is not routinely obtained pre-operatively for vaginal or laparoscopic surgery so, in addition to a full blood count, one should be obtained when excessive blood loss occurs. If haemorrhage recurs, repacking or return to theatre for cautery of bleeding points may be necessary. Silver nitrate sticks can be used by medical staff to cauterise persistent bleeding points following colposcopic cervical treatment.

Drains inserted peri-operatively during abdominal hysterectomy should be regularly monitored; drainage exceeding 200 ml frank blood in 24 hours could indicate internal bleeding. If drains are not inserted it is more difficult to observe for signs of internal haemorrhaging – the abdomen becomes tense, but pain is masked by post-operative analgesia. Hypovolaemia causes tachycardia and hypotension. Pulse rate exceeding systolic blood pressure in the absence of pyrexia suggests concealed blood loss and requires immediate medical or even surgical intervention. If blood pressure falls, with mean arterial pressure (MAP) below 65 mmHg, kidney perfusion is compromised. Urine should be measured hourly to monitor renal function. In acute situations either colloids or crystalloids can sustain circulating blood volume until blood is available for transfusion.

Wounds and post-operative infections

Observation of surgical wounds is a fundamental role of gynaecology nurses. Surgical site infections can cause serious post-operative febrile morbidity and increase hospital length of stay and readmission rates. Wounds healing by primary intention are usually sealed with fibrin within 24–48 hours (Prosser and McArthur-Rouse, 2007). Dressings should remain until the second post-operative day, unless wound examination is necessary due to excessive exudate or bleeding. Pelvic fluid collections and haematomas, common following a hysterectomy, may cause post-operative pyrexia. Ultrasound scans can detect and guide drainage of fluid collections to resolve suspected sources of infection. Many post-operative fluid collections resolve in time without risk of morbidity (Hasson *et al.*, 2007). Prophylactic antibiotics administered following abdominal hysterectomy decrease infection risk from 21 to 9 per cent (Eason *et al.*, 2004).

Other sources of sepsis should be investigated before commencing invasive treatment. Urinalysis excludes urinary tract infection. Catheters provide a convenient portal for bacteria to track up to the bladder, so good catheter care is imperative. Visual infusion phlebitis (VIP) scores for intravenous cannulae can indicate possible insertion-site infection. Post-operative chest infections are common, so assessment of respiratory rate, oxygen saturation levels and evidence of sputum production can prompt quick diagnosis. Early mobilisation post-operatively, deep-breathing exercises and effective analgesia help full expansion of lungs, reducing susceptibility to chest infection.

Clips or sutures remain in situ for 5–10 days, depending on incision type or consultant preferences. Dehiscence of sutures after removal indicates infection. Formation of a natural sinus allows pus to discharge from the wound. A hydrofibre packing agent like Aquacel© absorbs exudate to assist healing by secondary intention. Sinus packing should be changed at least daily, according to volume of exudate.

Ovarian cysts: acute events (rupture, haemorrhage and torsion)

Ovulation predisposes the ovary to cyst formation, from cyclical development of follicles that do not burst and release an egg. They often remain undetected unless discovered incidentally via ultrasound or they cause an acute event. Functional cysts are rare in users of oral contraceptive pills due to the ovulatory action of the hormone preparations.

The ovary is also susceptible to pathological cysts from endometriosis (endometrial tissue deposited outside the uterus) or malignancy. If the cyst is loculated, irregular, has solid components or abnormal blood vessels on ultrasound, further investigations are necessary to rule out ovarian malignancy. Pre-existing ovarian cysts can undergo rupture, haemorrhage or torsion initiating an acute onset of severe pain requiring admission to hospital for analgesia and observation.

Rupture of cyst content into the peritoneal cavity triggers sudden unilateral adnexal pain followed by generalised tenderness. Ultrasound shows free fluid in the Pouch of Douglas. Conservative treatment is recommended as reabsorption of fluid and resolution of symptoms occur naturally. Rupture of an endometriotic (chocolate) cyst may require emergency laparoscopy and surgical lavage, as contents irritate the peritoneum.

Severe unilateral adnexal pain can also be affected by haemorrhaging cysts. Haemorrhage into the peritoneal cavity is occasionally severe enough to cause hypovolaemic shock (Impey, 2004; see Chapter 27) so close observation and intravenous access is imperative. Haemorrhagic cysts are usually managed conservatively with analgesia to preserve ovarian tissue.

Torsion of the pedicle causes infarction and severe colicky pain. If left untreated the ovary becomes necrotic. If torsion is suspected, urgent diagnostic laparoscopy is required to untwist the pedicle to preserve ovarian tissue by restoring its blood supply. Removal is required if necrotic.

Ovarian hyperstimulation syndrome (OHSS)

OHSS is a systemic, iatrogenic condition caused by excessive luteinisation of ovaries. It most commonly occurs following IVF treatment, with high-dose gonadotrophins used to elicit a high number of oocytes for collection. Symptoms and complications of OHSS result from vasoactive products released by hyperstimulated ovaries, leading to increased capillary permeability and extravasation of fluid from intravascular to extravascular spaces (RCOG, 2006). This increases circulating blood viscosity and risk of developing deep vein thrombosis (DVT). Renal perfusion is impaired by hypovolaemia, but acute renal failure is rare. Extravascular accumulation of fluid such as ascites and pleural effusions are present in moderate to severe cases. Up to one-third of women undergoing IVF treatment experience mild OHSS and can be managed as outpatients. 3 to 8 per cent of IVF cycles are complicated by moderate or severe OHSS (RCOG, 2006), requiring management in specialist units. Presenting symptoms of moderate to severe OHSS following ovarian stimulation via IVF include:

- abdominal distension
- abdominal pain
- nausea and vomiting
- breathlessness
- oliguria.

Management of OHSS in hospital is concerned with rehydration, fluid balance (see Chapter 29), reducing risk of thromboembolism and providing reassurance. Guidelines for management include (RCOG, 2006; RCN, 2006):

- Rehydration with 2–3 litres of fluids per day (intravenous normal saline if unable to tolerate oral fluids) with strict fluid input/output recorded.
- Analgesics and anti-emetics to reduce pain and nausea.
- Daily girth and weight measurements.
- Anti-thromboembolic stockings and daily enoxaparin injections to reduce risk of thrombosis.
- Monitor urea and electrolytes, liver function, clotting and haemoconcentration (haematocrit and haemoglobin).
- Four-hourly observations.
- If tense ascites present, patients may be breathless and ultrasound-guided drainage is recommended, only 1 litre at a time to prevent excessive protein loss (Trew, 2007). Twenty per cent albumin can be infused to replace depleted protein. Intravenous colloid infusion can be considered for large-volume drainage (RCOG, 2006).

Moderate to severe OHSS primarily occurs in patients who are pregnant as the ovarian luteinising process is sustained by production of hCG. They should be reassured that the condition does not adversely affect pregnancy, and resolves in time. There is no evidence of increased risk of congenital abnormalities or miscarriage in women with OHSS (RCOG, 2006). Couples should liaise with their assisted conception unit if they have any further concerns.

Chronic gynaecological disease

Advanced cervical carcinoma commonly causes hydronephrosis, from tumours extending into the pelvis obstructing one or both kidneys. This often causes considerable pain, uraemia and significant rises in creatinine as kidney function is impaired. Treatment is referral to a urologist, for stent insertion to reopen the ureters. If this fails, palliative urinary diversion by insertion of percutaneous nephrostomies may be considered. When concerned about renal function a strict fluid chart should be maintained and electrolytes monitored.

The four most common complications of advanced ovarian cancer are ascites, bowel obstruction, pleural effusions and malnutrition (Errikson and Frazier, cited RCN, 2005d).

- Bowel obstruction – medical management includes keeping patient nil-by-mouth to rest the bowel, provide adequate intravenous fluids, and possibly commencing steroids. If this fails, palliative surgery may be performed to divert the bowel into a stoma to bypass the obstruction.
- Ascites – tense ascites can be drained by paracentesis. This, however, causes protein loss.
- Pleural effusion – needle aspiration of fluid relieves breathlessness.
- Malnutrition – anxiety, depression, nausea and poor pain control are appetite suppressants, and can be treated. Referral to a dietician and regular weight recording helps prevent further deterioration.

Women living with gynaecological cancer may experience temporary or permanent loss of sexual functioning and femininity. Loss of function and sexual desire can greatly affect self-esteem and much emotional support may be needed. Cancer affects the patient, family and friends. Pain and other symptoms often cause psychological distress (Regnard and Hockley, 2004). Forging a relationship with the patient and family helps to identify these issues so they can be addressed. The palliative care team can support patients, relatives and nurses regarding pain and nausea relief and psychological care. The chaplain is also an invaluable resource.

Implications for practice

- Nurses should have a fundamental knowledge of gynaecological emergencies.
- Prompt recognition of symptoms is necessary for ensuring effective management.
- Problems in early pregnancy can be life-threatening.
- Close monitoring of observations, vaginal blood loss, blood test results and patient comfort level is required.
- Allow time to explain tests/test results and answer questions to alleviate anxiety and empower patients.
- Make sure patients are seen in an area that promotes privacy and dignity.

Summary

Acute gynaecological events can occur in women who are otherwise healthy, and can compensate for long periods before showing clinical signs of being unwell. It is important to establish if a woman is pregnant on admission to the unit. If ectopic pregnancy or OHSS is suspected, the woman should be treated in a specialist unit as soon as possible as these are potentially life-threatening conditions that require prompt intervention. Nurses should closely monitor vital signs and fluid balance, be aware of abnormal blood results and ultrasound reports, and act upon them.

Clinical scenario

Jane Almond is 38 years old, and presents in A&E with abdominal pain and distension, nausea and oliguria. She underwent embryo transfer seven days ago during IVF treatment at a private hospital. Blood tests show a raised haematocrit and urea. The on-call gynaecology Senior House Officer is new to his post and has diagnosed OHSS but is unsure of the current management protocol.

1   What would you advise him as being his first priorities in A&E?

2   A third-year nursing student asks you to explain OHSS. Write a paragraph explaining the syndrome in a way a student nurse is able to understand.

3   Jane is feeling very anxious about the baby as she has had a positive pregnancy test. Jane and her husband have been trying to conceive for eight years. How would you reassure Jane?

4   Identify the main aspects of care for monitoring the syndrome over the next few days on a general ward.

Bibliography

Key reading

Authoritative guidelines are provided by RCOG Green-top guidelines (www.rcog. org.uk/index.asp?PageID=1042), RCN (2006) and NICE (2007c), while Regnard and Hockley's (2004) is a classic textbook for symptom management in palliative care, and includes more in-depth information on symptoms experienced with advanced gynaecological malignancies.

Further reading

Johnson (2005) provides a psychosocial perspective on fundamental aspects of gynaecology nursing. Symonds and Symonds (2004) provide a medical overview of gynaecological disorders.

Support groups and useful contacts

Stillbirth and Neonatal Death Society (SANDS): 0207 4365881
Child Bereavement Trust: 08453 571000
The Miscarriage Association www.miscarriageassociation.org.uk/ma2006/index. htm.

Part 6

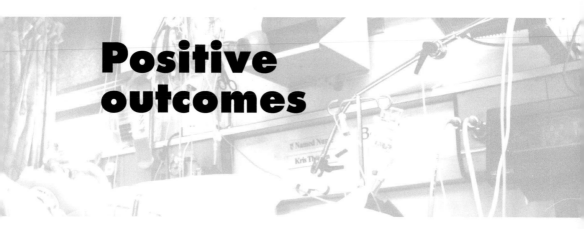

Positive
outcomes

Chapter 36

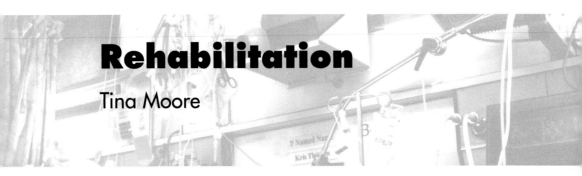

Rehabilitation

Tina Moore

Contents

Learning outcomes

After reading this chapter you will be able to:

- understand the concept of rehabilitation and associated strategies;
- analyse current practice in relation to health promotion and rehabilitation;
- appreciate the importance of partnership within the acute care setting;
- acknowledge opportunities with your own practice setting to implement concepts of rehabilitation.

Fundamental knowledge

Stress (Chapter 13); psychological disturbances (Chapter 11); health promotion models.

Introduction

As part of routine clinical activities there is an expectation that nurses undertake and participate in health promotion/rehabilitation activities. Studies suggest that intervention/strategies aiding recovery are sparse (Jones *et al.*, 2003; Robinson *et al.*, 2006). This intervention should be viewed as an integral part of most care activities rather than as a separate and 'add on' activity (Jones *et al.*, 2003). Rehabilitation should start as early as possible, even if it means within the intensive care unit (ICU) (Gutenbrunner *et al.*, 2007).

Anecdotal evidence within acute/critical care suggests that health promotional activities are usually limited by their unstructured, haphazard, ad hoc approaches, and are far more likely to be opportunistic and limited to information-giving. This may be influenced by the critical nature of the patient's history and the perceived lack of time. Today, in most wards discharge planning starts with admission, although this may inevitably become a paper exercise. Although the need for physical rehabilitation is well established substantive evidence to guide rehabilitation services is lacking (Baker and Mansfield, 2008).

Health promotion can start before the onset of critical illness (where possible) as some patients undergo planned treatment that will make them acutely or critically ill afterwards. So, pre-planned visits to a critical care unit (by ward nurses) or pre-assessment clinic can provide health promotion opportunities both before and after treatment.

Due to the severity of their illness, patients may not have the capacity or desire to be involved in rehabilitation. The nurse must set priorities that place immediate physical and psychological safety above rehabilitation. However, once the patient has passed the 'critical phase' of their illness and are assessed as competent (Chapter 41) rehabilitation should begin/resume. Opportunities for health promotion/rehabilitation within critical care exist, but are often missed, possibly resulting in some patients feeling unprepared for discharge to general wards.

This particular chapter will discuss rehabilitation in relation to the acutely ill. Particular emphasis is made on creating a culture to enable this to happen. Strategies to help achieve this will also be discussed.

Time out 36.1

1 Write down your own definition of rehabilitation.
2 What does it mean to you?
3 Now read the following section and compare your definition with those given below.

Health promotion

Health promotion is an integral part of rehabilitation. Health promotion is the process of enabling people to increase control over, and to improve, their health (WHO, 1986). Definitions of health promotion remain broad and potentially unhelpful within clinical practice due to their lack of strategic direction, particularly in relation to the acutely or critically ill patient.

Conceptualisation of health in its broadest sense must occur if a health promotion model is to be followed adequately. This should incorporate a holistic view (physical, mental, social and spiritual) and is required to be a developmental process. Patients suffering from the acute effects of diabetic ketoacidosis (newly diagnosed) will need to accept the fact that they are now diabetic (this initially involves exploring belief and values). Social values and how diabetes may affect their current lifestyle should be considered before educating them about diet, education regarding blood glucose monitoring, insulin administration and avoiding hypoglycaemia.

Foundations of health promotion are built upon empowerment and partnership. These features include holism, equity, participation, collaboration, individualisation, negotiation, facilitation and support. A 'sick-nursing' approach is distinguished by interactions that are dominating, generalised, prescriptive, reassuring and directive (Jonsdottir *et al.*, 2004). All nursing interactions have the potential to be health promoting; however, the culture of the clinical setting should foster a facilitative environment before health promotion activities can begin.

Initially, acutely ill patients will require a 'sick-nursing' approach. However, unhealthy dependency is encouraged if this approach continues when patients are in the recovery phase of their illness.

Rehabilitation

Rehabilitation is a dynamic process that facilitates the process of enabling an individual re-establish and regain optimal functioning as is possible. It involves re-education and retraining; re-learning skills and learning new skills in an attempt to restore the individual to an optimal level of health and in doing so restoring their sense of worth and dignity.

Rehabilitation is defined as a process of active change by which a person who has become disabled requires the knowledge and skills needed for optimal physical, psychological and social function (Gutenbrunner *et al.*, 2007).

Therefore, rehabilitation strategies should be active and dynamic with assumed committed involvement from the patient. It is designed to enable the patient to regain lost essentials of their life, e.g. physical functioning and psychological sense of well-being. Strategies are designed to promote optimal functioning for the patient and, therefore, enhancing quality of life that is meaningful. This could incorporate: physical, mental, social, emotional and productive well-being.

Skills required

Features of rehabilitation include:

- holism
- equity

- participation
- collaboration
- individualisation
- negotiation
- facilitation
- support.

These skills may be the same as in any other area of nursing but it is the application of those skills in rehabilitation that make it unique. Skills require commitment to the concept of health promotion and rehabilitation. The ultimate aim is the empowerment of the patient (discussed later). In order to achieve this, nurses must be flexible, adopt an individualised approach, providing a therapeutic environment, where the patient can flourish and having specialised knowledge and understanding of the rehabilitation process. They should also have the ability to offer constant support and positive reinforcement not only to the patient but also the family.

In order to empower others, nurses need such attributes as courage, commitment, intuitive understanding, flexibility, an appreciation of diversity, tolerance, co-operativeness, willingness to compromise and empathy (Ralph and Taylor, 2005).

Rehabilitation should be actively promoted with acute care. To achieve this collaboration between other healthcare professionals is essential (Ball, 2008).

Rehabilitation strategies

Strategies are currently unco-ordinated (Ball, 2008; Strahan and Brown, 2005) and are not routinely provided, particularly after hospital discharge (Jones *et al.*, 2003). After illness patients can suffer reduced physical function and quality of life up to 12 months post discharge (Herridge *et al.*, 2003; Orme *et al.*, 2003). Measures must be in place to prevent avoidable physical and non-physical morbidity. The NICE draft guidelines (due 2009) suggest at least a six-week rehabilitation plan together with a co-ordinated approach.

An assessment of learning needs and readiness to learn from both the patient and family should be performed. Short- and medium-term rehabilitation goals should be identified and agreed. An educational plan of care (rehabilitation care pathway) that is individualised should be developed, implemented and evaluated. This should occur for rehabilitation to be effective.

Where possible, the patient's education process should place responsibility on the individual for health and rehabilitating behaviours. The goal is to promote the individual to their optimum in terms of health.

More guidance will be available from NICE in relation to rehabilitation and the critically ill patient currently in draft form for consultation, due for publication 2009. This is a much needed guidance, not only to provide strategic direction (currently lacking in the draft), but also to remind nurses of the importance of rehabilitation as part of the overall care package. It will remain to be seen how much strategic direction will be given.

Empowerment

1   Think about your own beliefs and values, and those of the staff you work with, in relation to rehabilitation within your area of practice. Write down your thoughts.
2   Does your list relate towards empowering patients or a paternalistic approach?

Approaches to care can be paternalistic, where healthcare professionals think they know what was in the best interests of 'their' patient. Paternalistic care is often characterised by authoritarian, prescriptive, persuasive and generalised information given by the 'expert' to 'ignorant' laypersons. There is a need for an empowering, client-centred and collaborative approach. There will always be situations in acute/critical care that indicate paternalistic actions, and in some situations acting paternalistically is regarded as a duty, e.g. consider, a patient who is in hypovolaemic shock, requiring invasive monitoring and aggressive fluid replacement, while very anxious and still suffering from the psychological trauma of being admitted to the ward as an emergency. Physical safety is a priority and, therefore, the physiological status of the patient requires urgent attention. There is a thin dividing line between respecting a person's autonomy on the one hand and being open to the charge of negligence or failure of duty to care on the other (Tingle and Cribb, 2000).

A nurturing and caring environment is necessary for the promotion of health/ rehabilitation, not one of inappropriate paternalism. There must also be willingness and consent of both the nurse and the patient. Nurses need to respect the patient's individual capacity for growth and self-determination. The process of empowerment is a developmental one, increasing the shift of power and control of patients by increasing their knowledge and skill, and ability to participate. These include characteristics such as trust, openness, honesty, genuineness, communication and interpersonal skills, acceptance of people as they are, mutual respect, value of others, courtesy and shared vision. There must also be willingness of consent of both the nurse and the patient. The nurse must possess and use professional skills, e.g. teaching skills, facilitation.

Empowerment requires improving and increasing the patient's control. Reports from the Government repeatedly emphasise this process. Within practice the term 'empowerment' could be used inappropriately, influenced by perceptions/ understanding of the concept. The process of empowerment is a developmental one, increasing the shift of power and control to patients by increasing their knowledge and skill and ability to participate.

The above have implications for nursing practice, in that nurses must trust the patient's (who are assessed as competent and able to undergo rehabilitation) ability to make decisions, accept responsibility and act for themselves. Equally, for many patients, health might not be an important concern; some might choose

> **Box 36.1 Key features of empowerment**
>
> ■ Clarification of individuals' beliefs and values about themselves, health and health-influencing behaviour (Liimatainen *et al.*, 2001), e.g. patients who are admitted with uncontrolled hypertension should be encouraged to articulate what hypertension means to them, what affect it has on them, and how they can change their lifestyle and dietary habits.
> ■ A requirement to foster empowerment through raising self-esteem, beliefs about self-efficacy and the acquisition of life skills (Tones, 1991) in patients, e.g. by constant reassurance and by allowing them time to make decisions relating to how they will adapt or change their lifestyle. Nurses should not dictate to patients what they should be doing unless requested by the patient.
> ■ A partnership approach to communication – i.e. communicating *with* patients, not *at* them.

not to heed the advice given for attaining better health, therefore, nurses need to assess the patient's potential for requiring health promotion information.

Power versus control

Before attempting to be involved in rehabilitation, nurses must be willing to relinquish their control of the nurse–patient relationship and allow the patient to make more decisions. The attitude that the 'nurses know best' fosters a sense of dependency. Patient participation should be encouraged (at any level) and nurses need to be prepared to accept that patients may make decisions that are different from those that might be decided for them. This can only occur if the nurse assumes that health belongs to the individual (i.e. the patient) who is, therefore, responsible for his or her own health. Owing to the nature of acute care, this may in some instances be difficult to achieve.

Passive patients should be actively encouraged to participate in healthcare. This may prove to be difficult, as some patients are socialised in the tradition of the medical model and expect to be told what to do by the 'expert'. There are some patients who do not want to be involved in decisions about their care. In these situations, gradual facilitation by constant involvement in the decision-making process should be encouraged. Despite this, it must be remembered that individuals have the right to accept, adopt, or reject the information provided.

Partnership

While the idea of a nurse–patient partnership is appealing, nursing literature has been unclear about the elements and processes in such a partnership. This lack of clarity is hardly surprising as definitions of partnership differ in scope and vary according to the context of the partnership and types of partners (Gallant *et al.*, 2002). Such inconsistent use makes it difficult to find common ground to communicate about partnership.

Once the patient's condition permits, the nurse should assume a facilitative role, acting as a resource person and facilitating rehabilitation in a non-judgemental way. For success, both patient and nurse must commit to the role required in partnership. In partnership, the nurse brings nursing knowledge and clinical experiences, while the patient brings experiential knowledge about health and managing health concerns.

Nurses can promote patient partnership by

- maintaining the relationship;
- having positive attitudes towards patients and be willing to relinquish the status and privilege associated with being a nurse (Munro *et al.*, 2000);
- reinforcing patient progress;
- supporting decision-making;
- assisting the patient to learn new knowledge and skills.

Implications for practice

- Nurses need to assess the patient's potential for requiring rehabilitation.
- Nurses must trust the patient's ability to make decisions and accept reasonability to act for themselves.
- Rehabilitation might not be an important concern for many patients, either through severity of illness or lack of interest or motivation.

Summary

Rehabilitation activities should start as soon as the patient's condition allows and does not have to involve complicated processes. Prerequisites to facilitate partnership and empowerment need to be in place before rehabilitation attempts are successful.

Clinical scenario

Linda Thomas, a 44-year-old single mother with three pre-teen children, was admitted with bowel obstruction and underwent small bowel surgery involving colectomy and formation of a temporary colostomy. She was admitted for stabilisation and was intubated for less than 24 hours. She progressed from level 3 to level 2 care after two days. Linda is still very weak; her main complaints were poor appetite, lack of sleep and abdominal discomfort.

1 Outline the assessment you would perform before writing a rehabilitation plan for her.

2 What strategies will you employ to aid her recovery?

3 What criteria would you use to monitor success?

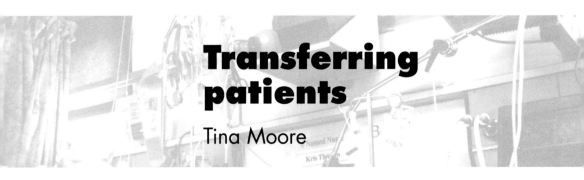

Chapter 37

Transferring patients

Tina Moore

Contents

Learning outcomes

After reading this chapter you will be able to:

- understand the needs of the patient before, during and after transfer from critical care units to the ward and from the ward to the critical care unit;
- recognise actual and potential problems relating to the critically ill following transfer and suggest strategies for resolution/coping;
- identify educational requirements of self and others;
- transfer a patient safely.

Introduction

The aim of transferring a critically ill patient to the critical care unit is to improve prognosis. Critically ill patients have a high risk of morbidity and mortality during transportation. Patients who have been transferred within departments have received sub-optimal care (Gray *et al.*, 2003). Through better preparation for the transfer and improved communication, many of the problems that occurred could be avoided (Ligtenberg *et al.*, 2005).

Transferring a patient from the critical care unit to the ward is also not without its problems. Trust guidelines on transferring patients to and from departments should now be readily available. Equally, guidance for patients being transferred to other hospitals (mainly from critical care units and accident and emergency) should also be accessible.

This chapter will discuss procedures in transferring critically ill patients from the ward to a critical care unit and the ward receiving acutely ill patients from critical care units.

Transfer of patients from the ward to a critical care unit

Publications (DOH, 2000a; ICS, 2002; NICE, 2007a) have documented the necessity for, and importance of, appropriate standards, equipment, procedures and staff training when dealing with the transfer of critically ill patients. These publications, while intending to provide guidance on inter-hospital transfers may, in some parts, be useful for intra-hospital transfers. The following discussions are not restricted to general ward areas but include areas such as accident and emergency departments and out-patient departments.

It is the duty of the referring ward to ensure that a safe transfer takes place. It is also their responsibility to inform the relatives prior to transfer (wherever possible). It is the duty of the receiving area to ensure that they are ready to accept the patient. Patients will require psychological preparation, including an awareness of the reasons for transfer (if patients are able). Bed managers should be informed of patients needing to be transferred. Once a bed is agreed by the critical care consultant, transport must be arranged immediately. The receiving unit should be called prior to the departure. Some hospitals have special transfer trolleys for the critically ill, while other hospitals transfer patients via their bed. Where Outreach is in place transfers are usually assisted by a member of the Critical Care Outreach Team (CCOT) (Chapter 38).

Assessment and physiological optimisation *before* transfer should be attempted for all transfers (Dunn *et al.*, 2007). This aims to help achieve optimum recovery for the patient, though it must be remembered that ward transfers are a combination of achievability and the need for urgent transfer. This means that there has to be a balance between achieving physiological optimisation and movement to the critical care unit (as much as possible), as delays may be harmful to some patients. Yet for others, longer pre-transfer times will not adversely affect outcome and pre-transfer optimisation may be beneficial (ICS, 2002).

Monitoring capabilities are limited during transportation. The patient's resuscitation and stabilisation should follow the ABCDE approach (Chapter 6). If airway or ventilation is compromised, this must be dealt with by intubation. The transfer should be carried out by competent individuals (qualified nurse and the patient's doctor).

The role of the nurse in transferring a patient is to

- monitor the patient's ABCDE;
- act as the patient's advocate;
- maintain respect of the patient's privacy, dignity and confidentiality;
- ensure that the correct documentation has been completed;
- provide nursing handover.

Box 37.1 Examples of documentation required

- A completed written transfer (summary) report – chief complaint; allergies; medical history; reason for transfer; age; vital signs and treatment already performed together with the outcome
- Up-to-date observation charts, medical and nursing documentation
- X-rays
- Laboratory results

An additional verbal handover is required.

Transfer from critical care areas to general wards

NICE clinical guideline 50 (NICE, 2007a) provides guidance in transferring acutely ill patients aiming for a safe and efficient transition from the critical care area to general wards. It does not provide recommendations for the transfer from ward areas.

Recommendations include:

A. Transfer 'within' hours as much as possible. Between the times of 22.00 and 7.00 should be avoided and if inevitable should be documented as an adverse incident.

(NICE, 2007a)

Studies conclude that the timing of transfer from ICUs to general wards was associated with increased hospital mortality (Tobin and Santamaria, 2006; Beck *et al.*, 2002), together with an influence on the ICU re-admission rate and could also be linked to premature transfer. In Finland it was established that there was no association between times of transfer and death (Uusaro *et al.*, 2003). Reliability of the study could be questioned or it may be that the results reflect excellent care provision. Box 37.2 shows the result of poor discharge planning.

> **Box 37.2 Reasons for poor discharge planning**
>
> - Discontinuity of care
> - Delayed recovery
> - Adverse health outcomes
> - Readmission to critical care
>
> (NICE, 2007a)

B. The critical care area transferring team and the receiving ward team should take shared responsibility for the care of the patient being transferred. They should jointly ensure:

- the use of a formal structured handover of care from critical care area staff and ward staff (medical and nursing) to ensure continuity of care;
- that the receiving ward, with support from critical care if required, can deliver the agreed plan.

(NICE, 2007a)

The formal structured handover of care should include:

- a summary of critical care stay including diagnosis and treatment;
- a monitoring and investigation plan;
- a plan for ongoing treatment, including drugs, therapies, nutrition and infection status together with any agreed limitations of treatment;
- physical and rehabilitation needs;
- psychological and emotional needs;
- specific communication or language needs.

(NICE, 2007a)

Transfer from the security of critical care (usually nursing 1:1 or 1:2) to the general ward areas where a nurse could be caring for up to 12 patients can be stress provoking for the patient and indeed relatives (Chapters 4 and 13). Patients can experience a reduction in the degree of care provision in the ward areas. This can prove to be worse if nurses on general wards are not fully aware of the patient's physical, emotional and psychological needs.

Many patients will experience a follow-up from the CCOT. While NICE recommends that all acute hospitals should have a CCOT there are still some Trusts where this provision is not available. It is, therefore, up to the general ward nurses to try and maintain continuity of care.

C. When patients are transferred to the general ward from a critical care area, they should be offered information about their condition and encouraged to actively participate in decisions that relate to their recovery. The information should be tailored to individual circumstances. If they (patient) agree, their family and carers should be involved.

(NICE, 2007a)

Patients found that a lack of continuity of care was due to poor communication between ICU and ward staff (Strahan and Brown, 2005). Critical care nurses should discuss the transfer with the patient, highlighting differences in care provision, e.g. less monitoring equipment and higher nurse:patient ratio than 1:1. In an ideal situation a nurse from the receiving ward should visit the patient, aiming for a smooth transition between critical care and the ward. In preparing the patient for transfer, critical care nurses should reduce the amount of monitoring the patient requires, e.g. two-hourly observations, a reduction in the monitoring equipment (i.e. arterial blood pressure monitoring, possibly central venous pressure monitoring).

The experience of being transferred from critical care areas to the ward

Patients can and do suffer physical and emotional experiences on transfer (relocation stress). Physical symptoms include gross physical weakness, possibly frailty; lack of mobility; sleep deprivation; minor to moderate pain; bowel complications; feelings of sickness and nausea leading to loss of appetite (McKinney and Deeny, 2002; Strahan and Brown, 2005). Some physical symptoms could last up to three months (McKinney and Deeny, 2002). Some patients believe that being transferred out of critical care areas is a step towards physical progression (McKinney and Deeny, 2002), a feeling of being able to take more control and a desire for normality.

Emotional experiences included: anxiety, loneliness and isolation on the wards, leading to depression; feelings of insecurity, exhaustion and confusion. They also observed different levels of care (McKinney and Deeny, 2002). Ward staff were found to have a lack of understanding about the patient's weak physiological status (McKinney and Deeny, 2002; Strahan and Brown, 2005). While patients acknowledge the differences in staffing levels they still experienced feelings such as abandonment.

D. Staff working with acutely ill patients on general wards should be provided with education and training to recognise and understand the physical, psychological and emotional needs of patients who have been transferred from critical care areas.

(NICE, 2007a)

Patients discharged from critical care units are at greater risk of clinical deterioration (DOH, 2000a). It is important that patients are followed up from either critical care staff or CCOT. Ward nurses must also have the appropriate knowledge, skill and attitude to care for such patients. This should be reflected in their appraisal with their manager.

Needs of the patient

According to the literature the patient requires

- continuity of care between critical care area and ward staff;
- high-quality individualised care;
- realistic expectations from ward staff and help with managing their physical and emotional experiences;
- help with managing the transition from one-to-one care;
- information tailored to their individual needs.

(Strahan and Brown, 2005)

Implications for practice

- Nurses need to be aware of the patient's needs in relation to information of their condition and about the transfer.
- The patient has a right to experience a safe and uneventful transfer.
- Nurses should attempt to understand/appreciate the perspective of the patient and attempt to address their needs.
- Receiving nurses should continue the plan of care identified by the critical care nurses.

Summary

It is noted that all studies did not consider the use of intermediate levels of care, i.e. HDU, and, therefore, it is unknown whether some of the documented experiences would have been different. Patients should not be transferred from critical care areas unless the receiving ward has the resources to be able to deliver the agreed care plan (NICE, 2007a). This is also seen to include the knowledge and skill of the nurses. Patients should be prepared for transfer from critical care areas as early as the patient's condition allows. Preparation and information should be tailored to the individual needs. A formal structured handover of care should address the patient's needs (NICE, 2007a).

Clinical scenario

Abdool Dervish, 18 years old, is admitted to your ward from A&E after sustaining a head injury. He was playing rugby and suffered a head collision with another player. He has no other suspected injuries (including neck). Neurological observations have been recorded and are uneventful.

Three hours after admission his condition deteriorates. GCS score shows signs of increasing intracranial pressure (Chapter 9) and he is becoming progressively more agitated.

After being examined by the doctor a CT scan is requested.

1   Consider what could go wrong with this transfer.

2   List your priorities in transferring this patient (including equipment required).

3   Write down how you would ensure a safe and efficient transfer for Abdool.

Bibliography

Further reading

Gray *et al.* (2004) provide a comprehensive guide for transporting critically ill patients; while its orientation is more medical, nurses will find it very useful.

Chapter 38

Critical Care Outreach and the early detection of acute illness

Debbie Higgs

Contents

Learning outcomes

After reading this chapter you will be able to:

- understand and appreciate the concept of Outreach, its aims and objectives;
- understand how the early warning score is applied to the acutely ill patient.

Introduction

The aim of this chapter is to explore the subject of Critical Care Outreach services and the use of physiological track and trigger systems to detect developing critical illness. Outreach is part of an innovative approach to critical care, which is based on a patient's needs, rather than their location in the hospital. In recent years Critical Care Outreach services have become a popular choice for NHS Acute hospitals in helping manage acutely ill patients outside the traditional boundaries of intensive care units (ICU).

Background to Outreach services

Patients who are, or become, acutely unwell in hospital require prompt intervention by experienced, healthcare professionals. Unfortunately an increasing body of evidence has emerged suggesting that some hospital patients exhibit premonitory signs of cardiac arrest which may be observed by nursing and medical staff, but which frequently are not acted upon (Franklin and Mathew, 1994; Rich, 1999). Similar findings have been observed in relation to deterioration in patients' conditions prior to admission to ICUs (Goldhill *et al.*, 1999a; McQuillan *et al.*, 1998; McGloin *et al.*, 1999). More recently the National Confidential Enquiry into Patient Outcome and Death (NCEPOD, 2005) reviewed the care given to medical patients referred for level 3 care. They identified the prime causes for the substandard care of the acutely ill in hospital as being delayed recognition and institution of inappropriate therapy that subsequently culminated in a late referral. The study found that on a number of occasions these factors were aggravated by poor communication between the acute and critical care medical teams. These studies suggest that early recognition and treatment of these signs may prevent the necessity for some ICU admissions, thus reducing morbidity and mortality, and making better use of costly intensive care resources. As patients admitted from hospital wards have a higher overall percentage mortality than patients admitted from other areas of the hospital (Goldhill and Sumner, 1998) an improvement in the management of seriously ill patients prior to ICU admission could potentially improve outcome.

A frequently cited study by McQuillan *et al.* (1998) examined the quality of care received by 100 patients prior to admission to intensive care. Their results indicated that 54 per cent of the cohort received sub-optimal care. The main reasons for staff failing to manage basic vital signs were attributed to delays in seeking advice, failure to recognise clinical urgency, lack of knowledge and skills in resuscitation and organisational problems within the hospital. The assessors believed that this had a significant impact on individual morbidity and mortality. A similar study by McGloin *et al.* (1999) confirmed these findings: 37 per cent of their patients received sub-optimal care with a significantly increased mortality. These papers provoked widespread discussion.

While much of the cited literature supports and highlights the view that seriously ill ward patients are often missed or inappropriately managed, it must be acknowledged why this phenomenon has arisen. In recent years the technological developments led to an increase in the number of procedures that are carried out in day surgery. Those patients who are now cared for in acute general wards are often older, undergoing major surgical procedures, or are acutely ill. Advancements in anaesthetic and critical care techniques have enabled higher-risk patients to undergo major surgical procedures that previously would have been inappropriate, additionally a reduction in the number of hospital beds (a result of shorter length stays) has led to an increase in the acuity of illness of hospital patients. The ability of critical care units to cope with this influx of sick patients continues to be a problem with capacity far outstripped by demand. In addition, the demand on critical care beds not infrequently results in significantly reduced stays for certain patients because of the need to make the bed available for the next admission. This practice, as highlighted by Daly *et al.* (2001), can put patients at risk, with early discharges in certain groups of patients causing an increase in mortality. The net effect of these occurrences is an increase in the acuity and dependency of patients being cared for in acute general wards (Coad and Haines, 1999). Meanwhile, difficulties in the recruitment and retention of qualified staff have led to a dilution of the skill mix in many areas. Therefore, inexperienced junior staff may frequently be expected to care for more highly dependent patients.

Several strategies for reducing the occurrence of sub-optimal care and to improve the early identification of sick patients have been proposed. These focus predominantly on the identification of patients at risk of critical illness and the provision of a graded response strategy to provide expert advice in the management of these patients (Audit Commission, 1999; Daffurn *et al.*, 1994; DOH, 2000a; Goldhill, 1997; Goldhill *et al.*, 1999b; Lee *et al.*, 1995; Morgan *et al.*, 1997; NCEPOD, 2005; NICE, 2007a). Lee *et al.* (1995) in an attempt to prevent cardio-pulmonary arrest and improve outcome introduced the concept of a medical emergency team (MET) in Australia. This involved a team built around multidisciplinary staff that responded to pre-defined physiological criteria. This innovation became the foundation for the implementation of Critical Care Outreach teams in the UK.

Critical Care Outreach teams

The introduction of Outreach teams was part of the innovative approach to the early detection and treatment of deterioration in ward-based patients. If treatment of patients experiencing deterioration in their condition is delayed they could die or require emergency admission to the ICU. It is thought that if staff could identify and manage patients earlier, then patient safety would be improved and poor outcomes avoided. Outreach teams are able to respond to calls when a patient is deteriorating and provide expert support at the bedside.

Acute hospitals have generally embraced the concept of Outreach. McDonnell *et al.* (2007) reported that in a recent survey of NHS acute hospitals in England that routinely provide level 1 care, 139 (73 per cent) have an Outreach team. This approval has been influenced by the changes introduced several years ago through the Audit Commission Report (Audit Commission, 1999) and *Comprehensive Critical Care* (DOH, 2000a). The Audit Commission Report set out a number of recommendations for staff to consider when reviewing critical care provision. One such approach was to reduce cost through flexibility using resources effectively. Improving ward care and recognising critical illness it suggested, as it develops, would potentially prevent admissions or make them much timelier, resulting in shorter stays. This view was echoed in *Comprehensive Critical Care* (DOH, 2000a) and resulted in the development of a framework for the future organisation and delivery of adult critical care services. The document also reclassified patients' dependencies. This has since been expanded in agreement with the Department of Health and the Intensive Care Society (ICS, 2002), in order to provide greater clarity between levels. Their vision for future critical care services included the establishment of an Outreach team to provide and support the care of level 1 patients on general wards and critical care facilities to meet the needs of level 2 and 3 patients.

This reinforced the view that it is the patients who hold the dependency level and not the beds. It also called for the flexible use of beds and provision of support services for long-term patients and those requiring follow-up. It stated that Outreach services are an integral part of comprehensive critical care and have three essential objectives:

- to avert admissions by identifying patients who are deteriorating and either helping to prevent admission or ensuring that admission to a critical care bed happens in a timely manner to ensure best outcome;
- to enable discharges by supporting the continuing recovery of discharged patients on wards and post discharge from hospital and their relatives and friends;
- to share critical care skills with staff in wards and the community-ensuring enhancement of training opportunities and skills practice and to use information gathered from the ward and community to improve critical care services for patients and relatives.

(DOH, 2000a)

Time out 38.1

Reflecting on the objectives above, consider as a member of a ward team what support you would need to manage an acutely ill or deteriorating patient in your care. Where would you get this support from?

Since this time Outreach services have continued to evolve, primarily to meet local requirements. Due to the differing priorities, needs and resources of individual hospitals, the teams themselves vary considerably in the way they deliver services. Some are nurse led, others are multidisciplinary and some are simply individuals charged with the task of delivering all the demands of an Outreach service. Nationally, Critical Care Outreach teams have worked collaboratively to promote the role of teams across the country. The National Outreach Forum and the Critical Care Stakeholders Forum have joined together to produce a document, which described the role of Outreach in supporting patient care.

They suggested that the objectives of any service should be to:

- improve the quality of acute patient care, patient experience and reduce adverse clinical events;

- enhance clinical staff confidence, competence and experience through training and the sharing of skills;
- improve organizational agility and resilience by delivering comprehensive care across organisational and professional boundaries, directorates or locations.

(National Outreach Forum and Critical Care Stakeholders Forum, 2007)

Outreach teams have been pivotal in sharing critical care skills. Evidence produced in the report by the National Critical Care Outreach Forum (2003) indicated that 94 per cent of respondents reporting Critical Care Outreach services include educational activity as part of their services. Such provision ranges from bedside teaching to multidisciplinary courses such as Acute Life Threatening Events – Recognition and Treatment (ALERT; Smith, 2000). Many authors also report the setting up of ward-based courses for the management of critically ill patients within the ward environment (Haines and Coad, 2001; O'Riordan *et al.*, 2003). Such courses provide information and training on a wide range of clinical practices, such as tracheostomy care, central line management and non-invasive ventilation.

Track and trigger systems

Many authors have developed track and trigger systems based on pre-defined physiological criteria. In many cases Outreach teams have been pivotal in the introduction of these in acute hospitals. These systems are designed to help nursing and medical staff, based in ward areas, to identify quickly, patients at risk of developing critical illness. This view is based on the assumption that those sick patients demonstrate changes in their physiological status sometimes hours before they require admission to the ICU. Vital signs measurement is an important aspect of in-patient care. Observations provide a trend of the patient's progress, which allow for the prompt detection of deterioration or improvement in their condition. One of the first scoring systems to be introduced was the Modified Early Warning Scoring System (Morgan *et al.*, 1997), which focused on five physiological parameters: pulse rate, respiratory rate, systolic blood pressure, temperature and AVPU score. The majority of acute hospitals in the UK have adopted such a system in an effort to reduce adverse events relating to the deteriorating patient (Table 38.1). The National Institute for Clinical Excellence has produced guidance on the recognition of and response to acute illness in adults in hospital. This clinical guideline makes evidence-based recommendations on the recognition and management of acute illness in acute hospitals and provides key priorities for implementation by acute hospitals (NICE, 2007a). Much emphasis was attributed to the importance of physiological observations. As with other national bodies (NPSA, 2007; NCEPOD, 2005) a key recommendation was for every hospital to have a track and trigger system that allows rapid detection of the signs of early clinical deterioration and an early and appropriate response. As with the variability in Outreach services there are many track and trigger systems, with no consistency regarding their physiological components (Smith *et al.*, 2008). NICE have not recommended one particular system; instead they recommend a multi-parameter or aggregated weighted score which allows a graded response and includes the monitoring of heart rate, respiratory rate, systolic blood pressure, level of consciousness, oxygen saturation and temperature (NICE, 2007a).

Table 38.1 Modified Early Warning System (MEWS)

A score of 3 or more requires a referral

Score	3	2	1	0	1	2	3
HR		<40	41–50	51–100	101–110	111–130	130
SBP	<70	71–80	81–100	101–199	>200		
RR		<8		9–14	15–20	21–29	>30
TEMP		<35	35.1–36.5	36.6–37.4	>37.5		
CNS				A	V	P	U

A = alert
P = response to pain
V = response to verbal stimulus
U = unconscious

Source: reproduced from Morgan *et al.* (1997).

Time out 38.2

Reflect on patients currently in your care.

1 Should any show signs of deterioration what would you do?
2 At what point would you contact out-of-hours support?

Physiological track and trigger systems should be used to monitor all adult patients in acute hospital settings.

■ Physiological observations should be monitored at least every 12 hours unless a decision has been made at a senior level to increase or decrease this frequency for an individual patient.
■ The frequency of monitoring should increase if abnormal physiology is detected as outlined in the recommendation on graded response strategy.

(NICE, 2007a)

Box 38.1 Modified Early Warning System (MEWS)

Queen's Hospital, Burton on Trent, has developed a Modified Early Warning System (MEWS – see Table 38.1) to provide an early accurate predictor of clinical deterioration. 'At risk' patients are scored and additionally any members of the multidisciplinary team (doctors, nurses, physiotherapists) can trigger MEWS for any other patients.

(DOH, 2000a)

The ability to recognise critical illness must not be underestimated. All the other systems of support mentioned rely on staff being able to identify sick patients. It should not be presumed that nurses or doctors do this well. Arguably, if early detection and intervention occurred, patients could be either prevented from moving to a critical care area, or could receive clinical management intervention early.

Implications for practice

- Outreach can support the care of critically ill patients throughout the hospital.
- Outreach offers ward staff the opportunities to develop skills and knowledge further.
- Some critically ill patients being cared for on wards will inevitably become more sick, necessitating admission to intensive care and other specialist areas; Outreach teams can help identify patients at risk, and hasten the transfer of patients to more appropriate areas.
- Outreach services should be easily available and accessible to wards.

Summary

The concept of Outreach appears to have been embraced enthusiastically by many acute hospitals throughout the country. Instinct tells us that it must be a good idea. Early recognition of potential or actual critical illness and the consequent correction of abnormalities should improve the patient experience and outcome. The collaboration between the Outreach team (whatever its model definition) and the multidisciplinary team actively contributes to the concept of 'seamless care' supported by *Comprehensive Critical Care* (DOH, 2000a), bridging the gap between critical care and the ward areas. In the past few years a significant amount of work has been directed towards improving the care given to patients at risk of or experiencing acute illness. While the model of delivering a robust response to patients experiencing acute illness has not been clearly articulated, NICE recommend that there should be a graded response by appropriately trained staff, competent in acute care skills (NICE, 2007a). Outreach fulfils this remit and as such appears to remain a key driver in the continued efforts to improve care for some of the sickest patients.

As the interest and adoption of Outreach teams has increased nationally, studies relating to their effectiveness have been undertaken. Gao *et al.* (2007) undertook a multi-centre interrupted time-series analysis of the impact of Critical Care Outreach. Unfortunately, in part due to the wide variability in service models, there was no clear evidence that Outreach has an impact on improved patient outcome. However, it was recognised that there was a reduction in the proportion of admissions receiving CPR before admission, admission out of hours and severity of illness for patients admitted to the ICU from the ward. Additionally, these changes in admission characteristics may be attributable to the use of track and trigger warning systems. In a systematic review of Outreach services, McGaughey *et al.* (2007) found that the evidence to determine the effectiveness of Critical Care Outreach and early warning scores on hospital mortality, unplanned ICU admissions and readmissions, length of stay and adverse events is inconclusive. Such information highlights the need for further high-level research. However, until we fully appreciate the problems faced by ward teams and are able to standardise measures of outcome, demonstrating the effectiveness of Outreach teams will be difficult.

As the National Outreach Forum report indicates, Outreach is more than just a service to help identify sick patients. Many teams provide significant support in terms of education and training for both nursing, junior medical staff and the allied professions. They may work in close co-operation with the resuscitation team, involving decisions about resuscitation status. Many teams support the respiratory teams in delivering ward-based non-invasive ventilation. Others are involved with providing follow-up services for patients discharged from the critical care units and the hospital. In addition many Outreach teams have been instrumental in providing guidelines and protocols for clinical practice within their own areas.

Such activities support the continuum of care for patients, staff and relatives.

Clinical scenario

Tracy Lewis, aged 68, a patient on your ward for two days, suddenly complains of dizziness and shortness of breath, while by her bedside. She is known to have Crohn's disease and has been admitted to hospital with anaemia.

1   What would your immediate response be?

2   Consider the observations you routinely undertake. What interventions might you include for a patient experiencing acute clinical deterioration?

3   Consider how you would determine the severity of the situation and communicate this to other members of the multidisciplinary team.

Bibliography

Key reading

The key text on Outreach remains the Department of Health's *Comprehensive Critical Care* (DOH, 2000a), which both reviewed the evidence and promoted national availability of Outreach. NICE (2007a) strongly supports and develops acute/critical care, and the value of Critical Care Outreach.

Further reading

McGaughey *et al.* (2007) provides the most up-to-date review of what is known from research about Outreach services for patients on general wards.
www.nice.org.uk/nicemedia/pdf/CG50FullGuidance.pdf
www.dh.gov.uk/en/Publicationsandstatistics/publications/PublicationsPolicy
AndGuidance/DH_4091873

Chapter 39

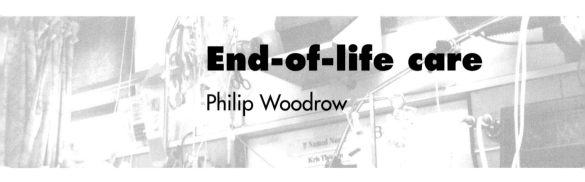

End-of-life care

Philip Woodrow

Contents

Learning outcomes

After reading this chapter you will be able to:

- identify the human needs (patients, families, friends and staff) involved when caring for patients dying in acute hospitals;
- promote individualised care which meets patients' needs;
- increase awareness of when and how treatment should be withdrawn;
- understand the value of follow-up care.

Introduction

Acute care aims to provide treatments and cures for people with potentially life-threatening illness. But inevitably not all patients will survive. Hospice care is often viewed as optimal for the terminally ill, yet most people die in acute hospitals (Fisher, 2006), where preoccupations with treatment can too often result in terminal care we would not wish for ourselves or our loved ones (Willard and Luker, 2006). This chapter explores three main themes surrounding death in acute hospitals:

1 Attitudes of nurses and other staff towards death. Some staff need support following death of patients. While patients may not be admitted for terminal care, life-saving treatment can become futile, unethical and unkind.
2 Treatment, including:

  ■ when and how such decisions should be made;
  ■ what should be withdrawn and what should remain or be provided as part of palliative care;

3 Needs of patients, family and friends during and after terminal care.

While hospices have improved bereavement care, death in acute wards may be sudden, leaving people little time to adjust to impending loss. This creates unique needs that cannot always be met by theory and practice drawn from areas specialising in palliative care. Many issues and needs discussed do not significantly change, so although much literature cited is relatively old, it remains largely relevant.

A century ago, people were usually exposed to death at an early age; life expectancy was generally lower, people usually died at home, and dead bodies would usually remain at home until the funeral. Western societies have sanitised death. It is largely a taboo subject, with few people being willing to discuss it or face their own mortality. Most professional courses develop scant time to bereavement. When death becomes likely, prolonging life (or death) with futile heroics may become cruel.

Many researchers are understandably cautious about approaching bereaved families in case they increase or revive distress. Research-based evidence is, therefore, limited both in quantity and sample sizes, making findings more often tentative.

Death: a medical failure?

Prolonging life, rather than allowing patients to die, sometimes becomes the unreasonable option. However, when to alter from life-sustaining to life-withdrawing treatment is debatable, value-laden and fraught with ethical moral and sometimes legal dilemmas. Death has traditionally been viewed as a medical failure (Stringer, 2007). Medical and nursing values have traditionally been contrasted as cure versus care. While potentially over-simplistic, nurses may consider prolonging a person's life is immoral/unethical, and consider that their own status and professionalism are undermined if their views are ignored or overridden.

The patient

For some, death is the beginning of an afterlife. But for many, death may bring psychological and/or spiritual traumas and regrets that many staff may feel uncomfortable discussing. Palliative care teams and chaplains are usually more experienced in supporting people facing death than most nurses on general wards. Some patients wish to sort out their affairs before dying, such as making their will. It is unwise for nurses to witness patients' wills, and most employers discourage this.

Where possible, patients should be informed of their prognosis, and participate in discussion about end-of-life care. Advance directives ('living wills') indicate patients' wishes, but advance directives are often either not made or not obviously available. Patients have a right to dignified care; they do not, however, have a right to futile treatment.

Unfortunately, acute illnesses causing terminal conditions may prevent people understanding explanations, or being able to make decisions. The five key principles of the Mental Capacity Act (Parliament, 2005) provide good guidance for patient involvement in end-of-life issues:

- presumed capacity – everyone is presumed to have capacity to make decisions until proven otherwise;
- individuals are supported in decision-making – all practical help is given before treating patients as lacking capacity to make decisions;
- unwise decisions – individuals retain the right to make what may seem unwise or eccentric decisions;
- best interest – any decision made for or on behalf of a person must be done in their best interest;
- least restrictive option – any action or decision made on behalf of someone else should be the least restrictive of their basic rights and freedom.

In Scotland, the Adults with Incapacity Act (Parliament, 2000) has similar requirements.

Withdrawing treatment

When further life-prolonging treatment becomes inappropriate, comfort and dignity should become the focus of care. The decision to withdraw life-prolonging treatment should be made by a team, ideally including the patient. The decision not to resuscitate ultimately rests with the most senior clinician currently in charge of the patient's care, which could be an appropriately experienced senior nurse (BMA, 2007b), but all staff caring for the patient should, where reasonably possible, contribute to the decision. Nurses, therefore, need sufficient knowledge and confidence to participate appropriately. Decisions to withdraw treatment involve individual values, morals and ethics.

Practices of withdrawing treatment vary between hospitals, doctors, and, sometimes, demand on beds (Cook *et al.*, 1995; Ravenscroft and Bell, 2000).

Nurse advocacy requires nurses to ensure that decisions in which patients cannot (or do not) participate are in the patient's best interests and reflect the patient's, rather than someone else's, values.

Time out 39.1

Imagine you are acutely ill. You have been diagnosed as having life-threatening illness. Your doctor informs you that you have only a 20 per cent chance of survival.

1 Would you wish life-prolonging treatment to be given?
2 At what point would life change from being acceptable to unacceptable? Identify an appropriate percentage figure.
3 List any factors that might alter your decision.
4 Discuss this exercise with some colleagues at work and compare differing values.

Science cannot ultimately *know* chances in each individual case. Assuming life is worse than death is also value-laden, as no one knows what death is like (Aksoy, 2000).

Withdrawing life-prolonging treatment does not mean withdrawing care. Treatments that provide comfort should be continued, and are often escalated.

Pain

A good death is usually described as pain-free (Stringer, 2007). Pain is the main reason euthanasia is requested (Emmanuel *et al.*, 2000). If there is any doubt about the patient's comfort, pain relief should be provided (BMA, 2007a). But nurses' assessment and management of pain is often poor (see Chapter 10), and many bereaved families consider analgesia needs of their loved one could have been improved (Danis, 1998). Pain relief often necessitates opioids, which can cause nausea, so anti-emetics should be given. Opioid doses may be larger than those prescribed for most patients. This is not to hasten their death, which would be both illegal and unethical. As long as the primary intention is to relieve pain and not hasten death, morally, opioids may be given in whatever quantities are needed to relieve pain. There is, however, a significant difference between being pain-free and lacking consciousness, so Gallagher and Wainwright (2007) warn about the ethical minefield of terminal sedation.

Depression

One-quarter of patients receiving palliative care are depressed, a figure likely to apply to palliative care in acute hospitals (Taylor and Ashelford, 2008). Depression is not a normal part of grief, so should be alleviated.

Not for resuscitation

Where death is likely, or successful resuscitation would be unlikely, attempting resuscitation would be cruel. Yet too often futile resuscitations are attempted, sometimes through lack of foresight but more often through temerity to instigate a DNR CPR (do not resuscitate with cardiopulmonary resuscitation). This should be a team decision, although currently the final order has to be signed by a medical consultant. Decisions not to resuscitate should be clearly recorded, following local policies. Most hospitals have proformas for 'do not attempt cardiopulmonary resuscitation' orders.

Liverpool Care Pathway

Most acute hospitals use the Liverpool Care Pathway (LCP), a plan for providing terminal care in the last 48–72 hours of life, although in practice sometimes used for considerably longer. Patients suitable for the LCP should meet at least two of the following criteria:

■ bed-bound
■ comatose
■ no longer able to take oral tablets
■ only able to take sips of fluid.

(Ellershaw and Wilkinson, 2003)

In acute care, there is often reluctance to acknowledge that patients are dying, and so to initiate terminal care, creating a potential gap between the start of terminal decline and commencing a LCP.

Spiritual care

Patients' spiritual values should be considered at all times, but spiritual values often become especially important when facing death. Most hospitals have chaplains, but also have access to information on faiths likely to be followed by their patients. Responses to death may be affected by cultural influences, such as religion. Nurses should, therefore, be sensitive to cultural and religious needs of patients and their families. There are hundreds of different faiths, so staff cannot be expected to be familiar with all, and covering all possibilities would require a book by itself. For example, Buddhist families may wish to stay with their departed for prolonged lengths of time, while Hindi often prefer to perform last offices themselves, keeping jewellery or 'sacred threads' on the body, and Muslims often wish to die facing Mecca. Unfortunately, assessment and recording of spiritual needs in nursing records are often poor (Swift *et al.*, 2007).

The family

Whatever the personal beliefs and values of each nurse, death of patients is an inevitable part of nursing in almost any speciality. Family and friends of each patient are unlikely to have seen as many people die, but would have known the patient longer and more intimately than the nurse. So however caring nurses are, experiencing bereavement is likely to be unique to family in a way it cannot be to the nurse. This almost inevitably places nurses outside the intimate circle of grieving.

Breaking bad news, and other sensitive interviews, should occur away from the bedside, preferably in a comfortable room where you will not be disturbed – hang a notice on the door; if possible, switch off any telephones. Do not obstruct the door, in case relatives unable to handle the situation need to rush out. Offering tea and other comforts can help to humanise an inevitably distressing situation.

Breaking bad news and witnessing suffering can cause stress (Wright, 1996; Farrell, 1999), so understandably many staff are uncomfortable doing this. Doctors' communication with families is often inconsistent (Ravenscroft and Bell, 2000) and could be improved (Danis, 1998). Nurses' communication is probably similarly variable. Staff should, therefore, try and find out what the family have already been told, both to avoid inconsistencies, and to try and ensure families are given sufficient information to meet their needs. Staff trained in counselling skills are more likely to be able to support family more effectively. However, family often trust particular members of staff, and may value that member of staff speaking with them – for families, interpersonal skills are more important than their professional rank (Finlay and Dallimore, 1991).

Guilt is probably the most painful aspect of grief (Kubler-Ross, 1970). Bereaved family often seek reasons for the death. However irrational, they often blame themselves for causing or contributing to the death. Nurses can profoundly affect how family respond to bereavement (Coolican, 1994). Whenever possible, families should be informed honestly and clearly about impending death of their loved one so that they may begin grieving (Eastland, 2001).

Sudden death makes relatives feel helpless (Wright, 1991). Suddenly bereaved family may need more support, but often receive less (Yates et al., 1990). Nurses should, therefore, help family to regain control and power while giving them the freedom to express their feelings and face the pain of death (Wright, 1991). The time immediately surrounding sudden death is crucial in determining the family's ability to accept death and deal with the crisis (Lindermann, 1994), partly because disbelief can be very strong (Jackson, 1996). Family need both practical advice/ information, such as how to make funeral arrangements, and someone to talk to (Hall and Hall, 1994). Providing printed information, such as the Department of Social Services' booklet *What to Do after Death*, can be particularly helpful, as grieving family may not remember everything they are told. Many hospitals provide information booklets giving details such as local places to register the death.

Anticipating events, or imaging what happened if not present, is often worse than reality (Kent and McDowell, 2004). Because reactions are unpredictable, it is usually best to inform relatives of sudden death after they have arrived in the hospital (Kent and McDowell, 2004). Viewing the body after death helps grieving (Ashdown, 1985; Cathcart, 1988), providing an opportunity to say 'goodbye'. Family may feel 'cheated' if they are not allowed to see and touch their loved one (Ellison, 1992). Unfortunately the busyness of acute hospitals may undermine opportunities to support bereaved relatives. Up to half of people contacting a branch of CRUSE (a voluntary group for bereaved family) did so because of feelings of anxiety and anger towards hospitals, doctors and nurses (Ewins and Bryant, 1992).

Grief is a process, family needs continuing support. Bereaved family usually value being contacted by nurses who cared for their loved one (Jackson, 1998), and some nurses may wish to attend funerals of those they have cared for, although a significant minority do not (Jackson, 1998). Many wards have bereavement programmes, such as sending condolence cards (Burke and Seeley, 1994), ideally sent two to six weeks after the death (Kubler-Ross, 1991; Wright, 1991; Jackson, 1996).

The nurse

Few nurses can avoid witnessing death. Death of patients can be distressing to nursing staff as well as family (Stringer, 2007), reviving unresolved grief from personal losses, or reviving fears about their own mortality. Many healthcare staff dislike being with dying people (Ellershaw and Ward, 2003).

Being with people in emotional pain is distressing, but the pain is caused by death, not the nurse. Nurses have the opportunity to help ease the pain by providing quality end-of-life care. Emotions are often raw, but nurses should not try and hide their tears – most families find it comforting to see staff are also upset (Finlay and Dallimore, 1991).

Support from peers or professional counsellors may help nurses cope (Spencer, 1994). Peer support could be informal, or structured through debriefing or reflective sessions. Peer support should be mutual – offer support to others when they are caring for dying patients. End-of-life care is often included in pre- and post-registration courses, although being an emotionally fraught topic can be difficult to facilitate and participate in. Many hospitals and other organisations also offer study days on bereavement.

Implications for practice

- Nurses should be actively involved in decisions about whether to prolong or withdraw active treatment.
- Whenever possible, patients should be involved with decision-making.
- Withdrawing active treatment does not mean withdrawing care; terminal care should provide comfort and maintain dignity.
- During and following death the family, friends and often staff need support, individualised to each person's needs.
- Family value follow-up support from wards where their loved one died.

- A system should be maintained for contacting family two to six weeks following bereavement.
- Be aware of your own, and your colleagues' needs for peer and other support.

Summary

Acute hospitals are designed to provide life-supporting treatments, but not all patients survive. Death is not a medical failure, but the inevitable end of each person's life. Nurses should strive to meet the needs of patients and their families. Nurses should actively participate in decisions about prolonging or withdrawing active treatment. Once active treatment is withdrawn care should focus on comfort and dignity.

Bereavement is likely to be traumatic for family, friends, and sometimes staff. Nurses should, therefore, provide support to families during bereavement, including practical information and space to express their emotions. Family value being able to see the body of their loved one. Needs of staff should also be supported.

Quality bereavement care can ease the trauma, but not remove it. Family usually need prolonged support, which hospitals can often initiate. Because reactions to loss are individual, any of the supports identified in this chapter may be valuable for both staff and family.

Clinical scenario

Albert Jones was admitted following a myocardial infarction and thrombolysis in A&E. Since taking early retirement three years ago at the age of 58, he and his wife have been able to travel more, including visits to their only son and his family, who live 350 miles away.

Albert's condition has stabilised sufficiently to return to a medical ward. However, his cardiac function is poor, and he becomes very breathless on exertion. His chances of survival to discharge are estimated at best to be 10–20 per cent. The medical team have suggested withdrawing treatment.

1   Identify your role as nurse advocate for Albert. What factors would influence your views of whether treatment should be withdrawn?

2   Consider the likely needs of Albert's family up to the time of his death.

3   Reflect on follow-up facilities available in your ward, hospital and local area. How far do these meet the needs suggested by evidence-based practice?

Bibliography

Key reading

The BMA (2007a) provides authoritative guidelines for doctors about withholding and withdrawing treatment. The Marie Curie website (www.mcpcil.org.uk/liverpool_care_pathway) has information about, and examples of, the Liverpool Care Pathway. Neuberger (2004) provides a guide for end-of-life care for widely encountered religions. Classic texts about bereavement include Kubler-Ross (1970), Buckman (1988), Parkes (1996) and Wright (1996). Kent and McDowell (2004) provide a useful nursing review. Stringer (2007) reviews what makes a 'good' death, while Taylor and Ashelford (2008) review depression in palliative care.

Further reading

Farrell (1999) discusses breaking bad news. Ellershaw has written widely about palliative care, including co-editing *Care of the Dying* with Wilkinson (2003). Mootoo (2005) provides a useful overview of religious needs.

Chapter 40

Tissue retrieval

Philip Woodrow

Contents

Learning outcomes

After reading this chapter you will be able to:

- identify main tissues that can be retrieved from patients who die in hospital wards;
- understand potential benefits to donors, their families, and recipients;
- recall resources that can be used to facilitate the process of donation.

Introduction

For half a century patients with end-stage (fatal) organ failure have increasingly benefited from organ transplantation. Some types of tissue (as opposed to solid organ) transplantation have been established for many years – notably corneas and heart valves. But tissues transplanted were largely retrieved from organ donors, and for organs to be retrieved, the donor needed to be certified dead while the organs remained perfused. This largely limited donation to people dying on intensive care units. Advances in technique have enabled tissues (not organs) to be retrieved hours after cessation of circulation. This means that patients dying on wards can now become tissue donors, retrieval occurring in the mortuary.

Currently, about 400 people on UK waiting lists die each year (Pace, 2006), and the number of patients needing transplants in the UK is expected to rise (Long and Sque, 2007). While many of these people need organs rather than tissues, tissue transplantation can improve quality of life, and may avert death. Yet many ward staff remain unaware of the possibility of tissue donation, so inadvertently deny their patient's wishes, while depriving those needing tissues of possible donors (Magrath and Boulstridge, 2005).

This chapter outlines the main 'tissues' that can be donated, with some guidelines for donation; bone is included as, although arguably not 'tissue', post-mortem retrieval is possible. Most tissues can be retrieved from children as well as adults, as waiting lists include children with end-stage organ failure. Some adult tissues may also be used for children. With most tissues, upper age limits exist for donation. Upper age limits are determined by likely viability of tissue for recipient. However, as technique or knowledge advance, age (and other) limits are frequently revised, and limitations can also vary between regions and countries. So guidelines may be out of date by the time they are read. If in doubt, nurses should always seek advice from the local transplant co-ordinators.

The term 'harvest' is often used to describe the process of retrieval. However, it does imply a dehumanising process that may deter potential donors or families. This chapter, therefore, uses the equally meaningful, but more humane, term 'retrieval'.

The main tissues that can be retrieved are:

- eye tissue
- heart valves
- skin
- bone
- tendons
- trachea
- pericardium
- brain and spinal cord.

These tissues can usually be retrieved 24–72 hours after death. After discussing each tissue, this chapter will list probable contraindications for all tissues.

Eye tissue

Corneal grafts have saved sight for many years. The whole eye is usually retrieved, and more than the cornea may be needed. Scleral tissue is used for reconstructive surgery. Healthy eye tissue of any age may benefit recipients; the oldest corneal donor was aged 103, and the oldest recipient 104 (Gumbley and Pearson, 2006). Eye tissue can be retrieved up to 24 hours after death.

Many people are squeamish about eyes, and might refuse donation because they envisage the body being left with a disfiguring empty eye socket. An artificial eye will be placed in the corpse, so that the body appears 'normal' in the mortuary. Staff explaining to patients or relatives should mention the lack of disfigurement.

Heart valve

Incidence of heart valve disease has decreased, and most UK valve replacements are artificial (Chikwe *et al.*, 2004). However, artificial valve replacement condemns the recipient to long-term, often life-long, anticoagulation therapy. So for some patients, tissue valves are preferable. Although xenotransplantation (animal tissue) is used, human tissue is preferable. Heart valves can be retrieved up to 48 hours after death. Because incidence of heart valve disease significantly increases in later decades of life, donors over the age of 60 are unlikely to be considered.

Myocardial infarction causes death of heart muscle, not heart valves, so is not an exclusion for donation. However, diseases that may cause valve disease, such as rheumatic fever or congenital conditions, are exclusions to donation.

Pericardium

Pericardium can be used as a 'patch graft' for atrial/septal defects in adults. Pericardium must be retrieved within 72 hours of death. Donors must usually be aged 16 to 60 years.

Skin

Skin is essential to human life, separating the body's internal and external environments. Its many vital functions include preventing dehydration by keeping body water inside, and preventing infection by providing a barrier to micro-organisms. Extensive skin loss, such as from burns, necessitates replacement. Where possible, autologous skin-grafts are used (skin from the person's own body), but where this is not possible, skin grafted from a donor may prove life-saving, or at least superior to artificial alternatives. Composite allografts – skin from more than one donor – is also possible (Ravindra, 2008). Among other advantages, using skin usually improves cosmetic results and reduces need for further reconstructive surgery.

Skin can be retrieved up to 48 hours after death. The main limitation on skin donation is size. Only a fine layer of skin is retrieved, leaving an intact skin surface on the body, so a large body surface area is needed. Typical criteria are that donors must be over 1.7 metres tall, more than 70 kilograms *and* below 85 years of age.

Bones

Although not strictly a tissue, bone can be retrieved from the mortuary. Donated bone is used for reconstructive/orthopaedic surgery, not as a total bone transplant, but as the base for a paste used as part of the repair. Bone from one donor can help up to 20 people. Bone can be retrieved up to 48 hours after death. Because of age-related degeneration, there are upper age limits for donors, typically of 75 years for men and 60 years for women (the female age limit being lower due to post-menopausal osteoporosis).

Tendons

Recovery from tendons damage can be very prolonged, so donor tendons can replace damaged ones, typically for athletes suffering sports injuries. Due to tissue degeneration, donor age is typically limited to below 45 years.

Trachea

Tracheal tissue can be useful to treat tracheal stenosis in infants. Diseases affecting the trachea, such as pneumonia or bronchitis, are contraindications to tracheal donation, but asthma is not an exclusion. Tracheal tissue must be retrieved within 72 hours of death. Donors must usually be aged 16 to 60 years.

Brain and spinal cord

Compared with other main organs, understanding of the brain, and so ways to treat central nervous system disease, is relatively limited. It is hoped in the future that cures for currently incurable neurological diseases can be achieved through transplantation. For example, transplanting dopamine-producing cells of the substantia nigra may provide a cure for Parkinson's disease. However, at present such attempts are limited to the laboratory, and are not clinically available. So donated brain and spinal cords are currently used only for research. This should be explained clearly to potential donors.

Because tissue will only be used for research, there are virtually no exclusions, except

- retrieval must be within 24 hours of death;
- donors must be adult – ethics of paediatric retrieval precludes considering donation where there is no therapeutic benefit to others;
- hepatitis, primarily to protect the health of researchers.

Probable contraindications

Transplanting tissues into recipients can also transplant disease. So any suspected source for transmitting the disease, or with diseases of unknown aetiology, usually prevents donation. At the time of writing, the only absolute contraindications to donation are HIV and new variant CJD (nvCJD), but relative and absolute contraindications have varied significantly over recent years, so if in doubt staff should check with their regional transplant co-ordinator.

Legal aspects

In UK law, a dead person cannot own anything. As this includes their own body, until recently the dead body was viewed as the 'property' of the next-of-kin, and so the next-of-kin were asked to give consent for any retrieval. If the person had clearly expressed a wish about donation, this meant that their next-of-kin could over-rule their wishes after their death. Increasing concern about wishes being over-ruled led to the Human Tissues Act (2004), which made the person's wishes paramount. People could now donate their body, and body parts, in the same way as their estate would be distributed according to their wishes. If the dead person did not express a wish about donation, the next-of-kin retains the right to decide.

Ethical and professional aspects

Some staff are understandably reluctant to ask about donation. At a time when patients, and their family, are facing death, discussing donation may seem cruel. However, once death becomes inevitable, it is unlikely that any discussion about donation will make things worse. Failing to discuss donation may deprive people of their right to choose. Few people facing death or bereavement will think about donation, but families may think about it some time after bereavement, by which time it is usually too late. The NMC Code (2008) states that nurses must act as advocates for those in their care. A core ethical principle of healthcare is non-malefecence (not doing any harm). Depriving patients of their right to choose, or failing to fulfil their wishes, is not in their best interests, but is doing harm.

While next-of-kin, and other relatives/significant others, can no longer over-rule the dead person's wishes about donation, bereavement is usually a traumatic time for family, so it remains good practice to inform the family about the donation. For many families, the thought that unavoidable death of their loved one at least brought others benefit, and that a part of their loved one 'lives on' in other people brings some comfort, refusal or absence of opportunity to donate often leaves regret (Ormrod et al., 2005).

Patients or, in the absence of expressed wishes, their next-of-kin, may choose not to donate. Accepting the principle of autonomy, their choice should be respected, whether or not we agree with it. Healthcare professionals should enable people to make informed choices, not coerce.

Consent

Repeated surveys in the UK show that while most people are willing to be donors, only a minority indicate their wishes in writing. Like most countries, the UK currently has an 'opting-in' system – people actively choose to be donors, and donation is viewed as a gift. Some countries operate an 'opting-out' system, whereby the person is presumed to be a donor unless they actively choose not to be. Continuing shortfalls between supply and demand of organs and tissues has generated demands for the UK to change to an 'opt-out' system, notably by the Department of Health (DOH, 2008). DOH (2008) also suggests hospital staff should be required to refer patients who die. Although this report concerns organ, rather than tissue, donation, changes would probably apply to both areas.

Despite widespread availability of donor cards, including on UK driving licences, most people dying in hospital have not completed one, or it is not evident if they did. The UK, therefore, operates an NHS Organ Donor Register, which can be accessed by health professionals nationally by telephoning 0117 975 7580. This helps ensure that people's wishes are respected rather than being lost through lack of evidence. To protect patient confidentiality, a hospital (not direct line) number must be left for the centre to telephone back with relevant details. When approaching families, it is useful to know whether or not their loved one is on the donor register.

Process of donation

The UK currently employs regional transplant co-ordinators, both for advice and to facilitate the process. If current (DOH, 2008) proposals are implemented, there could be a facilitator in each hospital. It is best to contact co-ordinators as soon as a potential donor, who is dying, has been identified. Hospital switchboards should have details of how to contact co-ordinators.

Even if the patient has expressed a choice, families should be informed of their loved one's wishes, and the process of donation. Approaching already distressed/ grieving families can be traumatic. Co-ordinators are skilled in all aspects of the process of donation, including liaising with family. However, before they arrive, initial approaches may have to be made by local staff, and family may prefer to talk to someone with whom they have already built up a rapport. Any staff may be involved with the approach, and in some support staff they may have developed confidence and skills to approach this delicate topic. Whoever approaches family, there should be two members of staff, and all discussions should be documented and signed by both staff, in case of later disputes.

Conversations should ideally be in a quiet, comfortable room, away from the patient's bedside. Any distractions, such as telephones, should be removed, and a 'do not disturb' notice placed on the door. Skills of good communication include:

- placing yourself at the listener's level;
- maintaining eye contact;
- using a non-threatening tone of voice;

- allowing time to absorb information;
- providing the opportunity to ask questions;
- not obstructing any exits with yourself, others or furniture.

It is often helpful to open by asking a question such as 'Did you ever discuss organ donation?' This enables the family to focus on their loved one's wishes.

Implications for practice

- Since the Human Tissues Act, patients' wishes are paramount.
- Refusal should be respected ('no is OK').
- Not to offer donation denies choice.
- Suddenly bereaved relatives are unlikely to think about donation.
- Tissues can be retrieved (in the mortuary) 24–72 hours following death.
- If adopted, DOH (2008) could cause significant changes.

Summary

Donating tissues can be life-saving or improve the quality of life for others. Patients may wish to donate tissues, and if they are imminently dying, or dead, ward staff should do their best to enable patients' wishes to be fulfilled. Ward staff should, therefore, have a working knowledge of likely criteria, and check whether dying/dead patients who meet these criteria are on the NHS Organ Donor Register. In the UK, regional transplant co-ordinators facilitate the process, and should be contacted as soon as possible.

Clinical scenario

Evelyn Hopkins, aged 56, is transferred to your ward for rehabilitation following evacuation of a subarachnoid haemorrhage. On arrival, her overall condition and prognosis are poor. Despite optimal therapy, her condition continues to deteriorate. One week after her transfer, the team agree to commence a Liverpool Care Pathway (see Chapter 39). Her only significant medical history is atrial fibrillation and a corneal abrasion, which was diagnosed six months previously.

1 List the possible ways you might find out whether Evelyn wished to become a tissue donor.

2 What tissues might Evelyn be able to donate? What resources could provide you with more information (include any locally available resources)?

3 Discuss this scenario with your work colleagues. Would they have considered suggesting donation? Why (not)? What problems might deter or worry them? How would they approach families and discuss issues?

Bibliography

Key reading

Gumbley and Pearson (2006) provide one of the few nursing reviews since the Human Tissues Act was passed. Wilkinson (2000) provides valuable ethical debate. Some hospitals have compiled guidance for staff about tissue donation. Staff should be aware of DOH (2008).

UK Transplant provide many resources on their website: www.uktransplant. org.uk/ukt/default.jsp

Further reading

Hadingham (1997) offers useful insights, albeit before the Human Tissues Act was passed. Pace (2006) discusses ethical issues, although largely from intensive care perspectives.

Chapter 41

Professional issues

Tina Moore

Contents

Learning outcomes

After reading this chapter you will be able to:

- understand the implications of professional accountability and role expansion;
- understand the doctrine of informed consent and how it relates to the acutely/critically ill;
- appreciate the complexities of informed consent in relation to acute care provision;
- demonstrate knowledge of the impact of the Mental Capacity Act (2005) for the nurse.

Fundamental knowledge

Ethics (Chapter 3).

Introduction

Since the beginning of the nineteenth century nursing has experienced a widening of role boundaries. Today, nurses are involved in more complex decision-making processes regarding care delivery and as a result must understand the professional and legal implications of their role.

This chapter will discuss the issues and implications of professional accountability. Advocacy (although a professional role) will not be discussed as this is addressed in Chapter 1.

Role expansion

Expanded roles are now seen as a natural progression of the nurse's existing role, this is coupled with increased accountability under the guidance of *The Code: Standards of Conduct, Performance and Ethics for Nurses and Midwives* (NMC, 2008).

On consenting to role expansion, nurses should consider issues relating to professional accountability. There is no defence in criminal or civil law that allows a nurse to say that someone ordered them to do a potentially harmful or unlawful act. Nurses should challenge practices and decisions that they believe are improper, for their own as well as the patient's benefit.

Taking on additional tasks should be accepted with caution and only if it is in the best interests of the patient. There is still concern that vital aspects of nursing will be lost if nurses begin to undertake functions that were once considered to be the domain of doctors, e.g. basic nursing care (hygiene needs, prevention of pressure ulcers) may be neglected. Despite this, role expansion is an accepted aspect of nursing.

Thus, expanded role requires appropriate education and clinical support mechanisms in place. There should be opportunities for Continuous Professional Development (CPD). Taking on the role expansion is seen to make care more personal, effective and holistic. Clinical supervision should now be operationalised in all practice settings, as this is on the government's agenda with clinical governance (DOH, 1997).

Professional accountability

Accountability is an integral part of professional practice, requiring the nurse to give explanation and justification for actions and omissions in relation to care. Definitions of accountability reflect the expectation that justification should be evidence-based.

Accountability implies that a situation has been assessed, a plan has been made and carried out, and the results evaluated. Accountability assumes the nurse has the necessary knowledge, skill, experience and subsequent authority to carry out the plan.

Arenas of accountability include:

- *Patient*: Nurses are primarily accountable to the patients within their care; they have a legal and professional duty to act in the best interest of the patient (Civil liability).
- *Professional body*: Nursing and Midwifery Council – Professional Conduct Committee (Professional liability).
- *Employers*: Nurses in breach of employment contract may face an industrial tribunal.
- *Public*: Nurses can be tried in the Criminal Law Courts (Criminal liability), if a crime is suspected of being committed.

Professional practice demands that the nurse be competent and has mastery in the chosen field of nursing. This mastery should also hold a genuine passion and vision for nursing, coupled with an endeavour towards excellence and quality. If a qualified nurse fails to follow the Code (NMC, 2008), they may be reported to the NMC for an investigation into their 'fitness to practice'.

Mental Capacity Act (2005)

This Act is a code of practice designed to protect vulnerable adult patient groups. It is a protection of the patient's autonomy. This act should be viewed as guidance rather than instructional as it provides a code of practice. It is aimed at anyone who is in contact with people who lack (or have the potential to lack) capacity. While the act does not refer to the acutely/critically ill specifically, this has huge implications for this patient group. It is directed towards those who are classified as incompetent (see p. 421 for the criteria for competence). The contents of this Act may have implications in terms of clinical decision-making.

The Act is aimed to:

- provide *empowerment* for adults who may lack capacity (enabling them to enhance their autonomy);
- provide *protection* for adults who lack capacity and for those who care for them;
- provide *choice* – by allowing adults to appoint those they trust to take decisions for them if they should lose capacity.

Key principles of this Act include:

1 The healthcare professional should assume that a person has capacity unless proved otherwise (a thorough assessment should be undertaken regularly as patient's capacity may fluctuate).
2 All practicable steps should be undertaken to help the patient make decisions before rendering them incapable.
3 Patients' decisions should be respected even if they are not agreed with or thought to be unwise.
4 For patients without capacity clinical decision-making should be done in *their* best interest.

5   Before acting on behalf of someone, ensure that all practical steps are taken to enable the patient to make the decision for themselves. Even if the patient does not have capacity they should be encouraged to make what decisions they can.

Patients have the right to appoint someone of their choice to make decisions on their behalf (when they lack capacity), but this decision must be made when they are competent. Healthcare professionals cannot interfere with an adult's body unless they have their consent (this does not apply to those who lack capacity). There is also the Court of Protection designed to be informal and quick for such disputes.

Advanced decisions set out what treatment would be unacceptable to them (the patient) and in what circumstances that it would be valid and applicable (for a person who has lost capacity these should be respected).

It is a criminal offence for wilfully neglecting or ill-treating a person who lacks capacity, carrying a maximum sentence of five years (Mental Capacity Act, 2005).

Informed consent

> **Time out 41.1**
>
> 1 List the different types of consent available. Which mode do you mainly use?
> 2 What type of patients do you gain consent from? What set of criteria do you use?

Acutely/critically ill patients may present a challenge for nurses in terms of balancing the respect for patient autonomy and the duty of care. Conflict arises when on the one hand nurses may wish to make a decision and respect the patient's autonomy, and on the other, there is the possibility of being open to the charge of negligence or failure of duty of care (Tingle and Cribb, 2002). Conflict could arise where the patient is harmed from the effects of pain (resultant from refusal to receive analgesia). For instance, a competent patient who develops severe pain post-operatively following an invasive procedure refuses analgesia. The patient's coping mechanisms fail, demonstrating signs of neurogenic shock. As a result the patient is harmed by the effects of pain (resulting from refusal to receive analgesia).

There is the risk of assuming that the majority of acutely ill patients are unlikely to understand the implications of treatment. Therefore, healthcare professionals should adopt the advocacy role, often providing care in a manner they feel would be most beneficial to the patient. This approach, where consent is not actively obtained implies indirect paternalism.

Consent means a voluntary, uncoerced decision, made by a sufficiently competent or autonomous person on the basis of adequate information and deliberation, to accept rather than reject some proposed course of action that will affect them.

For consent to be valid it must comply with the following:

1   *Be voluntary without any form of coercion or influence from others.* This may at times be difficult to achieve. Being acutely/critically ill creates a stressful situation for the patient. As a result, they have poor concentration and often are unable to recall information received. This could be due to the degree of illness, anxiety, medication or sleep/sensory deprivation. Some patients will exercise their autonomy not to be autonomous and select an advocate.

2   *The person must be competent in order to make an autonomous decision.* When patients are competent to give their informed consent they have all the qualities and abilities necessary to make autonomous decisions about their care management. Whether any patient can achieve this is debatable. There is an inconsistent approach to gaining consent and a lack of accepted standards of the principle of competence (Welie and Welie, 2001).

3   *Specific to the treatment proposed.* Generally, simple treatments require the absorption and analysis of simple concepts, whereas more complex treatments will require greater comprehension. There may be a number of factors influencing the patient's ability to perceive and retain information, e.g. environmental stress, medication, anxiety about their illness.

4   *Assessment of the patient's decision-making competence must also be specific to this situation.* For consent to be valid a patient must be mentally competent, if the competence of a patient is in doubt, the following criteria should be applied:

   ■   evidencing choice
   ■   'reasonable' outcome of choice
   ■   choice based on rational reasons
   ■   ability to understand
   ■   actual understanding (comprehension)
                     (Roth *et al.*, 1983 cited in Beauchamp and Childress, 2008)

Establishing a patient's competence (determined through understanding) is a subjective process and is open to assessor variability. Generalised labelling of a patient as incompetent (or lacking capacity) must be avoided.

5   *Patients should be provided with information of sufficient quality, scope and choice to enable them to make an informed autonomous decision.* This must include all risks and hazards associated with the procedure, in addition to disclosure of alternatives. Patients will vary on the amount and type of information they want. Nurses should be present when the patient is being given information, in order to be in a position to clarify and expand upon that information.

Nurses have an obligation to provide information and the opportunity for consent. A patient/client who is legally competent can understand and retain treatment information and can use it to make an informed choice (NMC, 2008).

The principle of informed consent is in place to respect the patient's right to be autonomous and the recognition that healthcare professionals have a duty to provide the patient with sufficient information.

Common Law Tort clearly states that the professional has a right to withhold some or all information, if it is in the patient's best interest to do so (Dimond, 2008). This is known as therapeutic privilege.

Acutely/critically ill patients require the use of simple, easy-to-understand language. This should help to prevent confusion and aid actual understanding. A patient can withdraw consent at any time. It is considered good practice to explore the reasons with the patient (if possible) before terminating treatment.

Consent should be viewed as a continuous process rather than an outcome to be achieved; therefore, constant reassessment of the patient's level of competence is required as this can change intermittently.

Failure to obtain patient consent or to provide information fully of the reasons for a procedure can result in a legal case of assault, trespass and battery. Exceptions include emergency situations where a patient is (possibly) treated against their will (healthcare professionals may not know the patient's decisions).

Defences to not giving informed consent could include:

- consent (i.e. consenting not to be informed);
- necessity;
- making a lawful arrest;
- acting under a statutory power, e.g. Mental Health Act (1983).

Failure to provide information according to the Bolam Test (1957) could, if harm were to occur, leave the individual/Trust open to litigation.

Time out 41.2

Consider Mrs Brown who has been admitted following bowel surgery. Pre-operatively she was in a debilitated state. Post-operatively she has developed hypovolaemic shock. The nurse assigned to care for Mrs Brown was busy helping another nurse with a patient; she was also in charge of the unit. During the course of the shift, Mrs Brown's condition deteriorates. Subsequently she suffers a cardiac arrest. During the resuscitation procedure the wall suction is found not to be working, and the portable machine is in use. Finally, she dies.

1 Do you consider negligence to have occurred?
2 Give reasons for your answer.
3 Write down your understanding of negligence.

Negligence

There are occasions when patients sue the Trust for damages from harm that they have suffered. The law of negligence is the most commonly used legal concept in maintaining standards. It is based on Tort Law, and refers to a Civil wrong. Patients have a range of rights that will be protected by the Civil Courts.

When an individual considers suing for damages for harm suffered, the burden of proof, according to law, lies with that individual. This burden of proof depends on a balance of probabilities.

The law of negligence can be used in two different ways:

1   to sue another person for compensation, harm or damage;
2   to indicate that behaviour has fallen below required standards.

To succeed in an action, the plaintiff must show:

1   the existence of a duty to care was owed to him by the defendant;
2   breach of that duty by the defendant;
3   that as a result the plaintiff had suffered damage (and the harm suffered must have been reasonably foreseeable).

Duty of care

A duty of care to someone in the law of negligence is to be obliged to take his or her interest into account. This person must take reasonable care to avoid acts or omissions that can reasonably foresee which will cause injury/harm.

A duty of care is owed when:

■   any person is voluntarily attended by a nurse in an emergency situation, whether on or off duty (*Kent v. Griffiths and others*, 2002);
■   any patients present themselves to hospital and nurses have knowledge of that patient.

In the case of Mrs Brown, because of the contractual agreement between patient and nurse, a legal duty of care is owed.

Breach of duty of care

The standard of care owed to the patient needs to be identified and examined. Patients depend upon nurses and their standards of professional conduct. The standard of care provided by any professional person must be of a higher level than that of a novice. The courts require an acceptable reasonable standard to be followed; a standard that would be supported by competent professional opinion and practice (Dimond, 2008). The nurse is expected to exhibit the expertise normally demonstrated by a competent nurse, i.e. to comply with the Bolam Test (Box 41.1).

Courts rely on expert evidence to give an opinion of what is deemed to be a reasonable action and the accepted practice in a given situation. It is assumed that their opinions will be based on current evidence in order to provide a logical reason. Documentation for consultation in regarding acceptable standard of performance would be NMC documentation, policies, procedures and national/ local guidelines.

In the case of role expansion, a medical standard of care may be looked for (Tingle, 2002). The law would not find it acceptable to say that doing a medical activity a nurse would be legally expected to perform at a lower standard of care. Some situations require deviation from the normal accepted procedures. Nurses can deviate from accepted standards, but need to clearly document why (Dimond, 2008).

Box 41.1 The Bolam Test

- Ordinary skilled person exercising and professing to have that skill
- A reasonable competent practitioner
- Acting in accordance with practice accepted at that time as proper by a reasonable body of professional opinion

(Bolam v. Friern Barnet, 1957)

With regards to Mrs Brown, it needs to be established whether the nurse involved was suitably qualified and experienced to provide unsupervised care and whether current guidance was followed.

Causation

Causation seeks to examine the casual link between the failure of the defendant to follow the approved practice and the harm suffered by the patient that must be reasonably foreseeable (Dimond, 2008). There is a need to establish a causal link between the breach of duty to care by the nurse and the harm suffered by the patient.

In the case of Mrs Brown, it could be argued that there was no causal link between the actions of the nurse and the suction machine not working. Mrs Brown's condition was so critical that even if the suction machine was in working order she may have died anyway. Therefore, while there may be evidence of poor practice, the criteria for negligence are not fulfilled.

Implications for practice

- Nurses should undertake role expansion with caution and be assessed as competent.
- Nurses will be judged in accordance with their actions (reasonable professional standard).
- Professional practice should be within the designated boundaries of the discipline.

- Before gaining consent patients should know the nature, purpose, risks and benefit of the proposed procedure before (where possible).
- Nurses should be in a position to assess whether the patient has the mental capacity to be involved in clinical decision-making.

Summary

If nurses are going to continue to expand their professional role, they will need to accept the increases in accountability and professional implications. All clinical decisions made should be in the best interest of the patient. CPD is required in order to maintain and enhance standards of care. By doing so, nurses will be in a strong position to defend practices.

Bibliography

Further reading

Dimond (2008) provides useful discussions/information relating to the legal aspects of nursing. Current cases provide interesting illustrations.

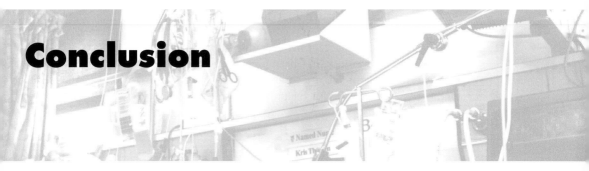

Conclusion

Approaches to the provision of acute care continue to grow and develop. Due to the diversity of patients with level 2 care needs, nurses working outside of critical care areas continue to experience the challenges of looking after such patients. All efforts should be directed at making the patient's experience/journey through acute/critical care as uneventful as is possible. Guidelines exist, to (in part) ensure that this happens, for example, NCEPOD (2007) offers comprehensive guidance for the emergency admission of acutely ill adults, particularly to the ward care areas.

There has been a more visible emphasis on patient safety within this edition. We believe that patient outcomes can be improved through early recognition of deterioration and the initiation of prompt, appropriate intervention. This can be achieved through a vigilant, comprehensive and systematic assessment of the patient. With an understanding (through evidence) nurses are able to provide rationale for the patient's data collected, enabling a pro-active rather than a reactive approach to care delivery. Nurses have a moral, professional and legal obligation to provide competent, safe and sensitive care. *High Dependency Nursing Care* has provided a comprehensive text (with critical appraisal of available information) to enable nurses to meet these expectations.

While technology is made available to benefit patients, the humanistic theme continues to be important within this edition. Proficient care requires the nurse to carefully balance not only knowledge and skill but also attitude when attending to vulnerable patients and their family.

High Dependency Nursing Care persists in adopting a holistic style to help you identify components of competent, safe and sensitive practice. There are still limitations to this holistic approach, notably rehabilitation and cultural competence (these are aspects of care that have been developed from the first edition). While the area of rehabilitation is currently being addressed (NICE guidance due in 2009) there continues to be a deficit in new knowledge.

As clinical developments grow within acute care, it is hoped that this book has contributed to such developments, in addition to identifying topics where there are opportunities for nurses to explore and critically appraise related practice. Through a rigorous education process (theory and practice), nurses will be capable of retaining, developing and maintaining their clinical competence within acute care. It is anticipated that this book offers some input on the various strategies that can be undertaken to facilitate nurses developing their practice, thus enabling them to accept the demands ahead.

This particular edition has been a challenge, as we faced so many obstacles – but we firmly believe and are committed to making a contribution to enhance the quality of care provision for the patients with level 2 care needs.

Glossary

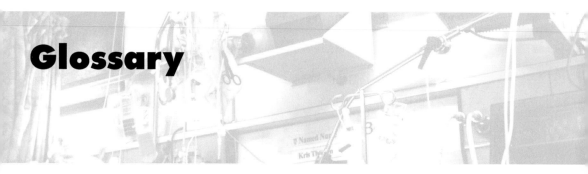

adnexal anatomical region either side of pelvis

atelectasis collapse of alveoli

cardioversion restoring normal sinus rhythm – can be chemical (drugs) or electrical (defibrillation)

collateral circulation blood vessels which develop to bypass complete or incomplete obstruction to bloodflow. Collateral blood vessels are weak, tortuous and friable, so liable to rupture

D-dimers a fibrin degradation product (FDP), released when clot breakdown (lysis) occurs. Normal levels are <250 nanograms per millilitre or micrograms (μ) per litre. Normal levels are sometimes reported as 'negative'

deadspace space between where air or gas enters the airway and the alveoli where gas exchange occurs (average physiological adult deadspace = 150 ml)

ejection fraction the percentage of blood ejected from the (usually left) ventricle in relation to total ventricular blood volume. Usually measured by echocardiogram, normal ejection fraction is 60–70 per cent

endometriosis endometrial tissue deposited outside the uterus

glycolysis breakdown of glucose in the presence of oxygen

gonadotrophin protein hormones

haematocrit proportion of blood volume occupied by red cells

haematemesis blood in vomit

haemoptysis blood in sputum

hypercapnia high (arterial) blood carbon dioxide (>6.0 kPa)

joule measurement of energy: the work involved by one Newton moving one metre

kilocalorie (kcal) measurement of energy: energy needed to warm 1 kilogram of water by 1°C. 1 kcal = 4.184 kJ

luteinisation mature follicles discharging their egg and transforming into a corpus luteum

melaena black, tar-like stools, containing blood

myocyte   cardiac muscle cell

pulse pressure   the difference between arterial systolic and diastolic pressure. High pulse pressure indicates poor vessel compliance (e.g. atherosclerosis), while narrow pulse pressure (e.g. 20) indicates hypovolaemia

respiratory failure Type 1   failure of oxygen exchange ($PaO_2 < 8.0$, $PaCO_2 < 6.0$ kPa)

respiratory failure Type 2   failure of oxygen exchange ($PaO_2 < 8.0$, $PaCO_2 > 6.0$ kPa)

rhabdomyolosis   rare cause of acute kidney injury, secondary to extensive muscle damage (e.g. from trauma)

stroke volume   amount of blood ejected with each contraction of the left ventricle

suppurate   form pus

tachypnoea   fast breathing

trophoplast   outer layer of cells surrounding blastocyst

xenotransplantation   transplantation of tissues from other species (e.g. baboon heart valves)

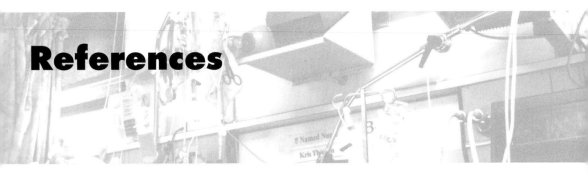

References

3M Health Care (2003) Website www.3m.com/uk/littmann.

AARC (1993) Clinical practice guidelines: endotracheal suctioning of mechanically ventilated adults and children with artificial airways. *Respiratory Care* 38 (4): 500–504.

ACCP/SCCM (1992) Consensus conference: definitions for sepsis and organ failure and guidelines for the use of innovative therapies. *Critical Care Medicine* 20 (6): 864–874.

Adam, A., Nicholson, C., Owens, L. (2008) Alcoholic dilated cardiomyopathy. *Nursing Standard* 22 (38): 42–47.

Adam S., Osborne, S. (2005) *Critical Care Nursing: Science and Practice.* 2nd edition. Oxford. Oxford University Press.

Adams, S., Whitlock, M., Baskett, P., Bloomfield, P., Higgs, R. (1994) Should relatives be allowed to watch resuscitation? *BMJ* 308 (6945): 1687–1689.

Adgey, A.A.J., Walsh, S.J. (2004) Theory and practice of defibrillation: (1) atrial fibrillation and DC conversion. *Heart* 90 (12): 1493–1498.

Adjei, N. (2004) The sickle cell disease patient. *Nurse 2 Nurse* 2 (6): 16–18.

Adrogué, H.J. (2007) Sodium and potassium in the pathogenesis of hypertension. *NEJM* 356 (19): 1966–1978.

Agarwal, R. (2006) The low-flow or high-flow oxygen delivery system and a low-flow or high-flow nonrebreather mask. *American Journal of Respiratory Care Medicine* 174 (2): 171–177.

Ahern, J., Philpot, P. (2002) Assessing acutely ill patients on general wards. *Nursing Standard* 16 (47): 47–54.

Akgul, A. (2002) Effects of normal saline on endotracheal suctioning. *Journal of Clinical Nursing* 11 (6): 826–830.

Aksoy, S. (2000) Can the 'quality of life' be used as a criterion in health care services? *Bulletin of Medical Ethics* 162: 19–22.

Alchaghouri, S. (2004) Atrial fibrillation 2: management. *Hospital Medicine* 65 (9): 546–552.

Alderson, P., Schierhout, G., Roberts, I., Bunn, F. (2004) *Colloids Versus Crystalloids for Fluid Resuscitation in Critically Ill Patients (Cochrane Review)*. The Cochrane Library issue 2. Chichester. Wiley & Sons.

Aldred, H., Gott, M., Gariballa, S. (2005) Advanced heart failure: impact on older patients and informal carers. *Journal of Advanced Nursing* 49 (2): 116–124.

Allen, C.H., Ward, J.D. (1998) An evidence-based approach to management of increased intracranial pressure. *Critical Care Clinics* 14 (3): 485–495.

Allen, S. (2005) Prevention and control of infection in the ICU. *Current Anaesthesia and Critical Care* 16 (5): 191–199.

Allibone, L. (2006) Assessment and management of patients with pleural effusions. *Nursing Standard* 20 (22): 55–64.

Almerud, S., Alapack, R.J., Fridlund, B., Ekebergh, M. (2007) Of vigilance and invisibility – being a patient in technological intense environments. *Nursing in Critical Care* 13 (3): 151–158.

Almerud, S., Alapack, R.J., Fridlund, B., Ekebergh, M. (2008) Beleaguered by technology: care in technologically intense environments. *Nursing Philosophy* 9 (2): 55–61.

Almirante, B., Rodrýguez, D., Park, B.J., Cuenca-Estrella, M., Planes, A.M., Almela, M., Mensa, J., Sanchez, F., Ayats, J., Gimenez, M., Saballs, P., Fridkin, S.K., Morgan, J., Rodriguez-Tudela, J.L., Warnock, D.W., Pahissa, A., Barcelona Candidemia Project Study Group (2005) Epidemiology and predictors of mortality in cases of *Candida* bloodstream infection: results from population-based surveillance, Barcelona, Spain, from 2002 to 2003. *Journal of Clinical Microbiology* 43 (4): 1829–1835.

American Psychiatric Association (2000) *Diagnostic and Statistical Manual of Mental Disorders*. 4th edition. Washington, DC. American Psychiatric Association.

Anderson, F.A., Spencer, F.A. (2003) Risk factors for venous thromboembolism. *Circulation* 23 (supplement): I9–I16.

Andrew, C.M. (1998) Optimising the human experience: nursing the families of people who die in intensive care. *Intensive and Critical Care Nursing* 14 (2): 59–65.

Antunes, G., Neville, E., Duffy, J., Ali, N., BTS Pleural Disease Group. (2003) BTS guidelines for the management of malignant pleural effusions. *Thorax* 58 (supplement II): ii29–ii38.

APHO (2007) *Indications of Public Health in the English Regions*. Number 4. London. Association of Public Health Observatories.

Arboleya, L.R., de la Figuera, E., Soledad García, M., Aragón, B., VICOXX Study Group. (2003) Experience of rofecoxib in patients with osteoarthritis previously treated with traditional non-steroidal anti-inflammatory drugs in Spain: results of phase 2 of the VICOXX study. *Current Medical Research and Opinion* 19 (4): 288–297.

Arroyo-Novoa, C.M., Figueroa-Ramos, M., Puntillo, K.A., Stanik-Hutt, J., Thompson, C.L., White, C., Wild, L.R. (2008) Pain related to tracheal suctioning in awake acutely and critically ill adults: a descriptive study. *Intensive and Critical Care Nursing* 24 (1): 20–27.

Ash, D. (2005) Sustaining safe and acceptable bowel care in spinal cord injured patients. *Nursing Standard* 20 (8): 55–64.

Ashdown, M. (1985) Sudden death. *Nursing Mirror* 161 (18): 22–24.

Ashworth, P. (1980) *Care to Communicate*. London. Royal College of Nursing.

Ashworth, P. (1990) High technology and humanity for intensive care. *Intensive Care Nursing* 6 (3): 150–160.

Asthma UK. (2008) Website www.asthma.org.uk/all_about_asthma/asthma_basics/index.html (accessed 1 April 2008).

Audit Commission (1999) *Critical to Success: The Place of Efficient and Effective Critical Care Services within the Acute Hospital*. London. Audit Commission.

Auerbach, S.M., Kiesler, D.J., Wartella, J., Rausch, S., Ward, K.R., Ivatury, R. (2005) Optimism, satisfaction with needs met, interpersonal perceptions of the healthcare team and emotional distress in patient's family members during critical care hospitalisation. *American Journal of Critical Care* 14 (3): 202–210.

B v. *Secretary for Health* (2002) All ER 449.

Bach, P.B., Brown, C., Gelfand, S.E., McCrory, D.C. (2001) Management of acute exacerbations of chronic obstructive pulmonary disease: a summary and appraisal of published evidence. *Annals of Internal Medicine* 134 (7): 600–620.

Bader, M.K., Arbour, R. (2005) Refractory increased intracranial pressure in severe traumatic brain injury. *AACN Clinical Issues* 16 (4): 526–541.

Baird, M.S., Keen, J.H., Swearingen, P.L. (2005) *Manual of Critical Care Nursing*. 5th edition. St Louis. Elsevier.

Baker, C., Mansfield, B. (2008) Physical rehabilitation following critical illness. *JICS* 9 (2): 166–169.

Baldwin, M. (2003) Patient advocary: a concept anlaysis. *Nursing Standard* 17 (21): 33–39.

Ball, C. (2002) Editorial: the devil is in the detail. *Intensive and Critical Care Nursing* 18 (2): 71–72.

Ball, C. (2008) Improving rehabilitation following transfer from ICU. *Intensive and Critical Care Nursing* 24 (4): 209–210.

Ballantyne, J.C., McKenna, J.M., Ryder, E. (2003) Epidural analgesia: experience of 5628 patients in a large teaching hospital derived through audit. *Acute Pain* 4 (3–4): 89–97.

Banks, P.A. (1998) Acute and chronic pancreatitis. In Felman, M., Scharschmidt, B.F., Sleisenger, M.H. (eds) *Sleisenger and Fordtran's Gastrointestinal and Liver Disease*. Philadelphia. WB Saunders Co., pp. 809–862.

Bar-El, Y., Ross, A., Kablawi, A., Egenburg, S. (2001) Potentially dangerous negative intrapleural pressure generated by ordinary pleural drainage systems. *Chest* 119 (2): 511–514.

Barnard, A. (2004) Philosophy of technology and nursing. In Reed, P., Shearer, N., Nicoll, L. (eds) *Perspectives on Nursing Theory*. Philadelphia. Lippincott, Williams & Williams, pp. 613–627.

Barratt, J. (2007) What to do with patients with abnormal dipstick urinalysis. *Medicine* 35 (7): 365–367.

Baskett, P.J. (1994) Doctors need to be trained to work in public. *BMJ* 308 (6945): 1687–1689.

Bateman, D.N. (2007) Poisoning: focus on paracetamol. *Journal of the Royal College of Physicians of Edinburgh* 37 (4): 332–334.

Bateman, N.T., Leach, R.M. (1998) Acute oxygen therapy. *BMJ* 317 (7161): 798–801.

Baudouin, S.V. (2002) The pulmonary physician in critical care. 3: Critical care management of community acquired pneumonia. *Thorax* 57 (3): 267–271.

Beauchamp, T., Childress, F. (2008) *Principles of Biomedical Ethics*. 5th edition. New York. Oxford University Press.

Beck, D.H., McQuillan, P., Smith, G. (2002) Waiting for the break of dawn? The effects of discharge time, discharge TISS scores and discharge facility on hospital mortality after intensive care. *Intensive Care Medicine* 28 (9): 1287–1293.

Becker, J.U., Wira, C.R. (2008) Disseminated intravascular coagulation. *emedicine*. www.medicine.medscape.com/artcle/1779097-overview.

Beckett, N.S., Peters, R., Fletcher, A.E., Staessen, J.A., Liu, L., Dumitrascu, D., Stoyanovsky, V., Antikainen, R.L., Nikitin, Y., Anderson, C., Belhani, A., Forette, F., Rajkumar, C., Thijs, L., Banya, W., Bulpitt, C.J., HYVET Study Group. (2008) Treatment of hypertension in patients 80 years of age or older. *NEJM* 358 (18): 1887–1898.

Bell, R.L., Ovadia, P., Abdullah, F., Spector, S., Rabinovici, R. (2001) Chest tube removal: end-inspiration or end-expiration? *Journal of Trauma* 50 (4): 674–677.

Bench, S. (2004) Clinical skills: assessing and treating shock: a nursing perspective. *British Journal of Nursing* 13 (12): 715–721.

Bennett, M. (ed.) (2006) *Neuropathic Pain*. Oxford. Oxford University Press.

Berliner, N. (2004) Disorders of red blood cells. In Andreoli, T.E., Carpenter, C.C.J., Griggs, R.C., Loscalzo, J. (eds) *Cecil's Essentials of Medicine*. 6th edition. Philadelphia. Sanders, pp. 449–460.

Berthelot, P., Grattard, F., Mahul, P., Pain, P., Jospé, R., Venet, C., Carricajo, A., Aubert, G., Ros, A., Dumont, A., Lucht, F., Zéni, F., Auboyer, C.A., Bertrand, J.C., Pozzetto, B. (2001) Prospective study of nosocomial colonization and infection due to *Pseudomonas aeruginosa* in mechanically ventilated patients. *Intensive Care Medicine* 27 (3): 503–512.

Bertrand, M.E., Simoons, M.L., Fox, K.A., Wallentin, L.C., Hamm, C.W., McFadden, E., De Feyter, P.J., Speccia, G., Ruzyllo, W. (2002) Management of acute coronary syndromes in patients presenting *without* persistent ST segment elevation. The task force on the management of Acute Coronary Syndromes of the European Society of Cardiology. *European Heart Journal* 23 (23): 1809–1840.

Best, C. (2007) Nasogastric tube insertion in adults who require enteral feeding. *Nursing Standard* 21 (40): 39–43.

Blackwood, B. (1999) Normal saline instillation with end tracheal suctioning: primum non nocere (first do no harm). *Journal of Advanced Nursing* 29 (4): 928–934.

BMA (2007a) *Withholding and Withdrawing Life-Prolonging Medical Treatment*. 3rd edition. London. BMJ Books.

BMA (2007b) *Decisions Relating to Cardiopulmonary Resuscitation. A Joint Statement from the British Medical Association, the Resuscitation Council (UK) and the Royal College of Nursing*. London. British Medical Association.

Bodenham, A.R., Barry, B.N. (2001) The role of tracheostomy in ICU. *Anaesthesia and Intensive Care Medicine* 2 (9): 336–339.

Bolam v. *Friern Barnet* HMC (1957) All ER 118.

Bollen, T.L., van Santvoort, H.C., Besselink, M.G., van Leeuwen, M.S., Horvath, K.D., Freeny, P.C., Gooszen, H.G. (2008) The Atlanta Classification of acute pancreatitis revisited. *British Journal of Surgery* 95 (1): 448–449.

Bolliger, D., Steiner, L.A., Kasper, J., Aziz, O.A., Filopovic, M., Seeberger, M.D. (2007) The accuracy of non-invasive carbon dioxide monitoring: a clinical evaluation of two transcutaneous systems. *Anaesthesia* 62 (4): 394–399.

Bone, R.C., Balk, R.A., Cerra, F.B., Dellinger, R.P., Fein, A.M., Knaus, W.A., Schein, R.M., Sibbald, W.J.I. (1992). Definitions for sepsis and organ failure and guidelines for the use of innovative therapies in sepsis. *Chest* 110 (6): 1644–1655.

Booker, R. (2007) Peak expiratory flow measurement. *Nursing Standard* 21 (39): 42–43.

Booth, C., Heyland, D.K., Paterson, W.G. (2002) Gastrointestinal promotility drugs in the critical care setting: a systematic review of the evidence. *Critical Care Medicine* 30 (7): 1429–1435.

Borger, P., Tamm, M., Black, J.L., Roth, M. (2006) Asthma: is it due to an abnormal airway smooth muscle cell? *American Journal of Respiratory and Critical Care Medicine* 174 (4): 367–372.

Borthwick, M., Bourne, R., Craig, M., Egan, A., Oxley, J. (2006). *Direction, Prevention and Treatment of Delirium in Critically Ill Patients*. London. UK Clinical Pharmacy Association.

Bosch, J., Abraldes, J.G. (2005) Variceal bleeding: pharmacological therapy. *Digestive Diseases* 23 (1): 18–29.

Bradley, C. (2001) Stress ulcer prevention – the controversy continues. *Intensive and Critical Care Nursing* 17 (1): 58–60.

Branch, W.T., Kern, D., Haidef, P., Weissmann, P., Gracey, C.F., Mitchell, G., Inui, T. (2001) Teaching the human dimension of care in clinical setting. *JAMA* 286 (9): 1067–1074.

Breathnach, A. (2005) Nosocomial infections. *Medicine* 33 (3): 22–26.

Brenner, Z.R. (2006) Management of hyperglycaemic emergencies. *AACN Clinical Issues* 17 (1): 56–65.

British Society of Gastroenterology Endoscopy Committee (2000) Non-variceal upper gastrointestinal haemorrhage guidelines. *Gut* 51 (supplement IV): iv1–iv6.

Bromet, D.S., Klein, L.W. (2004) Cardiogenic shock: art and science. *Critical Care Medicine* 32 (1): 293–294.

Broomhead, R. (2002) Percutaneous tracheostomy. *Anaesthesia and Critical Care* 3 (6): 210–212.

Browning, G., Warren, N.A. (2006) Unmet needs of family members in the medical intensive care waiting room. *Critical Care Nursing Quarterly* 29 (1): 86–95.

BSRM/RCP (2003) *Rehabilitation Following Acquired Brain Injury*. London. British Society of Rehabilitation Medicine/Royal College of Physicians.

BTS (2002) Non-invasive ventilation in acute respiratory failure. *Thorax* 57 (3): 192–211.

BTS (2003) British Thoracic Society guidelines for the management of suspected acute pulmonary embolism. *Thorax* 58 (6): 470–484.

BTS (2004) Management of acute exacerbations of COPD. *Thorax* 59 (supplement 1): 1–232.

BTS (2006) *The Burden of Lung Disease*. 2nd edition. London. British Thoracic Society.

BTS (2008) BTS guideline for emergency oxygen use in adult patients. *Thorax* 63 (supplement VI): vi1–vi68.

BTS/SIGN (2008) British guidelines on the management of asthma. *Thorax* 63 (supplement IV): iv1–iv121.

Buckman, R. (1988) *I Don't Know What to Say*. London. Pan.

Burdette, S.D., Parilo, M. (2007). Systemic inflammatory response syndrome. *emedicine*. www.emedicine.com/MED/topic2227.htm (accessed 14 November 2008).

Burger, C.M. (2004) Hyperkalaemia. *American Journal of Nursing* 104 (10): 66–70.

Burglass, E. (1999) Tracheostomy care: tracheal suctioning and humidification. *British Journal of Nursing* 8 (8): 500–504.

Burke, C., Seeley, M.G. (1994) An oncology unit's initiation of bereavement support programme. Oncology Forum. *Nursing* 21 (10): 1657–1680.

Campbell, S., Monga, A. (2006) *Gynaecology by Ten Teachers*. 18th edition. London. Hodder Education.

Campbell, S.E., Avenell, A., Walker, A.E., TEMPEST Group (2002) Assessment of nutritional status in hospital in-patients. *QJM* 95 (2): 83–87.

Carper, B.A. (1978) Fundamental patterns of knowing in nursing. *Advances in Nursing Science* 1 (1): 13–23.

Carr, E.C.J. (2000) Exploring the effect of postoperative pain on patient outcomes following surgery. *Acute Pain* 3 (4): 183–191.

Carroll, P. (2000) Exploring chest drain options. *RN* 63 (10): 50–54.

Carroll, P. (2002) A guide to mobile chest drains. *RN* 65 (5): 56–60.

Cars, O., Högberg, L.D., Murray, M., Nordberg, O., Sivaraman, S., Lundborg, C.S., So, A.D., Tomson, G. (2008) Meeting the challenge of antibiotic resistance. *BMJ* 337 (7672): 726–728.

Carskadon, M. (2004) Sleep deprivation: health consequences and societal impact. *Medical Clinics of North America* 88 (3): 767–776.

Casey, G. (2001) Oxygen transport and the use of pulse oxymetry. *Nursing Standard* 15 (47): 46–53.

Cassel, C.K., Leipzig, R.M., Cohen, H.J., Larson, H.J. (2003) *Geriatric Medicine: An Evidence-Based Approach*. 4th edition. New York. Springer.

Cathcart, F. (1988) Seeing the body after death. *BMJ* 297 (6655): 997–998.

Celik, S.S., Elbas, N.O. (2000) The standard of suction for patients undergoing endotracheal intubation. *Intensive and Critical Care Nursing* 16 (3): 191–198.

Cely, C.M., Arora, P., Quartrin, A.A., Kett, D.H., Schein, R.M.H. (2004) Relationship of baseline glucose homeostasis to hyperglycaemia during medical critical illness. *Chest* 126 (3): 879–887.

Chadda, K., Louis, B., Benaïssa, L., Annane, D., Gajdos, P., Raphaël, J.C., Lofaso, F. (2002) Physiological effects of decannulation in tracheostomized patients. *Intensive Care Medicine* 28 (12): 1761–1767.

Chalmers, C., Straub, M. (2006) Standard principles for preventing and controlling infection. *Nursing Standard* 20 (23): 57–65.

Chapman, S.J., Davies, C.W.H. (2003) Non-invasive positive pressure ventilation in acute respiratory failure. *Care of the Critically Ill* 19 (5): 145–149.

Charnock, Y., Evans, D. (2001) Nursing management of chest drains. *Australian Critical Care* 14 (4): 156–160.

Chaudhuri, R., Livingston, E., McMahon, A.D., Lafferty, J., Fraser, I., Spears, M. (2006) Effects of smoking cessation on lung function and airway inflammation in smokers with asthma. *American Journal of Respiratory and Critical Care Medicine* 174 (2): 127–133.

Cherian, J., Thwaini, A., Rao, A., Arya, N., Shergill, I.S., Patel, H.R.H. (2005) Autonomic dysreflexia: the forgotten medical emergency. *Hospital Medicine* 66 (5): 294–296.

Chhajed, P.N., Heuss, L.T., Tamm, M. (2005) Cutaneous carbon dioxide monitoring in adults. *Current Opinion in Anaesthesiology* 17 (6): 521–525.

Chikwe, J., Walther, A., Pepper, J. (2004) The surgical management of mitral valve disease. *British Journal of Cardiology* 11 (1): 42–47.

Clark, A.M., Thompson, D.R. (2008) The future of management programmes for heart failure. *Lancet* 372 (9641): 784–785.

Clark, S. (1993) Psychological needs of the critically ill patients. In Clochesy, J.M., Cardin, S., Rudy, E.B., Whittaker, A.A. (eds) *Critical Care Nursing*. Philadelphia. W.B. Saunders.

Clifford, C. (1985) Helplessness: a concept applied to nursing practice. *Intensive Care Nursing* 1 (1): 19–24.

Coad, S., Haines, S. (1999) Supporting staff caring for critically ill patients in acute care areas. *Nursing in Critical Care* 4 (5): 245–248.

Cobley, M., Atkins, M., Jones, P.L. (1991) Environmental contamination during tracheal suction. *Anaesthesia* 46 (11): 957–961.

Coggrave, M. (2008) Neurogenic continence. Part 3: bowel management strategies. *British Journal of Nursing* 17 (15): 962–968.

Coia, J.E., Duckworth, G.J., Edwards, D.I., Farrington, M., Fry, C., Humphreys, H., Mallaghan, C., Tucker, D.R., Joint Working Party of the British Society of Antimicrobial Chemotherapy, the Hospital Infection Society, and the Infection Control Nurses Association (2006) Guidelines for the control and prevention of methicillin-resistant *Staphylococcus aureus* (MRSA) in healthcare facilities. *Journal of Hospital Infections* 63S: S1–S44.

Cole, E. (2007) Measuring central venous pressure. *Nursing Standard* 22 (7): 40–42.

Cole, E., Lynch, A., Cugnoni, H. (2006) Assessment of the patient with acute abdominal pain. *Nursing Standard* 20 (39): 67–75.

Collin, C., Daly, G. (1998) Brain injury. In Stokes, M. (ed.) *Neurological Physiology*. London. Mosby.

Collins, T. (2000). Understanding shock. *Nursing Standard* 23 (4): 35–38.

Conen, D., Pidker, P.M., Buring, J.E., Glynn, R.J. (2007) Risk of cardiovascular events among women with high normal blood pressure or blood pressure progression: prospective cohort study. *BMJ* 335 (7617): 432–436.

Connolly, D.L, Lip, G.Y.H., Chin, B.S.P. (2002) Antithrombotic strategies in acute coronary syndromes and percutaneous coronary interventions. *BMJ* 325 (7377): 1404–1407.

Conzalez, J.C.M. (2008) Gastric residuals: are they important in the management of enteral nutrition? *Clinical Nutrition Highlights* 4 (1): 2–8.

Cook, D., Guyatt, G., Marshall, J., Leasa, D., Fuller, H., Hall, R., Peters, S., Rutledge, F., Griffith, L., McLellan, A., Wood, G., Kirby, A. (1998) A comparison of sucralfate and ranitidine for the prevention of upper gastrointestinal bleeding in patients requiring mechanical ventilation. *NEJM* 338 (12): 791–797.

Cook., D.J., Guyatt, G.H., Jaeschke, R., Reeve, J., Spanier, A., Molloy, D.W., Willan, A., Streiner, D.L. (1995) Determinants in Canadian health care workers of the decision to withdraw life support from the critically ill. *JAMA* 273 (9): 703–708.

Cook, N. (2003) Respiratory care in spinal cord injury with associated traumatic brain injury: bridging the gap in critical care nursing interventions. *Intensive and Critical Care Nursing* 19 (3): 143–153.

Coolican, M.B. (1994) Families facing the sudden death of a loved one. *Critical Care Clinics of North America* 6 (3): 607–612.

Cooper, M.C. (1993) The intersection of technology and care in the ICU. *Advances in Nursing Science* 15 (3): 23–32.

Cornish, C.A., Kennedy, N.P. (2000) Protein-energy undernutrition in hospital in-patients. *British Journal of Nutrition* 83 (6): 575–591.

Cottingham, C.A. (2006) Resuscitation of traumatic shock and hemodynamic review. *AACN Advanced Critical Care* 17 (3): 317–326.

Coulling, S. (2005) Nurses' and doctors' knowledge of pain after surgery. *Nursing Standard* 19 (34): 41–49.

Covington, S. (2000) *Infertility Counselling: A Comprehensive Handbook for Clinicians*. New York. Taylor & Francis.

Cox, C., McGrath, A. (1999) Respiratory assessment in critical care units. *Intensive and Critical Care Nursing* 15 (4): 226–234.

Cox, M., Kemp, R., Anwar, S., Athey, V., Aung, T., Moloney, E.D. (2006) Non-invasive monitoring of CO_2 levels in patients using NIV for AECOPD. *Thorax* 61 (4): 363–364.

Cox, N., Roper, T. (2005) *Clinical Skills*. Oxford. Oxford University Press.

Crichton, B. (2007) Blood pressure control. *Geriatric Medicine* 37 (3): 75–80.

Crombie, I.K., Davies, H.T.O., Macrae, W.A. (1998) Cut and thrust: antecedent surgery and trauma among patients attending a chronic pain clinic. *Pain* 76 (1–2): 167–172.

Crosby, L., Parsons, C. (1992) Cerebrovascular response of closed head-injured patients to a standardized end tracheal tube suctioning and manual hyperventilation procedure. *Journal of Neuroscience Nursing* 24: 40–49.

Crowcroft, N.S., Catchpole, M. (2002) Mortality from methicillin resistant *Staphylococcus aureus* in England and Wales: analysis of death certificates. *BMJ* 325 (7377): 1390–1391.

Cunningham, J.B., Kernohan, W.G., Sowney, R. (2005) Bed occupancy and turnover interval as determinant factors in MRSA infections in acute settings in Northern Ireland: 1 April 2001 to 31 March 2003. *Journal of Hospital Infections* 61 (3): 189–193.

Cuthbertson, B.H., Hull, A., Strachan, M., Scott, J. (2004) Post-traumatic stress disorder after critical illness requiring general intensive care. *Intensive Care Medicine* 30 (3): 450–455.

Czarnik, R.E., Stone, K.S., Everhart, C.G., Preusser, B.A. (1991) Differential effects of continuous versus intermittent suction on tracheal tissue. *Heart and Lung* 20 (2): 144–157.

Daffurn, K., Lee, A., Hillman, K.M., Bishop, G.F., Bauman, A. (1994) Do nurses know when to summon emergency assistance? *Intensive and Critical Care Nursing* 10 (2): 115–120.

Daly, K., Beale, R., Chang, R.W.S. (2001) Reduction in mortality after inappropriate early discharge from intensive care unit: logistic regression triage model. *BMJ* 322 (7297): 1–5.

Danis, M. (1998) Improving end-of-life care in the intensive care unit: What's to be learned from outcomes research? *New Horizons* 6 (1): 110–118.

Darouiche, R. (2006) Spinal epidural abscess. *NEJM* 355 (19): 2012–2020.

Davenport, A., Stevens, P. (2008) *Clinical Practice Guidelines: Acute Kidney Injury.* 4th edition. London. UK Renal Association. Available at www.renal. org/guidelines (accessed 26 June 2008).

Davies, B. (2007) The chest. In Brooks, A., Mahoney, P., Rowlands, B. (eds) *ABC of Tubes, Drains, Lines and Frames.* Oxford. Wiley-Blackwell/BMJ Books.

Davies, C.W.H., Gleeson, F.V., Davies, R.J.O., BTS Pleural Disease Group. (2003) BTS guidelines for the management of pleural infection. *Thorax* 58 (supplement II): ii18–ii28.

Davidson, B. (1999) *What's All This About Stress?* Wirral. Tudor Business Publishing Limited.

Dawes, E., Lloyd, H., Durham, L. (2007) Monitoring and recording patients' neurological observations. *Nursing Standard* 22 (10): 40–45.

Day, C.P. (2002) Alcohol and the liver. *Medicine* 30 (11): 18–20.

Day, T., Farnell, S., Wilson-Barnett, J. (2002) Suctioning: a review of current research recommendations. *Intensive and Critical Care Nursing* 18 (2): 79–89.

Day, T., Wainwright, S., Wilson-Barnett, J. (2001) An evaluation of a teaching intervention to improve the practice of end tracheal suctioning in intensive care units. *Journal of Clinical Nursing* 10 (5): 682–696.

De, D. (2005) Sickle cell anaemia 1: background, causes and incidences in the UK. *British Journal of Nursing* 14 (28): 447–450.

De Beer, K., Micheal, S., Thacker, M., Wynne, E., Pattni, C., Gomm, M., Ball, C., Walsh, D. (2008) Diabetic ketoacidosis and hyperglycaemic hyperosmolar syndrome – clinical guidelines. *Nursing in Critical Care* 13 (1): 5–11.

Dellinger, R.P., Carlet, J.M., Masur, H., Gerlach, H., Calandra, T., Cohen, J., Gea-Banacloche, J., Keh, D., Marshall, J.C., Parker, M.M., Ramsay, G., Zimmerman, J.L., Vincent, J.-L., Levy, M.M. (2004) Surviving sepsis campaign guidelines for management of severe sepsis and septic shock. *Intensive Care Medicine* 30 (3): 536–555.

Dellinger, R.D., Levy, M.M., Carlet, J.M., Bion, J., Parker, M.M., Jaeschke, R. *et al.* (2008) Surviving sepsis campaign: international guidelines for management of severe sepsis and septic shock. *Critical Care Medicine* 36 (1): 296–327.

Detsky, A.S., McLaughlin, J.R., Baker, J.P., Johnston, N., Whittaker, S., Mendelson, R.A., Jeejeebhoy, K.B. (1987) What is subjective global assessment of nutritional status? *Journal of Parenteral and Enteral Nutrition* 11 (1): 8–13.

De Waele, J.J., Hoste, E.A.J., Baert, D., Hendricks, K., Rijckaert, D., Thibo, P., Van Biervliet, P., Blot, S.I., Colardyn, F. (2007) Relative adrenal insufficiency in patients with severe acute pancreatitis. *Intensive Care Medicine* 33 (10): 1754–1760.

Dimond, B. (2008) *Legal Aspects in Nursing.* 5th edition. Essex. Pearson Education Limited.

Dinges, D.F., Douglas, S.D., Zaugg, L., Campbell, D.E., McMann, J.M., Whitehouse, W.G. (1994) Leukocytosis and natural killer cell function parallel neurobehavioral fatigue induced by 64 hours of sleep deprivation. *Journal of Clinical Investigation* 93 (5): 1930–1939.

Distenfield, A., Woermann, U. (2002) Sickle cell anaemia. *emedicine.* www.emedicine.com/med/topic216htm.

Docherty, B., Bench, S. (2002) Tracheostomy management for patients in general ward settings. *Professional Nurse* 18 (2): 100–104.

Dodek, P.M., Heyland, D.K., Graeme, R.M. (2004) Translating family satisfaction data into quality improvement. *Critical Care Medicine* 32 (9): 1975–1976.

DOH (1997) *The New NHS: Modern, Dependable.* London. Department of Health.

DOH (2000a) *Comprehensive Critical Care: A Review of Adult Critical Care Services.* London. Department of Health.

DOH (2000b) *Heart Attacks and Other Acute Coronary Syndromes: Modern Standards and Service Models.* London. Department of Health.

DOH (2001) *National Service Framework for Diabetes: Standards.* London. Department of Health.

DOH (2007) *Dignity in Care.* London. Department of Health.

DOH (2008) *Organs for Transplants.* London. Department of Health.

Doig, C., Murray, H., Bellomo, R., Kuiper, M., Costa, R., Azoulay, A., Crippen, D. (2006) Ethics round table debate: patients and surrogates want 'everything done' – what does 'everything' mean? *Critical Care* 10 (5): 231–237.

Dougherty, L., Lister, S. (eds) (2008) *The Royal Marsden Hospital Manual of Clinical Nursing Procedures.* 7th edition. Oxford. Wiley-Blackwell.

Dowling, J., Wang, B. (2005) Impact on family satisfaction: the Critical Care Family Assistance Program. *Chest* 28 (3 supplement): 76S–80S.

Dreyer, A., Per Nortvedt, D. (2007) Sedation of ventilated patients in intensive care units: relatives' experiences. *Journal of Advanced Nursing* 61 (5): 549–556.

Driscoll, D.J. (2006) *Fundamentals of Pediatric Cardiology.* Philadelphia. Lippincott, Williams & Wilkins.

Druml, W. (2005) Nutritional management of acute renal failure. *Journal of Renal Nutrition* 15: 63–70.

Dunn, M., Gwinnutt, C., Gray, A. (2007) Critical care in the emergency department: patient transfer. *Emergency Medicine Journal* 24 (1): 40–44.

Dyer, C. (1997) Family accuses doctors of failing to warn of risk. *BJM* 314: 1217.

Dyer, I. (1991) Meeting the needs of visitors: a practical approach. *Intensive Care Nursing* 7 (3): 135–147.

Dyer, I. (1995) Preventing the ITU syndrome, or how not to torture an ITU patient! Part 1. *Intensive and Critical Care Nursing* 11 (3): 130–139.

Eason, E., Wells, G., Garber, G., Hemmings, R., Luskey, G., Gillett, P., Martin, M. (2004) Antisepsis for abdominal hysterectomy: a randomised controlled trial of povidone-iodine gel. *BJOG* 111 (7): 695–699.

Eastland, J. (2001) A framework for nursing the dying patient in ICU. *Nursing Times* 97 (3): 36–39.

Eckel, R.H., Grundy, S.M., Zimmet, P.Z. (2005) The metabolic syndrome. *Lancet* 365 (9468): 1415–1428.

Edwards, S. (1996) *Nursing Ethics: A Principle-Based Approach.* Basingstoke. Macmillan.

Edwards, S. (2001) Regulation of water, sodium and potassium: implications for practice. *Nursing Standard* 15 (22): 36–45.

Eggimann, P., Pittet, D. (1998) Central line sepsis in intensive care units: overview and update. *Current Anaesthesia and Critical Care* 10 (1): 14–20.

Eggimann, P., Pittet, D. (2001) Infection control in the ICU. *Chest* 120 (6): 2059–2093.

Eichorn, D. (1996) Opening the doors: family presence during resuscitation. *Journal of Cardiovascular Nursing* 10 (4): 59–70.

El-Ghariani, K., Unsworth, D.J. (2006) Therapeutic apheresis – plasmapheresis. *Clinical Medicine* 6 (4): 343–347.

Ellershaw, J., Ward, C. (2003) Care of the dying patient: the last hours or days of life. *BMJ* 326 (30): 30–34.

Ellershaw, J., Wilkinson, S. (2003) *Care of the Dying: A Pathway to Excellence.* Oxford. Oxford University Press.

Elliott, H. (2006) Epidemiology, aetiology and prognosis of hypertension. *Medicine* 34 (8): 286–289.

Ellison, G. (1992) A private disaster. *Nursing Times* 88 (52): 52–53.

Ely, E.W., Shintani, A., Truman, B., Speroff, T., Gordon, S.M., Harrell, F.E., Inouye, S.K., Bernard, G.R., Dittus, R.S. (2004). Delirium as a predictor of mortality in mechanically ventilated patients in the intensive care unit. *JAMA* 291 (14): 1753–1762.

Emanuel, E.J., Fairclough, D.L., Emanuel, L.L. (2000) Attitudes and desires related to euthanasia and physician-assisted suicide among terminally ill patients and their caregivers. *JAMA* 284 (19): 2460–2468.

English, P., Williams, G. (2004) Hyperglycaemic crisis and lactic acidosis diabetes mellitus. *Postgraduate Medicine Journal* 80 (493): 253–261.

Engström, A., Söderberg, S. (2007) Receiving power through confirmation: the meaning of close relatives for people who have been critically ill. *Journal of Advanced Nursing* 59 (6): 569–576.

Epstein, O., Perkin, D., de Bono, D., Cookson, J. (2003) *Clinical Examination*. 3rd edition. London. Mosby.

Epstein, R.M. (1999) Mindful practice. *JAMA* 282 (9): 833–839.

Eriksson, T., Bergbom, I. (2007) Visits to intensive care unit: frequency, duration and impact on outcome. *British Association of Critical Care Nurses* 12 (1): 20–26.

Essposito, K., Nappo, F., Marfella, R., Giugliano, G., Giugliano, F., Ciotola, M., Quagliaro, L., Ceriello, A., Giugliano, D. (2002) Inflammatory cytokine concentrations are acutely increased by hyperglycaemia I humans. Role of oxidative stress. *Circulation* 106 (16): 2067–2072.

European Resuscitation Council (2005) Guidelines for adult and paediatric basic life support and advanced life support. *Resuscitation* 48: 199–239.

Ewins, D., Bryant, J. (1992) Relative comfort. *Nursing Times* 88 (52): 61–63.

Eynon, C.A., Menon, K.D. (2002) Critical care management of head injury. *Anaesthesia and Critical Care* 3 (4): 135–139.

Fahey, S. (2007) Developing a nursing service for patients with hepatitis C. *Nursing Standard* 21 (43): 35–40.

Fallah, M.A., Prakah, C., Edmundowica, S. (2000) Acute gastrointestinal bleeding. *The Medical Clinics of North America* 84 (5): 1183–1208.

Farrell, M. (1989) Dying and bereavement. The role of the critical care nurse. *Intensive Care Nursing* 5 (1): 39–45.

Farrell, M. (1999) The challenge of breaking bad news. *Intensive and Critical Care Nursing* 15 (2): 101–110.

Fawcett, T., Smith, G. (2005) Acute pancreatitis: pathophysiology and patient care. *Gastrointestinal Nursing* 3 (8): 31–39.

Fearnhead, N.S. (2007) Acute lower gastrointestinal bleeding. *Medicine* 35 (3): 164–167.

Fearon, K.C.H., Ljunqvist, O., von Meyenfeldt, M., Revhaug, A., Dejong, C.H.C., Lassen, K., Nygren, J., Hausel, J., Soop, M., Andersen, J., Kehlet, H. (2005) Enhanced recovery after surgery: a consensus review of clinical care for patients undergoing colonic resection. *Clinical Nutrition* 24 (3): 466–477.

Fehrenbach, C. (2002) Chronic obstructive pulmonary disease. *Nursing Standard* 17 (10): 45–51.

Ferer, M., Esquinas, A., Leon, M., Gonzalez, G., Alarcon, A., Torres, A. (2003) Noninvasive ventilation in severe hypoxemic respiratory failure. *American Journal of Respiratory and Critical Care Medicine* 168 (12): 1438–1444.

Feiner, J.R., Severinghaus, J.W., Bick, L. (2007) Dark skin reduces the accuracy of pulse oximeters and low oxygen saturation: the effects of oxinate probe type and genda. *Anesthesia and Analgesia* 105 (6 supplement): S18–S23.

Finlay, I., Dallimore, D. (1991) Your child is dead. *BMJ* 302 (6791): 1524–1525.

Fiorentini, A. (1992) Potential hazards of tracheobronchial suctioning. *Intensive and Critical Care Nursing* 8 (4): 217–226.

Firth, P.G. (2005) Anaesthesia for peculiar cells: a century of sickle cell disease. *BJA* 95 (3): 287–299.

Fisher, K. (2006) Specialist palliative care for patients with non-cancer diagnosis. *Nursing Standard* 21 (4): 44–47.

Fitzgerald, G., Patrono, C. (2001) The Coxibs, selective inhibitors of cyclooxygenase-2. *NEJM* 345 (6): 433–442.

FitzGerald, M. (2001) Acute asthma. *BMJ* 323 (7317): 841–845.

Flanning, H. (2000) Fluid and electrolyte balance. In Manley, K., Bellman, L. (eds) *Surgical Nursing: Advancing Practice*. Edinburgh: Churchill Livingstone, pp. 538–555.

Flynn, J.B., Bruce, N.P. (1993) *Introduction to Critical Care Skills*. St. Louis. Mosby.

Forrester, D.A., Murphy, P.A., Price, D.M. (1990) Critical care family needs: nurse–family members confederate pairs. *Heart and Lung* 19 (6): 655–661.

Fotherby, M. (2006) Atrial fibrillation and heart failure. *Geriatric Medicine* 36 (9): 33–36.

Fox, M. (1999) The importance of sleep. *Nursing Standard* 13 (24): 44–47.

Foxton, J. (2003) CHD prevention: the importance of identifying dyslipidaemia. *British Journal of Nursing* 12 (16): 950–957.

Fox-Wasylyshyn, S., Maher, E.M., Williamson, K. (2005) Family perceptions of nurses' roles towards family members of critically ill patients: A descriptive study. *Heart and Lung: Journal of Acute and Critical Care* 34 (5): 335–344.

Franklin, C., Mathew, J. (1994) Developing strategies to prevent in-hospital cardiac arrest: analysing responses of physicians and nurses in the hours before the event. *Critical Care Medicine* 22 (2): 244–247.

Friedemann, M.L. (1989) The concept of family nursing. *Journal of Advanced Nursing* 14 (3): 211–216.

Fuccio, L., Laterza, L., Zagari, R.M., Cennamo, V., Grilli, D., Bazzoli, F. (2008) Treatment of *Helicobacter pylori* infection. *BMJ* 337 (7672): 746–750.

Fukatsu, K., Zarzaur, B.L., Johnson, C.D., Lundberg, A.H., Wilcox, H.G., Kudsk, K.A. (2001) Enteral nutrition prevents remote organ injury and death after a gut ischaemia insult. *Annals of Surgery* 233 (5): 660–668.

Fukuda, S., Warner, D.S. (2007) Cerebral protection. *BJA* 99 (1): 10–17.

Fulbrook, P., Bonkers, A., Albarran, J.W. (2007) A European survey of adult intensive care nurses' practice in relation to nutritional assessment. *Journal of Clinical Nursing* 16 (11): 2132–2141.

Fulbrook, P., Buckley, P., Mills, C., Smith, G. (1999) On the receiving end: experiences of being a relative in critical care (part 2). *Nursing in Critical Care* 4 (4): 179–1185.

Furlan, J.C., Urbach, D.R., Fehlings, M.G. (2007) Optimal treatment for severe neurogenic bowel dysfunction after chronic spinal cord injury: a decision analysis. *British Journal of Surgery* 94 (9): 1139–1150.

Gallagher, A., Wainwright, P. (2007) Terminal sedation: promoting ethical nursing practice. *Nursing Standard* 21 (34): 42–46.

Gallant, M.H., Beaulieu, M.C., Carevale, F.A. (2002) Partnership: an analysis of the concept within the nurse–client relationship. *Journal of Advanced Nursing* 40 (2): 149–157.

Galley, H.F., Webster, N.R. (2004) Physiology of the endothelium. *BJA* 93 (1): 105–111.

Gallon, A. (1998) Pneumothorax. *Nursing Standard* 13 (10): 35–39.

Ganong, W.F. (2005) *Review of Medical Physiology*. 22nd edition. San Francisco. McGraw-Hill.

Gao, H., Harrison, D., Parry, G., Daly, K., Subbe, C., Rowan, K. (2007) The impact of the introduction of critical care outreach services in England: a multicentre interrupted time-series analysis. *Critical Care* 11 (5): R113.

Garfield, M.J., Jeffrey, R., Ridley, S.A. (2000) An assessment of staffing level required for a high dependency unit. *Anaesthesia* 55 (2): 137–143.

Gavaghan, S.R., Carroll, D.L. (2002) Families of critically ill patients and the effect of nursing interventions. *Dimensions in Critical Care Nursing* 21 (2): 64–71.

Ghost, S., Watts, D., Kinnear, M. (2002) Management of gastrointestinal haemorrhage. *Postgraduate Medical Journal* 78 (915): 4–14.

Gines, P., Cardenas, A. (2008) The management of ascites and hyponatremia in cirrhosis. Seminars in Liver Disease. *Complications of Cirrhosis* 28 (1): 43–58.

Girou, E., Brun-Buisson, C., Taillé, S., Lemaire, F., Brochard, L. (2003) Secular trends in nosocomial infections and mortality associated with noninvasive ventilation in patients with exacerbation of COPD and pulmonary edema. *JAMA* 290 (22): 2985–2991.

Gladwin, M.T., Sachdev, V., Jison, M., Shizukuda, Y., Plehn, J., Minter, K., Brown, B., Coles, W.A., Nichols, J.S., Ernst, I., Hunter, L.A., Blackwelder, W.C., Schechter, A.N., Rodgers, G.P., Castro, O., Ognibene, F. (2004) Pulmonary hypertension as a risk factor of death in patients with sickle cell disease. *NEMJ* 350 (9): 886–895.

Glass, C., Grap, M. (1995) Ten tips for safe suctioning. *American Journal of Nursing* 5 (5): 51–53.

Godden, J., Hiley, C. (1998) Managing the patient with a chest drain: a review. *Nursing Standard* 12 (32): 35–39.

GOLD Executive Summary (2007) Global strategy for the diagnosis, management, and prevention of chronic obstructive pulmonary disease. *American Journal of Respiratory and Critical Care Medicine* 176 (6): 532–555.

Goldacre, M.J., Roberts, S.E. (2004) Hospital admission for acute pancreatitis in an English population, 1963–98: database study of incidence and mortality. *BMJ* 328 (7454): 1466–1469.

Goldhill, D.R. (1997) Introducing the postoperative care team: additional support, expertise and equipment for general postoperative patients. *BMJ* 314 (7078): 389.

Goldhill, D.R., Sumner, A. (1998) Outcome of intensive care patients in a group of British intensive care units. *Critical Care Medicine* 26 (8): 1337–1345.

Goldhill, D.R., White, S.A., Sumner, A. (1999a) Physiological values and procedures in the 24h before ICU admission from the ward. *Anaesthesia* 54 (9): 529–534.

Goldhill, D.R., Worthington, L., Mulcahy, A., Tarling, M., Sumner, A. (1999b) The patient-at-risk team: identifying and managing seriously ill ward patients. *Anaesthesia* 54 (9): 853–860.

Golembiewski, J.A., O'Brien, D. (2002) A systematic approach to the management of postoperative nausea and vomiting. *Journal of Perianesthesia Nursing* 17 (6): 364–376.

Gorman, K. (1999) Sickle cell disease: do you doubt your patient's pain? *American Journal of Nursing* 99 (3): 38–43.

Gould, D. (2008) Enterococcal infection. *Nursing Standard* 22 (27): 40–43.

Graham, A. (1996) Chest drain insertion. *Care of the Critically Ill* 12 (5): centre insert.

Granberg, A., Enberg, B., Lundberg, D. (1996) Intensive care syndrome: a literature review. *Intensive and Critical Care Nursing* 12 (3): 173–182.

Granberg-Axèll, A., Bergbom, I., Lunberg, D. (2001) Clinical signs of ICU syndrome/delirium: an observational study. *Intensive and Critical Care Nursing* 17 (2): 72–93.

Grap, M.J., Glass, C., Corley, M., Creekmore, S., Mellott, K., Howard, C. (1994) Effect of level of lung injury on HR, MAP, and SaO_2 changes during suctioning. *Intensive Critical Care Nursing* 10 (3): 171–178.

Gray, A., Bush, S., Whiteley, S., Williams, R. (2004) Secondary transport of the critically ill and injured adult. *Emergency Medicine Journal* 21 (3): 281–285.

Gray, A., Gill, S., Airey, M. (2003) Descriptive epidemiology of adult critical transfers from the emergency department. *Emergency Medicine Journal* 20 (3): 242–246.

Gray, A., Goodacre, S., Newby, D.E., Masson, M., Sampson, F., Nicholl, J., 3CPO Triallists (2008) Noninvasive ventilation in acute cardiogenic pulmonary edema. *NEJM* 359 (2): 142–151.

Gray, E. (2001) Pain management for patients with chest drains. *Nursing Standard* 14 (23): 40–44.

Grech, E. (2003) Pathophysiology and investigation of coronary artery disease. *BMJ* 326 (7397): 1027–1030.

Grech, E., Ramsdale, D. (2003) Acute coronary syndrome: unstable angina and non ST segment elevation myocardial infarction. *BMJ* 326 (7401): 1259–1261.

Gries, C.J., Curtis, R.J., Wall, R.J., Engelberg, R.A. (2008) Family member satisfaction with end-of-life decision making in the ICU. *Chest* 133 (3): 704–712.

Grieve, R.J., Finnie, A. (2002) Nutritional care: implications and recommendations for nursing. *British Journal of Nursing* 11 (7): 432–437.

Grundmann, H. (2006) Emergence and resurgence of methicillin-resistant *Staphylococcus aureus* as a public-health threat. *Lancet* 368 (9538): 874–885.

Guenter, P.A., Settle, R.G., Perlmutter, S., Marino, P.L., DeSimone, G.A.,

Rolandelli, R.H. (1991) Tube feeding-related diarrhoea in acutely ill patients. *Journal of Parenteral and Enteral Nutrition* 15 (3): 277–280.

Gumbley, E., Pearson, J. (2006) Tissue donation: benefits, legal issues and the nurse's role. *Nursing Standard* 21 (1): 51–56.

Gunning, K., Rowan, K. (1988) ABC of intensive care: outcome data and scoring systems. Influence of terbutaline on endotoxin-induced lung injury. *Circulatory Shock* 25: 153–163.

Gupta, N. (2001) Pneumothorax: is chest tube clamp necessary before removal? *Chest* 119 (4): 1292–1293.

Gutenbrunner, C., Ward, A., Chamberlain, M.A. (2007) White book on physical and rehabilitation medicine in Europe. *Journal of Rehabilitation Medicine.* www.medicaljournals.se/jm.

Guyton, A., Hall, J.C. (2005) *Textbook of Medical Physiology.* Philadelphia. Elsevier.

Guzman, J.A., Kruse, J.A. (2001) Targeting the gut in shock and organ failure. *Clinical Intensive Care* 12 (5,6): 203–209.

Gwinnutt, C. (2006) *Clinical Anaesthesia.* 2nd edition. Oxford. Blackwell Publishing.

Hadaway, L.C. (2005) Reopen the pipeline. *Nursing 2005* 35 (8): 54–61.

Haddadin, A.S., Fappiano, S.A., Lipsett, P.A. (2002) Methicillin resistant *Staphylococcus aureus* (MRSA) in the intensive care unit. *Postgraduate Medical Journal* 78 (921): 385–392.

Hadingham, J. (1997) Talking about tissue donation. *Professional Nurse* 12 (7): 473.

Hadley, M.N. (2002) Management of acute spinal cord injuries in an intensive care unit or other monitored setting. *Neurosurgery Online* 50 (3): S51–S57.

Haines, S., Coad, S. (2001) Supporting ward staff in acute care areas: expanding the service. *Intensive and Critical Care Nursing* 17 (2): 105–109.

Hairon, N. (2008) Action to prevent the spread of norovirus infection. *Nursing Times* 104 (2): 27–28.

Hajjeh, R.A., Sofair, A.N., Harrison, L.H., Lyon, G.M., Arthington-Skaggs, B.A., Mirza, S.A., Phelan, M., Morgan, J., Lee-Yang, W., Ciblak, M.A., Benjamin, L.E., Sanza, L.T., Huie, S., Yeo, S.F., Brandt, M.E., Warnock, D.W. (2004) Incidence of bloodstream infections due to *Candida* species and in vitro susceptibilities of isolates collected from 1998 to 2000 in a population-based active surveillance program. *Journal of Clinical Microbiology* 42 (4): 1519–1527.

Hale, A.S., Moseley, M.J., Warner, S.C. (2000) Treating pancreatitis in the acute care setting. *Dimensions of Critical Care Nursing* 19 (4): 15–21.

Hales, R.E., Yudofsky, S.C. (2004) *Essentials of Clinical Psychiatry.* 2nd edition. Washington, DC. American Psychiatric Publications.

Hall, A.P., Henry, J.A. (2006) Acute toxic effects of 'Ecstasy' (MDMA) and related compounds: overview of pathophysiology and clinical management. *BJA* 96 (6): 678–685.

Hall, B., Hall, D.A. (1994) Learning from the experience of loss: people bereaved during intensive care. *Intensive and Critical Care Nursing* 10 (4): 265–1709.

Hall, J., Horsley, M. (2007) Diagnosis and management of patients with *Clostridium difficile*-associated diarrhoea. *Nursing Standard* 21 (46): 49–56.

Hall, M., Jones, A. (1997) Reducing morbidity from insertion of chest drains: clamping may be appropriate to prevent discomfort and reduce risk of oedema. *BMJ* 315 (7103): 313.

Hampton, J.R. (2008a) *The ECG Made Easy*. 7th edition. Edinburgh. Churchill Livingstone.

Hampton, J.R. (2008b) *The ECG in Practice*. 5th edition. Edinburgh. Churchill Livingstone.

Hampton, J.R. (2008c) *150 ECG Problems*. 3rd edition. Edinburgh. Churchill Livingstone.

Hans-Geurts, I.J.M., Hop, W.C.J., Kok, N.F.M., Lim, A., Brouwer, K.J., Jeekel, J. (2007) Randomized clinical trial of the impact of early enteral feeding on postoperative ileus and recovery. *British Journal of Surgery* 94 (5): 555–561.

Hanson, C., Strawser, D. (1992) Family presence during cardiopulmonary resuscitation: Foote hospital emergency department's nine-year perspective. *Journal of Emergency Nursing* (182): 104–106.

Harbath, S., Sax, H., Gastmeier, P. (2003) The preventable proportion of nosocomial infections: an overview of published reports. *Journal of Hospital Infection* 54 (4): 258–266.

Hart, R.G., Halperin, J.L., Pearce, L.A., Anderson, D.C., Kronmal, R.A., McBride, R., Nasco, E., Sherman, D.G., Talbert, R.L., Marler, J.R., Stroke Prevention in Atrial Fibrillation Investigators (2003) Antithrombotic therapy to prevent stroke in patients with atrial fibrillation: a meta-analysis. *Annals of Internal Medicine* 138 (10): 831–838.

Harvey, L. (2008) *Management of Spinal Cord Injuries*. Edinburgh. Churchill Livingstone.

Harvey, M.G. (1992) Humanizing the intensive care unit experience. *Clinical Issues in Perinatal and Women's Health Nursing* 3 (3): 369–376.

Hasson, J., Maslovich, S., Har-Toov, J., Lessing, J.B., Grisaru, D. (2007) Post-hysterectomy pelvic fluid collection: is it associated with febrile morbidity? *BJOG* 114 (12): 1566–1568.

Hatchett, R. (1994) Should relatives watch resuscitation? A successful American programme. *BMJ* 309 (6951): 407.

Hawthorne, J., Redmond, K. (1998) *Pain: Causes and Management*. Oxford. Blackwell.

Hayes, C., Browne, S., Lantry, G., Burstal, R. (2002) Neuropathic pain in the acute pain service: a prospective survey. *Acute Pain* 4 (2): 45–48.

Helman, C. (2007) *Culture Health and Illness*. 5th edition. London. Hodder/Arnold.

HELP Booklet adapted from ALERT™ course manual (2002) *A Multi Professional Training Course in the Care of the Critically Ill Patient*. Portsmouth. University of Portsmouth.

Henrion, J., Schapira, M., Luwaert, R., Colin, L., Delannoy, A., Heller, F. (2003)

Hypoxic hepatitis: clinical and haemodynamic study in 142 consecutive cases. *Medicine* 82 (6): 392–406.

Henry, M., Arnold, T., Harvey, J., BTS Pleural Disease Group (2003) BTS guidelines for the management of spontaneous pneumothorax. *Thorax* 58 (supplement II): ii39–ii52.

Herridge, M.S., Cheung, A.M., Tansey, C.M. (2003) One year outcomes in survivors of the acute respiratory distress syndrome. *NEJM* 384 (8): 683–693.

Hewitt, J. (2002) A critical review of the arguments debating the role of the nurse advocate. *Journal of Advanced Nursing* 37 (5): 439–445.

Hewitt, J., Jordan, S. (2004) Prescription drugs: uses and effects. Opioids. *Nursing Standard* 19 (6): insert.

Heyland, D., Rocker, G.M., Dodek, P.M., Kusogiannis, D.J., Konopad, E., Cook, D.J. *et al.* (2002) Family satisfaction in the intensive care unit: results of a multiple centre study. *Critical Care Medicine* 30 (7): 1413–1418.

Hickey, J.V. (ed.) (2003a) *The Clinical Practice of Neurological and Neurosurgical Nursing.* 5th edition. Philadelphia. Lippincott, pp. 285–318.

Hickey, J.V. (2003b) Craniocerebral trauma. In Hickey, J.V. (ed.) *The Clinical Practice of Neurological and Neurosurgical Nursing.* 5th edition. Philadelphia. Lippincott.

Higgs, R. (1994) Relatives' wishes should be accommodated. *BMJ* 308 (6945): 1688.

Higgins, C. (2007) *Understanding Laboratory Investigations.* 2nd edition. Oxford. Blackwell.

Hillberg, R.E., Johnson, D.C. (1997) Noninvasive ventilation. *NEJM* 337 (24): 1746–1752.

Hinkelbein, J., Genzwuerker, H.V., Sogl, R., Fiedler, F. (2007) Effect of nail polish on oxygen saturation determined pulse oximetry in critically ill patients. *Resuscitation* 72 (1): 82–91.

Hipp, A., Sinert, R. (2008) Metabolic acidosis. *emedicine.* www.emedicine.com/emerg/topic312.htm (accessed 29 September 2008).

Ho, K.M., Sheridan, D.J. (2006) Meta-analysis of frusemide to prevent or treat acute renal failure. *BMJ* 333 (7565): 420–423.

Hoedema, R.E, Luchtefeld, M.A. (2005) The management of lower gastrointestinal hemorrhage. *Diseases of the Colon and Rectum* 48 (11): 2010–2024.

Hoffbrand, A.V., Modd, P.A.H., Petit, J.E. (2006) *Essential Haematology.* 5th edition. Oxford. Blackwell.

Hofhuis, J., Bakker, J. (1998) Experiences of critically ill patients in the ICU: what do they think of us? *International Journal of Intensive Care* 98 (5): 114–117.

Hogg, J.C., Senior, R.M. (2002) Chronic obstructive pulmonary disease C2: pathology and biochemistry of emphysema. *Thorax* 57 (9): 830–834.

Holgate, S.T., Polosa, R. (2006) The mechanisms, diagnosis, and management of severe asthma in adults. *Lancet* 368 (9537): 780–793.

Holmes, S. (2007) The effects of undernutrition in hospitalised patients. *Nursing Standard* 22 (12): 35–38.

Honkus, V. (2003) Sleep deprivation in critical care units. *Critical Care Nursing Quarterly* 26 (3): 179–189.

Horne, J. (1998) *Why We Sleep*. Oxford. Oxford University Press.

Hough, A. (2001) *Physiotherapy in Respiratory Care*. 3rd edition. Cheltenham. Nelson Thornes.

Houghton, A.R., Gray, D. (2008) *Making Sense of the ECG*. 3rd edition. London. Edward Arnold.

Howard, A., Zaccagnini, D., Ellis, M., Williams, A., Davies, A.H., Greenhalgh, R.M. (2004) Randomized clinical trial of low molecular weight heparin with thigh-length or knee-length antiembolism stockings for patients undergoing surgery. *British Journal of Surgery* 91 (7): 842–847.

Huether, S.E., McCance, K.L. (2004) *Understanding Pathophysiology*. St Louis. Mosby.

Hughes, E. (2004) Understanding the care of patients with acute pancreatitis. *Nursing Standard* 18 (18): 45–52.

Hughes, R.A.C., Wijdicks, E.F.M., Benson, E., Cornblath, D.R., Hahn, A.F., Meythaler, J.M., Sladky, J.T., Barohn, R.J., Stevens, J.C. (2005) Supportive care for patients with Guillain–Barré syndrome. *Archives of Neurology* 62 (8): 1194–1198.

Human Rights Act (1998) London. HMSO.

Humphreys, H. (2001) Infection control on the intensive care unit. In Galley, H.F. (ed.) *Critical Care Focus 5: Antibiotic Resistance and Infection Control*. London. BMJ Books, pp. 12–18.

Humphreys, M. (2002) Hyperkalaemia: a dangerous electrolyte disturbance. *Connect* 2 (1): 28–30.

Hunningher, A., Smith, M. (2006) Update on the management of severe head injury in adults. *Care of the Critically Ill* 22 (5): 124–129.

Hyers, T.M. (2003) Management of venous thromboembolism. *Archives of Internal Medicine* 163 (7): 759–768.

ICS (1997) *Standards for Intensive Care*. London. Intensive Care Society.

ICS (2002) *Guidelines for the Transport of the Critically Ill Adult*. London. Intensive Care Society.

ICS (2008) *Standards for Care of Adult Patients with Temporary Tracheostomies*. London. Intensive Care Society.

Impey, L. (2004) *Obstetrics and Gynaecology*. 2nd edition. Oxford. Blackwell Publishing Ltd.

Institute for Clinical Systems Improvement (2006) *Chronic Obstructive Pulmonary Disease*. Bloomington (MN). Institute for Clinical Systems Improvement.

International Association for the Study of Pain (1979) Pain terms: a list of definitions and usage. *Pain* 6: 249–252.

Jablonski, R.S. (1994) The experience of being mechanically ventilated. *Qualitative Health Research* 4 (2): 186–207.

Jackson, I. (1996) Critical care nurses' perception of a bereavement follow-up service. *Intensive and Critical Care Nursing* 12 (1): 2–11.

Jackson, I. (1998) A study of bereavement in an intensive care unit. *Nursing in Critical Care* 3 (3): 141–150.

Jackson, N., Wendon, J. (2000) The management of acute liver failure. *Clinical Intensive Care* 11 (3): 127–135.

Janssen, J.P., Collier, G., Astoul, P., Tassi, G.F., Noppen, M., Rodriguez-Panadero, F., Loddenkemper, R., Herth, F.J.F., Gasparini, S., Harquette, C.H., Becke, B., Froudarakis, M.E., Driesen, P., Bolliger, C.T., Tschopp, J.-M. (2007) Safety of pleurodesis with talc poudrage in malignant pleural effusion: a prospective cohort study. *Lancet* 369 (9572): 1435–1539.

Jarvis, C. (2008) *Physical Examination and Health Assessment*. 5th edition. Philadelphia. W.B. Saunders.

Jarvis, H. (2006) Exploring the evidence base of the use of non-invasive ventilation. *British Journal of Nursing* 15 (14): 756–759.

Jensen, L.O., Thayssen, P., Pedersen, K.E., Stender, S., Torben, H. (2004) Regression of coronary atherosclerosis by Simvastatin. *Circulation* 110 (3): 265–270.

Jeschke, M.G., Klein, D., Herndon, D.N. (2003) Insulin treatment improves the systemic inflammatory reaction to severe trauma. *Annals of Surgery* 239 (4): 553–560.

Jevon, P. (2003) *ECGs for Nurses*. Oxford. Blackwell Publishing.

Jevon, P., Ewens, B. (2007) *Monitoring the Critically Ill Patient*. 2nd edition. Oxford. Blackwell Publishing.

Joanna Briggs Institute (2008) Nursing interventions to minimise undernutrition in older patients in hospital. *Nursing Standard* 22 (1): 35–40.

Johnson, K., Rawlings, K., Anderson, K. (2007) *Oxford Handbook of Cardiac Nursing*. Oxford. Oxford University Press.

Johnson, S. (2005) *Fundamental Aspects of Gynaecology Nursing*. London. Quay Books Division, MA Healthcare Ltd.

Jolliet, P., Abajo, B., Pasquina, P., Chevrolet, J.-C. (2001) Non-invasive pressure support ventilation in severe community-acquired pneumonia. *Intensive Care Medicine* 27 (5): 812–821.

Jones, C., Skirrow, P., Griffiths, R.D., Humphris, G.H., Ingleby, S., Eddleston, J., Waldmann, C., Gager, M. (2003) Rehabilitation after critical illness: a randomized, controlled trial. *Critical Care Medicine* 31 (10): 2456–2461.

Jones, C., Skirrow, P., Griffiths, R.D., Humphris, G., Ingleby, S., Eddleston, J., Waldmann, C., Gager, M. (2005) Post-traumatic stress disorder-related symptoms in relatives of patients following intensive care. *Intensive Care Medicine* 30 (3): 456–460.

Jones, D.W., Appel, L.J., Sheps, S.G., Roccella, E.J., Lenfant, C. (2003) Measuring blood pressure accurately. *JAMA* 289 (8): 1027–1030.

Jones, I. (2003) Acute coronary syndromes: identification and patient care. *Professional Nurse* 18 (5): 289–292.

Jonsdottir, H., Litchfeild, M., Dexheimer Pharris, M. (2004) The relational care of nursing practice. *Journal of Advanced Nursing* 47 (3): 241–250.

Jubb, M., Shanley, E. (2002) Family involvement: the key to opening locked wards and closed minds. *International Journal of Mental Health Nursing* 11 (1): 47–53.

Kannan, S. (1999) Practical issues in non-invasive positive pressure ventilation. *Care of the Critically Ill* 15 (3): 76–79.

Keely, B.R. (1998) Preventing complications. Recognition and treatment of autonomic dysreflexia. *Dimensions in Critical Care Nursing* 17 (4): 170–176.

Keely, E.C., Boura, J.A., Grines, C.L. (2003) Primary angioplasty versus intravenous thrombolytic therapy for acute myocardial infarction: a quantitative review of 23 randomised trials. *Lancet* 361 (9351): 13–20.

Kehlet, H. (2001) Multimodal approach to control postoperative pathophysiology and rehabilitation. *BJA* 78 (5): 606–617.

Kelly, C.A., Upex, A., Bateman, D. (2004) Comparison of consciousness level assessment in the poisoned patient using the alert/verbal/painful/unresponsive scale and the Glasgow Coma Scale. *Annals of Emergency Medicine* 44 (2): 108–113.

Kelly, C.P., LaMont, T. (2008) *Clostridium difficile*: more difficult than ever. *NEJM* 359 (18): 1932–1940.

Kennedy, J.F. (1997) Enteral feeding for the critically ill patient. *Nursing Standard* 11 (33): 39–43.

Kent, H., McDowell, J. (2004) Sudden bereavement in acute care settings. *Nursing Standard* 19 (6): 38–42.

Kessenich, C. (2000) Teaching health assessment in advanced practice nursing programs. *Nurse Educator* 25 (4): 170–172.

Kent v. *Griffiths and others* (2002) 2 All ER 474.

Keyes, C.L., Shmotkin, D., Ryff, C.D. (2002) Optimizing well being: the empirical encounter of two traditions. *Journal of Personality and Social Psychology* 82 (6): 1007–1022.

Khan, N.U.A., Movahed, A. (2005) Pulmonary embolism and cardiac enzymes. *Heart and Lung* 34 (2): 142–146.

Kiely, J.L., Deegan, P., Buckley, A., Shiels, P., Maurer, B., McNicholas, W.T. (1998) Efficacy of nasal continuous positive airway pressure therapy in chronic heart failure: importance of underlying cardiac rhythm. *Thorax* 53 (11): 957–962.

Kings Fund (2006) Kings Fund briefing: access to healthcare and minority ethnic groups. London. Kings Fund.

Kingsnorth, A., O'Reilly, D. (2006) Acute pancreatitis. *BMJ* 332 (7549): 1072–1076.

Kinn, S., Scott, J. (2001) Nutritional awareness of critically ill surgical high-dependency patients. *British Journal of Nursing* 10 (11): 704–709.

Kisel, M., Perkins, C. (2006) Nursing observations: knowledge to help prevent critical illness. *British Journal of Nursing* 15 (19): 1052–1056.

Kissoon, N. (2005) Bench-to-bedside review: humanism in pediatric critical care medicine – a leadership challenge. *Critical Care* 9 (4): 371–375.

Kitabachi, A.E., Umpierrez, G.E., Murphy, M.B., Kreisberg, R.A. (2006) Hyperglycemic crisis in diabetes mellitus: diabetic ketoacidosis and hyperglycemic hyperosmolar state. *Journal of Endocrinology and Metabolism* 35 (4): 725–751.

Kligfield, P., Gettes, L.S., Bailey, J.J., Childers, R., Deal, B.J., Hancock, W., van Herpen, G., Jors, J.A., Macfarlane, P., Mirvis, D.M., Pahlm, O., Rautaharju,

P., Wagner, G.S. (2007) Recommendations for the standardization and interpretation of the electrocardiogram. *Circulation* 115 (10): 1306–1324.

Kogos Jr, S.C., Richards, J.S., Banos, J., Schmitt, M.M., Brunner, R.C., Meythaler, J.M., Salisbury, D.B., Renfroe, S.G., White, A.J. (2005) A descriptive study of pain and quality of life following Guillain–Barré syndrome: one year later. *Journal of Clinical Psychology in Medical Settings* 12 (2): 111–116.

Kokozides, G.E. (2006) Implementation of hemostatic techniques in the treatment of upper gastrointestinal hemorrhage. *Annals of Gastroenterology* 19 (4): 325–334.

Kolecki, P. (2008) Hypovolaemic shock. *emedicine.* www.emedicine.medscape.com/article/760145/overview.

Kosco, M., Warren, N.A. (2000) Critical care nurses' perceptions of family needs as met. *Critical Care Nursing Quarterly* 23 (2): 60–72.

Koti, R.S., Davidson, B.R. (2003) Portal hypertension. *Surgery* 21 (5): 113–117.

Kramer, N., Meyer, T.J., Meharg, J., Cece, R.D., Hill, N.S. (1995) Randomized, prospective trial on noninvasive positive pressure ventilation in acute respiratory failure. *American Journal of Respiratory and Critical Care Medicine* 151 (6): 1799–1806.

Kristensen, S.D., Anderson, H.R., Thuesen, L., Krussel, L.R., Botker, H.E., Lasses, J.F., Nielsen, T.T. (2004) Should patients with acute ST segment elevation MI be transferred for PCI? *Heart* 90 (11): 1358–1363.

Kruip, M.J.H.A., Leclercq, M.G.L., van der Heul, C., Prins, M.H., Büller, H.R. (2003) Diagnostic strategies for excluding pulmonary embolism in clinical outcome studies. *Annals of Internal Medicine* 138 (12): 941–951.

Krumberger, J. (2002) When the liver fails. *RN* 65 (2): 26–29.

Kubitz, T. (1999) Increase the muscular mass and lose corporeo fat during sleep (translated version). www.olypian.it/on/55.

Kubler-Ross, E. (1970) *On Death and Dying.* London. Routledge.

Kubler-Ross, E. (1991) *On Life after Death.* California. Celestial Arts.

Kudst, K.A. (2003) Effect of route and type of nutrition on intestine-derived inflammatory responses. *American Journal of Surgery* 185 (1): 16–21.

Kumar, P., Clark, M. (2006) *Acute Clinical Medicine.* 2nd edition. Oxford. Saunders Elsevier.

Kuwabara, S., Ogawara, K., Sing, J.-Y., Mori, M., Kanai, K., Hattori, T., Yuki, N., Lin, C.S.-Y., Burke, D., Bostock, H. (2002) Differences in membrane properties of axonal and demyelinating Guillain–Barré syndrome. *Annals of Neurology* 52 (2): 180–187.

Kyle, G., Brynn, P., Oliver, H. (2004) A procedure for the digital removal of faeces. *Nursing Standard* 19 (20): 33–39.

Lakasing, E., Francis, H. (2006) Diagnosis and management of heart failure. *Primary Health Care* 16 (5): 36–39.

Lanfear, J. (2002) The individual with epilepsy. *Nursing Standard* 16 (4): 43–53.

Langley, J., Adams, G. (2007) Insulin-based regimens decrease mortality rates in critically ill patients: a systematic review. *Diabetes/Metabolism Research and Reviews* 23 (3): 184–192.

Larsen, L., Neverett, S., Larsen, R. (2001) Clinical nurse specialist as facilitator of interdisciplinary collaborative program for adult sickle cell population. Nursing practice. *Clinical Nurse Specialist* 15 (1): 15–22.

Laws, D., Neville, E., Duffy, J., BTS Pleural Disease Group (2003) BTS guidelines for the insertion of a chest drain. *Thorax* 58 (supplement ii): ii53–ii59.

Lazarus, R.S. (1966) *Psychological Stress and Coping Process.* New York. McGraw-Hill.

Lee, A., Bishop, G., Hillman, K.M., Daffurn, K. (1995) The medical emergency team. *Anaesthesia and Intensive Care* 23 (2): 183–186.

Lee, K. (1997) An overview of sleep and common sleep problems. *American Nephrology Nurse's Association* 24: 614–677.

Lentine, K.L., Flavin, K.E., Gould, M.K. (2005) Variability in the use of thrombolysis and outcomes in critically ill medical patients. *American Journal of Medicine* 118 (12): 1373–1380.

Leske, J.S. (1992) Needs of adult family members after critical illness. Prescriptions for interventions. *Critical Care Nursing Clinics of North America* 4 (4): 587–595.

Levi, M.M. (2008) Disseminated intravascular coagulation: what's new? *Critical Care Clinic* 21 (3): 449–467.

Levy, S., Camm, A.J., Saksena, S., Aliot, E., Breithardt, G., Crijns, H., Davies, W., Kay, N., Prystowsky, E., Sutton, R., Waldo, A., Wyse, D.G. (2003) International consensus on nomenclature and classification of atrial fibrillation: a collaborative project of the Working Group on Arrhythmias and the Working Group on Cardiac Pacing of the European Society of Cardiology and the North American Society of Pacing and Electrophysiology. *Europace* 5 (2): 119–122.

Lewis, S.J., Egger, M., Sylvester, P.A., Thomas, S. (2001) Early enteral feeding versus 'nil by mouth' after gastro-intestinal surgery: systematic review and meta-analysis of controlled trials. *BMJ* 323 (7316): 773–776.

Lewis, T., Oliver, G. (2005) Improving tracheostomy care for ward patients. *Nursing Standard* 19 (19): 33–37.

LHO (2004) *Ethnic Disparities in Health and Health Care: A Focused Review of the Evidence and Selected Examples of Good Practice.* London. London Health Observatory.

Lightowler, J.V., Wedzicha, J.A., Elliott, M.W., Ram, F.S. (2003) Non-invasive positive pressure ventilation to treat respiratory failure resulting from exacerbations of chronic obstructive pulmonary disease: Cochrane systematic review and meta-analysis. *BMJ* 326 (7382): 185–187.

Ligtenberg, J., Arnold, L., Stienstra, Y., Van der Werf, T., Meertens, J., Tulleken, J., Zijistra, J. (2005) Quality of interhospital transport of critically ill patients: a prospective audit. *Critical Care* 9 (4): 343–344.

Liimatainen, L., Poskiparta, M., Sjögren, A., Kettunen, T., Karhila, P. (2001) Investigating student nurses' constructions of health promotion in nursing education. *Health Education Research* 16 (1): 33–48.

Lima, A., Bakker, J. (2005) Noninvasive monitoring of peripheral perfusion. *Intensive Care Medicine* 31 (10): 1316–1326.

Lim, S.-M., Webb, S.A. (2005) Nosocomial bacterial infections in intensive care units. I: Organisms and mechanisms of antibiotic resistance. *Anaesthesia* 60 (9): 887–902.

Lindahl, B., Sandman, P. (1998) The role of advocacy in critical care nursing: a caring response to another. *Intensive and Critical Care Nursing* 14 (4): 179–186.

Lindermann, E. (1994) Symptomatology and management of acute grief. *American Journal of Psychiatry* 151 (6): 155–160.

Lisse, J.R., Perlman, M., Johansson, G., Shoemaker, J.R., Schechtman, J., Skalky, C.S., Dixon, M.E., Polis, A.B., Mollen, A.J., Geba, G.P., ADVANTAGE Study Group. (2003) Gastrointestinal tolerability and effectiveness of Rofecoxib versus Naproxen in the treatment of osteoarthritis. *Annals of Internal Medicine* 139 (7): 539–546.

Liu, C.-M., Hang, L.-W., Chen, W.-K., Hsia, T.-C., Hsu, W.-H. (2003) Pigtail tube drainage in the treatment of spontaneous pneumothorax. *American Journal of Emergency Medicine* 21 (3): 41–44.

Lochs, H., Dejong, C., Hammarqvist, F., Hebuterne, X., Leon-Sanz, M., Schütz, M., van Gemert, W., van Gossum, A., Valentini, L., Lübke, H., Bischoff, S., Engelmann, N., Thul, P. (2006) ESPEN guidelines on enteral nutrition: gastroenterology. *Clinical Nutrition* 25: 260–274.

Long, T., Sque, M. (2007) An update on initiatives to increase organ donation: a UK perspective. *British Journal of Transplantation* 2 (2): 10–15.

Lower, J. (2003) Using pain to assess neurologic response. *Nursing2003* 33 (6): 56–57.

Lumb, A.B. (2005) *Nunn's Applied Respiratory Physiology*. 6th edition. Oxford. Butterworth and Heinemann.

McCaffery, M., Pasero, C. (1999) *Pain: Clinical Manual*. 2nd edition. St Louis. Mosby.

McCance, K.L., Huether, S.E. (2006) *Pathophysiology: The Biological Basis for Disease in Adults and Children*. St Louis. Elsevier.

McConnell, E.A. (1998) The coalescence of technology and humanism in nursing practice: it doesn't just happen and it doesn't come easy. *Holistic Nursing Practice* 12 (4): 23–30.

McDonnell, A., Esmonde, L., Morgan, R., Brown, R., Bray, K., Parry, G., Adam, S., Sinclair, R., Harvey, S., Mays, N. (2007) The provision of critical care outreach services in England: findings from a national survey. *Journal of Critical Care* 22 (3): 212–218.

McGaughey, J., Alderdice, F., Fowler, R., Kapila, A., Mayhew, A., Moutray, M. (2007) Outreach and Early Warning Systems (EWS) for the prevention of intensive care admission and death of critically ill adult patients on general hospital wards. Cochrane Database of Systematic Reviews.

McGloin, H., Adam, S., Singer, M. (1999) Unexpected deaths and referrals to intensive care of patients on general wards. Are some cases potentially avoidable? *Journal of the Royal College of Physicians of London* 33 (3): 255–259.

McGrath, A., Cox, C. (1998) Cardiac and circulatory assessment in intensive care units. *Intensive and Critical Care Nursing* 14 (5): 283–287.

Macintyre, P., Ready, L. (1996) *Acute Pain Management: A Practical Guide*. London. Saunders.

McKenna, W.J. (1996) Report of the 1995 World Health Organization/International Society and Federation of Cardiology Task Force on the definition and classification of cardiomyopathies. *Circulation* 93: 841–842.

McKinnell, J., Holt, S. (2007) Liver disease and renal dysfunction. *Medicine* 35 (9): 521–523.

McKinney, A., Deeny, P. (2002) Leaving the intensive care unit: a phenomenological study of the patients' experience. *Intensive and Critical Care Nursing* 18 (6): 320–331.

Mackintosh, C. (2007) Assessment and management of patients with post-operative pain. *Nursing Standard* 22 (5): 49–55.

McLafferty, E., Farley, A. (2008) Assessing pain in patients. *Nursing Standard* 22 (25): 42–46.

McLeod, G.A., Davies, H.T.O., Munnoch, N., Bannister, J., Macrae, W. (2001) Postoperative pain relief using thoracic epidural analgesia: outstanding success and disappointing failures. *Anaesthesia* 56 (1): 75–81.

McLuckie, A. (2003) Shock: an overview. In Oh, H., Bernsten, A.D., Soni, N. (eds) *Oh's Intensive Care Manual*. 5th edition. London. Butterworth-Heinemann, pp. 71–77.

McMahon, S., Koltzenburg, M. (eds) (2005) *Wall and Melzack's Textbook of Pain*. 5th edition. Edinburgh. Churchill Livingstone.

McMahon-Parkes, K. (1997) Management of pleural drains. *Nursing Times* 93 (52): 48–52.

McMahon-Parkes, K., Moule, P., Benger, J., Albarran, J.W. (2008) The views and preferences of resuscitated and non resuscitated patients towards family witnessed resuscitation: a qualitative study. *International Journal of Nursing* 46 (1): 12–21.

McPherson, K., Metcalfe, M.A., Herbert, A., Maresh, M., Casbard, A., Hargreaves, J., Bridgman, S., Clarke, A. (2004) Severe complications of hysterectomy: the VALUE study. *BJOG* 111 (7): 688–694.

McQuay, H., Moore, A. (1998) *An Evidence-Based Resource for Pain Relief*. Oxford. Oxford Medical.

McQuillan, P., Pilkington, S., Allan, A., Taylor, B., Short, A., Morgan, G., Nielsen, M., Barrett, D., Smith, G. (1998) Confidential inquiry into quality of care before admission to intensive care. *BMJ* 316 (7148): 1853–1858.

McWhirter, J.P., Pennington, C.R. (1994) Incidence and recognition of malnutrition in hospital. *BMJ* 308 (6934): 945–948.

MAG (2003) *Malnutrition Universal Screening Tool*. Worcestershire. Malnutrition Advisory Group, BAPEN.

Magarey, J., McCutcheon, H. (2005) Fishing with the dead: recall of memories from the ICU. *Intensive and Critical Care Nursing* 21: 344–345.

Magrath, H.P., Boulstridge, L.J. (2005) Tissue donation after death in the accident and emergency department: an opportunity wasted? *Journal of Accident and Emergency Medicine* 16 (2): 117–119.

Mahowald, M.W., Schenck, C.H. (2005) Review article insights from studying human sleep disorders. *Nature* 437 (7063): 1279–1285.

Mak, V., Davies, S.C. (2003) The pulmonary physician in critical care. Illustrative case 6: Acute chest syndrome of sickle cell anaemia. *Thorax* 58 (8): 726–728.

Malacrida, R., Bettelini, C.M., Degrate, A., Martinez, M., Marina, P.S., Badia, F., Plazza, J., Vizzardi, N., Wullschleger, R., Rapin, C.H. (1998) Reasons for dissatisfaction: a survey of relatives of intensive care patients who died. *Critical Care Medicine* 26 (7): 1187–1193.

Malangoni, M.A., Martin, A.S. (2005) Outcome of severe acute pancreatitis. *American Journal of Surgery* 189 (3): 273–277.

Mandelstam, M. (2007) *Betraying the NHS*. London. Jessica Kingsley.

Manias, E., Botti, M., Bucknall, T. (2002) Observation of pain assessment and management: the complexities of clinical practice. *Journal of Clinical Nursing* 11 (6): 724–233.

Mann, E., Carr, E. (2006) *Pain Management*. Oxford. Blackwell.

Mant, J., Hobbs, R., Fletcher, K., Roalfe, A., Fitzmaurice, D., Lip, G.Y.H., Murray, E., BAFTA Investigators, Midland Research Practice Network (2007) Warfarin versus asprin for stroke prevention in an elderly community population with atrial fibrillation (the Birmingham Atrial Fibrillation Treatment of the Aged Study, BAFTA): a randomised controlled trial. *Lancet* 370 (9586): 493–503.

March, A. (2005) A review of respiratory management in spinal cord injury. *Journal of Orthopaedic Nursing* 9 (1): 19–26.

Marieb, E.N. (2004) *Human Anatomy and Physiology*. 6th edition. San Francisco. Pearson/Benjamin Cummings.

Marieb, E.N. (2008) *Human Anatomy and Physiology*. 7th edition. San Francisco. Pearson/Benjamin Cummings.

Marik, P.E., Varon, J. (2004) The management of status epilepticus. *Chest* 126 (2): 582–591.

Marik, P.E., Zaloga, G.P. (2004) Meta-analysis of parenteral nutrition versus enteral nutrition in patients with acute pancreatitis. *BMJ* 328 (7453): 1407–1410.

Marini, J.J., Wheeler, A.P. (2006). *Critical Care Medicine: The Essentials*. 3rd edition. Philadelphia. Lippincott, Williams & Wilkins.

Marlowe, K.F., Chicella, M.F. (2002). Treatment of sickle cell pain. *Pharmacotherapy* 22 (4): 484–491.

Marret, E., Remy, C., Bonnet, F., Postoperative Pain Forum Group (2007) Meta-analysis of epidural analgesia *versus* parenteral opioid analgesia after colorectal surgery. *British Journal of Surgery* 94 (6): 665–673.

Marshall, A.P., West, S.H. (2006) Enteral feeding in the critically ill: are nursing practices contributing to hypocaloric feeding? *Intensive and Critical Care Nursing* 22 (2): 95–105.

Martinson, B.C., O'Connor, P.J., Pronk, N.P. (2001) Physical inactivity and short-term all-cause mortality in adults with chronic disease. *Archives of Internal Medicine* 161 (9): 1173–1180.

Mascini, E.M., Bonten, M.J.M. (2005) Vancomycin-resistant *enterococci*: consequences for therapy and infection control. *Clinical Microbiology and Infection* 11 (supplement 4), 43–56.

Masip, J., Roque, M., Sánchez, B., Fernández, R., Subirana, M., Expósito, J.A. (2005) Noninvasive ventilation in acute cardiogenic pulmonary edema. *JAMA* 294 (24): 3124–3130.

Mattson Porth, C. (2005) *Pathophysiology: Concepts of Altered Health State*. Philadelphia. Lippincott, Williams & Wilkins.

MDA (2001) *Tissue Necrosis Caused by Pulse Oximeter Probe – SN2001(08)*. London. Medical Device Agency.

Meagher, D. (2001) Delirium: the role of psychiatry. *The Royal College of Psychiatrists* 7 (6): 433–443.

Medford, A., Maskell, N. (2005) Pleural effusion. *Postgraduate Medical Journal* 81 (961): 702–710.

Mehanna, H.M., Moledina, J., Travis, J. (2008) Refeeding syndrome: what is it, and how to prevent and treat it? *BMJ* 336 (7659): 1495–1498.

Mehta, P.A., Cowie, M.R. (2006) Epidemiology and pathophysiology of heart failure. *Medicine* 34 (6): 210–214.

Mehta, R.L., Paascual, M.T., Soroko, S., Chertow, G.M., PICARD Study Group (2002) Diuretics, mortality, and nonrecovery of renal function in acute renal failure. *JAMA* 188 (19): 2547–2553.

Meier, R., Ockenga, J., Pertkiewicz, M., Pap, A., Milinic, N., MacFie, J., Löser, C., Keim, V. (2006) ESPEN guidelines on enteral nutrition: pancreas. *Clinical Nutrition* 25 (2): 275–284.

Meldon, S.W., Mion, L.C., Palmer, R.M., Drew, B.L., Connor, J.T., Lewicki, L.J., Bass, D.M., Emerman, C.L. (2003) A brief risk stratification to predict repeat emergency department visits and hospitalizations in older patients discharged from the emergency department. *Academic Emergency Medicine* 10 (3): 224–232.

Melzack, R., Wall, P. (1988) *The Challenge of Pain*. 2nd edition. London. Penguin.

Menon, D.K. (1999) Cerebral protection in severe brain injury: physiological determinants of outcome and their optimisation. *British Medical Bulletin* 55 (1): 226–258.

Mental Capacity Act (2005) London. HMSO.

Mental Health Act (1983) London. HMSO.

Merritt, S. (2000) Putting sleep disorders to rest. *RN* 63 (7): 26–31.

Messori, A., Trippoli, S., Vaiani, M., Gorini, M., Corrado, A. (2000) Bleeding and pneumonia in intensive care patients given ranitidine and sucralfate for prevention of stress ulcer: meta-analysis of randomised controlled trials. *BMJ* 321 (7269): 1103–1106.

Meyer, T.J., Eveloff, S.E., Bauer, M.S., Schwartz, W.A., Hill, N.S., Millman, R.P. (1994) Adverse environmental conditions in the respiratory and medical ICU settings. *Chest* 105 (4): 1211–1216.

MHRA (2008) *Medical Device Alert MDA/2008/028*. London. Medicine and Healthcare Products Regulatory Agency.

Michelet, P., Guervilly, C., Hélaine, A., Avaro, J.P., Blayac, D., Gaillat, F., Dantin, T., Thomas, P., Kerbaul, F. (2007) Adding ketamine to morphine for patient-controlled analgesia after thoracic surgery: influence on morphine consumption, respiratory function, and nocturnal desaturation. *BJA* 99 (3): 396–403.

Miller, A.C., Harvey, E. (1993) Guidelines for the management of spontaneous pneumothorax. *BMJ* 307 (6896): 114–116.

Miscarriage Association (2008) *We're Sorry You've Had a Miscarriage*. London. Miscarriage Association.

Mitchell, G.F., Vasan, R.S., Keyes, M.J., Parise, H., Wang, T.J., Larson, M.G., D'Agostino, R.B., Kannel, W.B., Levy, D., Benjamin, E.J. (2007) Pulse pressure and risk of new-onset atrial fibrillation. *JAMA* 297 (7): 709–715.

Mitchell, R.M.S., Byrne, M.F., Baillie, J. (2003) Pancreatitis. *Lancet* 361 (9367): 1447–1455.

Miyasaka, K. (2003) Do we really know how pulse oximetry works? *Journal of Anesthesia* 17 (45): 216–217.

Mokhlesi, B., Leikin, J.B., Murray, P., Corbridge, T.C. (2003) Adult toxicity in critical care. Part II: specific poisonings. *Chest* 123 (3): 897–922.

Molter, N.C. (1979) Needs of relatives of critically ill patients: a descriptive study. *Heart and Lung* 8 (2): 332–339.

Moore, T. (2007) Respiratory assessment in adults. *Nursing Standard* 21 (49): 48–56.

Mootoo, J.S. (2005) *A Guide to Cultural and Spiritual Awareness*. London. Nursing Standard (originally published as a booklet in volume 19, no. 1; available via the Nursing Standard website, www.nursing-standard.co.uk/resources/media/pdfs/v19n22culturalbooklet.pdf (accessed 7 January 2008).

Moppett, I.K. (2007) Traumatic brain injury: assessment, resuscitation and early management. *BJA* 99 (1): 18–31.

Morgan, M., Evans-Williams, D., Salmon, R., Hosein, I., Looker, D.N., Howard, A. (2000) The population impact of MRSA in a country: the national survey of MRSA in Wales, 1997. *Journal of Hospital Infection* 44 (3): 227–239.

Morgan, R.J.M., Williams, F., Wright, M.M. (1997) An early warning scoring system for detecting developing critical illness. *Clinical Intensive Care* 8 (2): 100.

Morris, F., Edhouse, J., Brady, W.J., Camm, J. (2003) *ABC of Clinical Electrocardiography*. London. BMJ Books.

Morris, R.J., Woodcock, J.P. (2004) Evidence-based compression: prevention of stasis and deep vein thrombosis. *Annals of Surgery* 239 (2): 162–171.

Morton, P.G., Fontaine, D. (2000) *Critical Care Nursing*. 9th edition. Philadelphia. Lippincott.

Morton, P.G., Fontaine, M. (2009) *Critical Care Nursing: A Holistic Approach*. 9th edition. Philadelphia. Lippincott, Williams & Wilkins.

Morton, P.G., Fontaine, M., Hudack, C.M, Gallo, B.M. (2006) *Critical Care Nursing: A Holistic Approach*. 8th edition. Philadelphia. Lippincott.

Moyle, J. (2002) *Pulse Oximetry*. London. BMJ.

Munoz-Price, L.S., Weinstein, R.A. (2008) Acinetobacter infection. *NEJM* 358 (12): 1271–1281.

Munro, M.F., Gallant, M., MacKinnon, M., Dell, G., Herbert, R., MacNutt, G., McCarthy, M.J., Murnaghan, D., Robertson, K. (2000) The Prince Edward Island conceptual model for nursing: a nursing perspective of primary health care. *Canadian Journal of Nursing Research* 32 (1): 39–55.

Murdoch, J., Larsen, D. (2004) Assessing pain in cognitively impaired older adults. *Nursing Standard* 18 (38): 33–39.

Murphy, T., Robinson, S. (2006) Renal failure and its treatment. *Anaesthesia and Intensive Care Medicine* 7 (7): 247–252.

Musco, S., Conway, E.L., Kowey, P.R. (2008) Drug therapy for atrial fibrillation. *Medical Clinics of America* 92 (1): 121–141.

Myers, T.A., Eichhorn, D.J., Guzzetta, C.E. (2000) Family presence during invasive procedures and resuscitation. *American Journal of Nursing* 100 (2): 32–41.

Nadzam, D.M., Mackles, R.M. (2001) Promoting patient safety: Is technology the solution? *Joint Commission Journal on Quality Improvement* 27 (8): 430–436.

Nathens, A.B., Curtis, J.R., Beale, R.J., Cook, D.J., Moreno, R.P., Romand, J.-A., Skerrett, S.J., Stapleton, R.D., Ware, L.B., Waldmann, C.S. (2004) Management of the critically ill patient with severe acute pancreatitis. *Critical Care Medicine* 32 (12): 2524–2536.

National Collaborating Centre for Acute Care (2007) *Head Injury: Triage, Assessment, Investigation and Early Management of Head Injury in Infants, Children and Adults.* London. National Clinical Guideline developed by the National Collaborating Centre for Acute Care at The Royal College of Surgeons of England.

National Critical Care Outreach Forum (2003) *Critical Care Outreach: Progress in Developing Services, Best Practice Guidance.* London. Department of Health.

National Outreach Forum and the Critical Care Stakeholders Forum (2007) *Critical Care Outreach Services: Indicators of Service Achievement and Good Practice.* London. Department of Health.

National Statistics Online (2003) www.statistics.gov.uk/cci/nugget.asp?id=273 (accessed 4 April 2008).

NCEPOD (2005) Emergency admissions: a journey in the right direction? London. National Confidential Enquiry into Patient Outcome and Death.

NCEPOD (2007) Emergency admissions: a journey in the right direction? London. National Confidential Enquiry into Patient Outcome and Death.

Nelson, R.A., Yu, H., Ziegler, M.G., Mills, P.J., Clausen, J.L., Dinsdale, J.E. (2001) Continuous positive airway pressure normalizes cardiac autonomic and hemodynamic responses to a laboratory stressor in apneic patients. *Chest* 119 (4): 1092–1101.

Neubauer, S. (2007) The failing heart: an engine out of fuel. *NEJM* 356 (11): 1140–1151.

Neuberger, J. (2004) *Caring for Dying People of Different Faiths.* 3rd edition. Abingdon. Radcliff Medical Press Ltd.

Newby, D.E., Grubb, N.R. (2005) *Cardiology*. Edinburgh. Elsevier/Churchill Livingstone.

Ng, A., Hall, F., Atkinson, A., Kong, K.L., Hahn, A. (2000) Bridging the analgesic gap. *Acute Pain* 3 (4): 194–199.

Nguyen, N.Q., Chapman, M.J., Fraser, R.J., Bryant, L.K., Holloway, R.H. (2007) Erythromycin is more effective than metoclopramide in the treatment of feed intolerance in critical illness. *Critical Care Medicine* 35 (2): 483–489.

NHS Quality Improvement Scotland (2007) *Caring for the Patient with a Tracheostomy*. Edinburgh. NHS Quality Improvement Scotland.

NICE (2003a) *Head Injury, Triage Assessment, Investigation and Early Management of Head Injury in Infants, Children and Adults – Clinical Guideline 4*. London. National Institute for Clinical Excellence.

NICE (2003b) *Chronic Heart Failure: Management of Chronic Heart Failure in Adults in Primary and Secondary Care. Clinical Guideline 5*. London. National Institute for Clinical Excellence.

NICE (2004a) *The Epilepsies: The Diagnosis and Management of the Epilepsies in Adults and Children in Primary and Secondary Care*. London. National Institute for Clinical Excellence.

NICE (2004b) *Chronic Obstructive Pulmonary Disease. Management of Chronic Obstructive Pulmonary Disease in Adults in Primary and Secondary Care. Clinical Guideline 12*. London. National Institute for Clinical Excellence.

NICE (2004c) *Diagnosis and Management of Type 1 Diabetes in Children, Young People and Adults*. London: National Institute for Health and Clinical Excellence.

NICE (2006a) *Nutrition Support for Adults*. London. National Institute for Clinical Excellence.

NICE (2006b) *Hypertension: Management of Hypertension in Adults in Primary Care*. London. National Institute for Clinical Excellence.

NICE (2007a) *Acutely Ill Patients in Hospital: Recognition of and Response to Acute Illness in Adults in Hospital*. London. National Institute for Clinical Excellence.

NICE (2007b) *Head Injury. Triage, Assessment, Investigation and Early Management of Head Injury in Infants, Children and Adults*. London. National Institute for Clinical Excellence.

NICE (2007c) *Heavy Menstrual Bleeding. Clinical Guideline 44*. London. National Institute for Health and Clinical Excellence.

NICE (2008) *Continuous Subcutaneous Insulin for the Treatment of Diabetes Mellitus: Review of Technological Appraisal Guidance 57*. London. National Institute for Health and Clinical Excellence.

NICE (2009) *Contemporary Management of Acute Exacerbations of COPD*. London. National Institute for Health and Clinical Excellence.

Nicholas, M. (2004) Heart failure: pathophysiology, treatment and nursing care. *Nursing Standard* 19 (11): 46–51.

Nicholson, C. (2007) Cardiovascular disease in women. *Nursing Standard* 21 (38): 43–47.

NMC (2008) *The Code: Standards of Conduct, Performance and Ethics for Nurses and Midwives*. London. Nursing and Midwifery Council.

Nolan, J.P., Hazinski, M.F., Steen, P.A., Becker, L.B. (2005) Controversial topics from 2005 International Consensus Conference on Cardiopulmonary Resuscitation and Emergency Cardiovascular Care Sciences with Treatment Recommendations. *Resuscitation* 67(2–3): 175–179.

NPSA (2002) *Patient Safety Alert. Ref PSA 01.* London. National Patient Safety Agency.

NPSA (2004) *Patient Safety Information, 15th September 2004.* London. National Patient Safety Agency.

NPSA (2007) Safer Care for the Acutely Ill Patient: Learning from Serious Incidents. London. National Patient Safety Agency.

NPSA (2008) Rapid Response Report: Risks of Chest Drain Insertion – Reference NPSA/2008/RRR003. London. National Patient Safety Agency.

Oal, H., Chugh, A., Good, E., Sankaran, S., Reich, S.S., Igic, P., Elmouchi, D., Tschopp, D., Crawford, T., Dey, S., Wimmer, A., Lemola, K., Jongnarangsin, K., Bogun, F., Pelosi, F., Morady, F. (2006) A tailored approach to catheter ablation of paroxysmal atrial fibrillation. *Circulation* 113 (15): 1824–1831.

Oats, J., Abraham, S. (2005) *Llewellyn-Jones Fundamentals of Obstetrics and Gynaecology.* 8th edition. London. Elsevier Mosby.

O'Grady, J. (1999) Acute liver failure. *Medicine* 27 (1): 80–82.

O'Hanlon-Nichols, T. (1996) Commonly asked questions about chest drains. *American Journal of Nursing* 96 (5): 60–64.

O'Hanlon-Nichols, T. (1998) Basic assessment series: the adult pulmonary system. *American Journal of Nursing* 98 (2): 39–45.

Oh, H., Seo, W. (2003) A meta-analysis of the effects of various interventions in preventing endotracheal suction-induced hypoxemia. *Journal of Clinical Nursing* 12 (6): 912–924.

O'Malley, P., Favaloro, R., Anderson, B. (1991) Critical care nurse perceptions of family needs. *Heart and Lung* 20 (2): 198–201.

O'Neill, D. (2003) Using a stethoscope in clinical practice in the acute sector. *Professional Nurse* 18 (7): 391–394.

O'Neill, L.J., Carter, D.E. (1998) The implications of head injury for family relationships. *British Journal of Nursing* 7 (14): 842-846.

Oppert, M., Schindler, R., Husung, C., Offermann, K., Graf, K.J., Boenisch, O., Barchow, D., Frei, U., Eckardt, K.U. (2005) Low-dose hydrocortisone improves shock reversal and reduces cytokine levels in early hyperdynamic septic shock. *Critical Care Medicine* 33 (11): 2457–2464.

O'Riordan, B., Gray, K., McArthur Rouse, F. (2003) Implementing a critical care course for ward nurses. *Nursing Standard* 17 (20) 41–44.

Orme, J., Romney, J., Hopkins, R.O. (2003) Pulmonary function and health related quality of the life in survivors of acute respiratory distress syndrome. *American Journal of Respiratory Critical Care Medicine* 167 (5): 690–694.

Ormrod, J.A., Ryder, T., Chadwick, R.J., Bonner, S.M. (2005) Experiences of families when a relative is diagnosed brain stem dead: understanding of death, observation of brain stem death testing and attitudes to organ donation. *Anaesthesia* 60 (10): 1002–1008.

Otter, H., Martin, J., Bäsell, K., von Heymann, C., Hein, O.V., Böllert, P., Jänsch,

P., Behnisch, I., Wernecke, K.D., Konertz, W., Loening, S., Blohmer, J.U., Spies, C. (2005) Validity and reliability of the DDS for severity of delirium in the ICU. *Neurocritical Care* 2 (2): 150–158.

Owen, A.R., Gibson, M.R. (2004) Pulmonary embolism: advances in diagnosis and treatment. *Care of the Critically Ill* 20 (3): 79–84.

Owen, S., Gould, D. (1997) Underwater seal chest drains: the patient's experience. *Journal of Clinical Nursing* 6 (3): 215–225.

Pace, N. (2006) Transplantation: ethical and legal consideration. *Anaesthesia and Intensive Care Medicine* 7 (6): 155–188.

Page, S.R., Hall, G.M. (1999) *Diabetes Emergency and Hospital Management*. London. BMJ Books.

Paley, J. (2000) Asthma and dualism. *Journal of Advanced Nursing* 31 (6): 1293–1299.

Palma, S., Cosano, A., Mariscal, M., Martinez-Gallego, G., Medina-Cuadros, M., Delgado-Rodriguez, M. (2007) Cholesterol and serum albumin as risk factors for death in patients undergoing general surgery. *British Journal of Surgery* 94 (3): 369–375.

Papadopoulos, I. (ed.) (2006) *Transcultural Health and Social Care: Development of Culturally Competent Practitioner*. Edinburgh. Churchill Livingstone/Elsevier.

Papadopoulos, I., Tilki, M., Taylor, G. (1998) *Transcultural Care: A Guide for Health Professionals*. Trowbridge. Quay Books.

Pareek, M., Stephenson, I. (2007) Clinical evaluation of vaccines for pandemic influenza H5N1. *British Journal of Hospital Medicine* 68 (2): 80–84.

Parkes, C. (1996) *Bereavement: Studies of Grief in Adult Life*. London. Penguin.

Parliament (2000) *Adults with Incapacity (Scotland) Act*. London. Stationary Office.

Parliament (2005) *Mental Capacity Act*. London. Stationary Office.

Parsons, C.L., Sole, M.L., Byers, J.F. (2000) Noninvasive positive-pressure ventilation: averting intubation of the heart failure patient. *Dimensions of Critical Care Nursing* 19 (6): 18–24.

Pasero, C. (1996) Pain during sickle-cell crises. *American Journal of Nursing* 96 (1): 59–60.

Patel, S.R., White, D.P., Malhotra, A., Stanchina, M.L., Ayas, N.T. (2003) Continuous positive airway pressure therapy for treating sleepiness in a diverse population with obstructive sleep apnea. *Archives of Internal Medicine* 163 (5): 565–571.

Patil, B.B., Dowd, T.C. (2000) Physiological functions of the eye. *Current Anaesthesia and Critical Care* 11 (6): 291–298.

Patterson, M.T., Begnoche, V.L., Graybeal, J.M. (2007) The effect of motion on pulse oximetry and its clinical significance. *Anaesthesia and Analgesia* 105 (6 supplement): 578–584.

Pattison, N. (2005) Psychological implications of admission to critical care. *British Journal of Nursing* 14 (13): 708–714.

Pearce, C.B., Duncan, H.D. (2002) Enteral feeding: nasogastric, nasojejunal, percutaneous endoscopic gastrostomy, or jejunostomy: its indications and limitations. *Postgraduate Medical Journal* 78 (918): 198–204.

Pedersen, C.M., Rosendahl-Nielsen, M., Hjermind, J., Egerod, I. (2008) Endotracheal suctioning of the adult intubated patient: what is the evidence? *Intensive and Critical Care Nursing* 25(1): 21-30.

Pépin, J., Valiquette, L., Cossette, B. (2005) Mortality attributable to nosocomial *Clostridium difficile*-associated disease during an epidemic caused by a hypervirulent strain in Quebec. *Canadian Medical Association Journal* 173 (9): 1037–1042.

Perkins, C., Kisiel, M. (2005) Utilizing physiological knowledge to care for acute renal failure. *British Journal of Nursing* 14 (14): 768–773.

Peters, R.J.G., Mehta, S., Yusuf, S. (2007) Acute coronary syndromes without ST segment elevation. *BMJ* 334 (7606): 1265–1269.

Pickworth, T. (2003) Acute pancreatitis. *Anaesthesia and Intensive Care* 4 (4): 106–107.

Pierce, L. (2007) *Management of the Mechanically Ventilated Patient*. 2nd edition. St Louis. Elsevier.

Pilcher, T., Odell, M. (2000) Position statement on nurse–patient ratios in critical care. *Nursing Standard* 15 (12): 38–41.

Pitt, T. (2007) Management of antimicrobial-resistant *Acinitobacter* in hospitals. *Nursing Standard* 21 (35): 51–56.

Plant, P.K., Owen, J.L., Elliott, M.W. (2001) Non-invasive ventilation in acute exacerbation of chronic obstructive pulmonary disease: long term survival and predictors of in-hospital outcome. *Thorax* 56 (9): 708–712.

Plant, P.K., Owen, J.L., Parrott, S., Elliott, M.W. (2003) Cost effectiveness of ward based non-invasive ventilation for acute exacerbations of chronic obstructive pulmonary disease: analysis of randomised controlled trial. *BMJ* 326 (7396): 956–959.

Polderman, K.H., Girbes, A.R.J. (2002) Central venous catheter use. Part 1: mechanical complications. *Intensive Care Medicine* 28 (1): 1–17.

Polkey, M.I. (2008) Chronic obstructive pulmonary disease. *Medicine* 36 (4): 213–217.

Poponcik, J.M., Renston, J.P., Bennett, R.P., Emerman, C.L. (1999) Use of a ventilatory support system (BiPAP) for acute respiratory failure in the emergency department. *Chest* 116 (1): 166–171.

Poxton, I.R. (2005) *Clostridium difficile*-associated disease: an increasing burden. *Journal of the Royal College of Physicians of Edinburgh* 36 (3): 216–219.

Prandoni, P., Lensing, A.W.A., Prins, M.H., Frulla, M., Marchiori, A., Bernardi, E., Tormene, D., Mosena, L., Pagnan, A., Girolami, A. (2004) Below-knee elastic compression stockings to prevent the post-thrombotic syndrome. *Annals of Internal Medicine* 141 (4): 249–256.

Pratt, R.J., Pellowe, C.M., Wilson, J.A., Loveday, H.P., Harper, P.J., Jones, S.R.L.J., McDougall, C., Wilcox, M.H. (2007) Epic 2: national evidence-based guidelines for preventing healthcare-associated infections in NHS hospitals in England. *Journal of Hospital Infection* 65 (supplement 1): S1–S64.

Priestley, J. (1999) How critical care nurses identify and meet the needs of visitors to intensive care units. *Nursing in Critical Care* 4 (1): 27–29.

Priestley, M.A. (2006) Respiratory failure. *emedicine*. www.emedicine.com/ped/topic1994.htm.

Pritchard, J. (2008) What's new in Guillain–Barré syndrome? *Postgraduate Medical Journal* 84 (996): 522–538.

Prosser, S., McArthur-Rouse, F. (2007) Post-operative recovery. In McArthur-Rouse, F., Prosser, S. (eds) *Assessing and Managing the Acutely Ill Adult Surgical Patient*. Oxford. Blackwell Publishing, pp. 39–59.

Pryor, J.A., Prasad, S.A. (2008) *Physiotherapy for Respiratory and Cardiac Problems*. 4th edition. Edinburgh. Churchill Livingstone/Elsevier.

Pulido, T., Aranda, A., Zevallos, M.A., Bautista, E., Martínez-Guera, M.L., Santos, L.E., Sandoval, J. (2006) Pulmonary embolism as a cause of death in patients with heart disease: an autopsy study. *Chest* 129 (5): 1282–1287.

Puntillo, K., McAdam, J. (2006) Communication between physicians and nurses as a target for improving end-of-life care in the intensive care unit: challenges and opportunities in moving forward. *Critical Care Medicine* 34 (11 supplement): S332–S340.

Puntillo, K.A., Smith, D., Arai, S., Stotts, N. (2008) Critical care nurses provide their perspectives of patient's symptoms in intensive care units. *Heart and Lung* 37 (6): 466–475.

Quinn, S., Redman, K., Begley, C. (1996) The needs of relatives visiting adult critical care units as perceived by relatives and nurses: Part 2. *Intensive and Critical Care Nursing* 12 (4): 239–245.

Rady, M.Y., Joseph, L., McGregor, J.L. (2008) Cardiopulmonary resuscitation at the end of life without patient consent: an ethical challenge to autonomy and self-determination. *Chest* 133 (1): 320.

Rahman, N.M., Chapman, S.J., Davies, R.J.O. (2004) Pleural effusion: a structured approach to care. *British Medical Bulletin* 72: 31–47.

Rahman, T.M., Treacher, D. (2002) Management of acute renal failure on the intensive care unit. *Clinical Medicine* 2 (2): 108–113.

Rakel, B., Herr, K. (2004) Assessment and treatment of postoperative pain in older adults. *Journal of Perianesthesia Nursing* 19 (3): 194–208.

Ralph, S.S., Taylor, C.M. (2005) *Nursing Diagnosis: Reference Manual*. Philadelphia. Lippincott, Williams & Wilkins.

Ravenscroft, A.J., Bell, M.D.D. (2000) 'End-of-life' decision making within intensive care: objective, consistent, defensible? *Journal of Medical Ethics* 26 (6): 435–440.

Ravindra, K. (2008) Composite tissue transplantation and recent advances in transplant immunology. *British Journal of Transplantation* 3 (2): 8–9.

RCN (2003a) *Defining Nursing*. London. Royal College of Nursing.

RCN (2003b) *Guidance for Nursing Skills in Critical Care*. London. Royal College of Nursing.

RCN (2005a) *Clinical Practice Guidelines: Perioperative Fasting in Adults and Children*. London. Royal College of Nursing.

RCN (2005b) *Methicillin-Resistant* Staphylococcus aureus *(MRSA). Guidance for nursing staff*. London. Royal College of Nursing.

RCN (2005c) *Guidance of Uniforms and Clothing Worn in the Delivery of Patient Care*. London. Royal College of Nursing.

RCN (2005d) *Gynaecological Cancer: Guidance for Nursing Staff*. London. Royal College of Nursing.

RCN (2006) *Caring for Patients with Ovarian Hyperstimulation Syndrome. RCN Guidance for Fertility Nurses*. London. Royal College of Nursing.

RCN (2008a) *Bowel Care, Including Digital Rectal Examination and Removal of Faeces*. London. Royal College of Nursing.

RCN (2008b) *Enhancing Nutritional Care*. London. Royal College of Nursing.

RCOG (2003) *Management of Acute Pelvic Inflammatory Disease: Green-Top Guideline No. 23*. London. Royal College of Obstetricians and Gynaecologists.

RCOG (2004) *The Management of Tubal Pregnancy: Green-Top Guideline No. 21*. London. Royal College of Obstetricians and Gynaecologists.

RCOG (2006) *The Management of Ovarian Hyperstimulation Syndrome: Green-Top Guideline No. 5*. London. Royal College of Obstetricians and Gynaecologists.

RCP/BTS/ICS (2008) *Chronic Obstructive Pulmonary Disease: Non-Invasive Ventilation with Bi-Phasic Positive Airways Pressure in the Management of Patients with Acute Type 2 Respiratory Failure*. London. Royal College of Physicians, British Thoracic Society, Intensive Care Society.

RCP/NICE (2006) *Atrial Fibrillation. National Clinical Guideline for Management in Primary and Secondary Care*. London. Royal College of Physicians/National Institute for Clinical Excellence.

Redeker, N.S. (2000) Sleep in acute care settings: an integrated review. *Journal of Nursing Scholarship* 32 (1): 31–38.

Redeker, N.S., Whykpis, E. (1999) Effects of age on activity–rest after coronary artery bypass surgery. *Heart and Lung* 28 (1): 5–14.

Rees, J., Kanabar, D. (2000) *ABC of Asthma*. 4th edition. London. BMJ Books.

Regnard, C., Hockley, J. (2004) *A Guide to Symptom Relief in Palliative Care*. 5th edition. Oxford. Radcliff Medical Press Ltd.

Reinke, L., Hoffman, L. (2000) Asthma education: creating a partnership. *Heart and Lung* 9 (3): 225–236.

Resuscitation Council (UK) (2006) *Advanced Life Support*. 5th edition. London. Resuscitation Council.

Revelley, J.P., Tappy, L., Berger, M.M., Gerbach, P., Cayeux, C., Chiolero, R. (2001) Early metabolic and splanchnic responses to enteral nutrition in postoperative cardiac surgery patients with circulatory compromise. *Intensive Care Medicine* 27 (3): 540–547.

Rich, K. (1999) In-hospital cardiac arrest: pre-event variables and nursing response. *Clinical Nurse Specialist* 13 (3): 147–153.

Richardson, C. (2008) Nursing aspects of phantom limb pain following amputation. *British Journal of Nursing* 17 (7): 422–426.

Ridwan, B., Mascini, E., van der Reijden, N., Verhoef, J., Bonte, M. (2002) What action should be taken to prevent spread of vancomycin resistant *Enterococci* in European hospitals. *BMJ* 324 (7338): 666–668.

Roach, S. (1987) *The Human Act of Caring.* Ottowa: Canadian Hospital Association.

Roberts, G.A. (1986) Burnout: psycho babble or valuable concept? *British Journal of Hospital Medicine* 36 (3): 194–197.

Robinson, K.L., Driedger, M.S., Elliott, S.J., Eyles, J. (2006) Understanding facilitators of and barriers to health promotion practice. *Health Promotion Practice* 7 (4): 467–476.

Ropper, A.H. (1993) Treatment of intracranial hypertension. In Ropper, A.H. (ed.) *Neurological and Neurosurgical Intensive Care.* New York. Raven Press.

Roskelly, L. (2008) Intrapleural drainage. In Dougherty, L., Lister, S. (eds) *The Royal Marsden Hospital Manual of Clinical Nursing Procedures.* 7th edition. Oxford. Wiley-Blackwell, pp. 428–433.

Rossi, S., Zanier, E.R., Mauri, I., Columbo, A., Stocchetti, N. (2001) Brain temperature, body core temperature, and intracranial pressure in acute cerebral damage. *Journal of Neurology, Neurosurgery and Psychiatry* 71 (4): 448–454.

Roy, D., Talajic, M., Nattel, S., Wyse, G., Dorian, P., Lee, K.L., Bourassa, M.G., Arnold, J.M.O., Buxton, A.E., Camm, A.J., Connolly, S.J., Dubuc, M., Ducharme, A., Guerra, P.G., Hohnloser, S.H., Lambert, J., Le Heuzey, J.-Y., O'Hara, G., Pedersen, O.D., Rouleau, J.-L., Singh, B.N., Stevenson, L.W., Stevenson, W.G., Thibault, B., Waldo, A.L., Atrial Fibrillation and Congestive Heart Failure Investigators (2008) Rhythm control versus rate control for atrial fibrillation and heart failure. *NEJM* 358 (25): 2667–2677.

Rucker, D.W. (2008) Diabetic ketoacidosis. *emedicine.* www.emedicine.com/emerg/topic135htm (accessed 29 October 2008).

Rushforth, H., Warner, J., Burge, D., Glasper, E. (1998) Nursing physical assessment skills: implications for UK practice. *British Journal of Nursing* 7 (16): 965–970.

Russell, C. (2005) Providing the nurse with a guide to tracheostomy care and management. *British Journal of Nursing* 14 (8): 428–433.

Russell, K. (2008) Observations: neurological. In Dougherty, L., Lister, S. (eds) *The Royal Marsden Hospital Manual of Clinical Nursing Procedures.* 7th edition. Oxford. Wiley-Blackwell, pp. 545–556.

Russo-Magno, P., O'Brien, A., Panciera, T., Rounds, S. (2001) Compliance with CPAP therapy in older men with obstructive sleep apnea. *Journal of the American Geriatrics Society* 49 (9): 1205–1211.

Saab, M. (2005) Thrombolysis versus PCI: Can cardiologists have their cake and eat it? *Cardiology News* 8 (2): 6–9.

Sagarin, J., McAfee, A. (2001) Diabetic ketoacidosis. *Endocrinology Metabolism Clinics of North America* 30 (4): 817–831.

Sandelowski, M. (2000) *Devices and Desires. Gender, Technology and American Nursing.* North Carolina. The University of North Carolina Press.

Sargent, S. (2007) Pathophysiology and management of hepatic encephalopathy. *British Journal of Nursing* 16 (6): 335–339.

Sarnak, J.W., Greene, I., Wang, X., Beck, G., Kusek, J.W., Collins, A.J. (2005)

The effect of a lower target blood pressure on the progression of kidney disease: long-term follow-up of the modification in diet in renal disease study. *Annals of Internal Medicine* 142 (5): 342–351.

Sawhney, N.S., Feld, G.K. (2008) Diagnosis and management of typical atrial flutter. *Medical Clinics of America* 92 (1): 65–85.

Scalea, T.M., Bochicchio, G.V., Bochicchio, K.M., Johnson, S.B., Joshi, M., Pyle, A. (2007) Tight glycemic control in critically injured trauma patients. *Annals of Surgery* 246 (4): 605–612.

Schafheutle, E.I., Cantrill, J.A., Noyce, P.R. (2001) Why is pain management suboptimal on surgical wards? *Journal of Advanced Nursing* 33 (6): 728–737.

Schilling, R.J. (1994) Should relatives watch resuscitation? *BMJ* 309 (6951): 406.

Schmaier, A.H. (2004) Disseminated intravascular coagulation: pathogenesis and management. *emedicine*.

Schulman, P., Fessler, E. (2001) Management of acute coronary syndromes. *American Journal of Respiratory and Critical Care Medicine* 164 (6): 917–922.

Scullion, J. (2008) Patient-focused outcomes in chronic obstructive pulmonary disease. *Nursing Standard* 22 (21): 50–56.

Searight, H.R., Gafford, J. (2005) Cultural diversity at the end of life: Issues and guidelines for the family physician. *American Family Physician* 71 (3): 515–522.

Seaton, A., Seaton, D., Leitch, A.G. (2000) *Croft and Douglas's Respiratory Diseases*. 5th edition. London. Blackwell Science.

Selye, H. (1956) *The Stress of Life*. New York. McGraw-Hill.

Serra, A. (2000) Tracheostomy care. *Nursing Standard* 14 (42): 45–55.

Sevransky, J.E., Haponik, E.F. (2003) Respiratory failure in elderly patients. *Clinical Geriatric Medicine* 19 (1): 205–224.

Shapiro, M. (1993) *The ABC of Sleep Disorders*. London: British Medical Association.

Sharara, A.I. (2001) Gastroesophageal variceal hemorrhage. *NEJM* 345 (9): 669–681.

Sharma, S. (2006) Respiratory failure. *emedicine*. www.emdicine.com/med/topic2011.htm (accessed 20 November 2008).

Sheerin, F. (2005) Spinal cord injury: causation and pathophysiology. *Emergency Nurse* 12 (9): 29–38.

Shiotani, A., Graham, D.Y. (2002) Pathogenesis and therapy of gastric and duodenal ulcer disease. *Medical Clinics of North America* 86 (6): 1447–1466.

Shutz, S.L. (2001). Oxygen saturation monitoring by pulse oximetry. *AACN Procedure Manual for Critical Care* 4 (11): 77–82.

SIGN (2007) *Management of Chronic Heart Failure*. Edinburgh. Scottish Intercollegiate Guidelines Network.

Sikes, D.H., Ahrawal, N.M., Zhao, W.W., Kent, J.D., Recker, D.P., Verburg, K.M. (2002) Incidence of gastroduodenal ulcers associated with valecoxib compared with that of ibuprofen and diclofenac in patients with osteoarthritis. *European Journal of Gastroenterology and Hepatology* 14 (10): 1101–1111.

Sim, K.M. (2002) Respiratory emergencies. *Anaesthesia and Intensive Care Medicine* 3 (11): 410–413.

Simpson, T., Lee, E.R., Camaron, S. (1996) Relationships among sleep dimensions and factors that impair sleep after cardiac surgery. *Research in Nursing and Health* 19 (3): 213–223.

Sin, D.D., Logan, A.G., Fitzgerald, F.S., Liu, P.P., Bradley, T.D. (2000) Effects of continuous positive airway pressure on cardiovascular outcomes in heart failure patients and without Cheyne–Stokes respiration. *Circulation* 102 (1): 61–66.

Singh, B.M., Mehta, J.L. (2003) Interactions between the renin-angiotensin system and dyslipidemia. *Archives of Internal Medicine* 163 (11): 1296–1304.

Sirodkar, M., Mohandas, K.M. (2005) Subjective global assessment: a simple and reliable screening tool for malnutrition among Indians. *Indian Journal of Gastroenterology* 24 (6): 246–250.

Sisodiya, S.M., Duncan, J. (2004) Epilepsy, epidemiology, clinical assessment and natural history. *Medicine* 32 (10): 47–51.

Siva, S., Pereira, S.P. (2007) Acute pancreatitis. *Medicine* 35 (3): 171–177.

Skipworth, R.J.E., Stewart, G.D., Ross, J.A., Guttridge, D.C., Fearon, K.C.H. (2006) The molecular mechanisms of skeletal muscle wasting: implications for therapy. *The Surgeon* 4 (5): 273–283.

Slota, M., Shearn, D., Potersnak, K., Haas, L. (2003) Perspectives on family-centred, flexible visitation in the intensive care unit setting. *Critical Care Medicine* 31 (5 supplement): S362–S366.

Smaha, D.A. (2001) Asthma emergency care: national guidelines summary. *Heart and Lung* 30 (6): 472–474. Introduction.

Smith, D.H. (2007) Managing acute acetaminophen toxicity. *Nursing 2007* 37 (1): 58–63.

Smith, G. (2000) ALERT: A multiprofessional course in care of the acutely ill patient. University of Portsmouth.

Smith, G., Prytherch, P., Schmidt, P., Feathersone, P. (2008) Review and performance evaluation of aggregate weighted 'track and trigger' systems. *Resuscitation* 77 (2): 170–179.

Smith, P.M. (2000) Portal hypertension. *Surgery* 18 (7): 153–156.

Smith, S.J. (1993) Suctioning the airway. *Emergency* 25 (3): 41–45.

Snell, C.C., Fothergill-Bourbonnais, F., Durocher-Henriks, S. (1997) Patient controlled analgesia and intramuscular injections: a comparison of patient pain experiences and postoperative outcomes. *Journal of Advanced Nursing* 25 (4): 681–690.

Snowball, J. (1996) Asking nurses about advocating for patients: 'reactive' and 'proactive' accounts. *Journal of Advanced Nursing* 24 (1): 67–75.

Somauroo, J.D., Wilkinson, M., White, V.J., Rodrigues, E., Connelly, D.T., Calverley, P.M.A., Angus, R.M. (2000) Effect of nasal bilevel positive airway pressure (BiPAP) and continuous positive airway pressure (CPAP) ventilation on cardiac haemodynamics in patients with congestive heart failure. *Heart* 83 (supplement II): A20.

Soni, N., Wagstaff, A. (2005) Fungal infection. *Current Anaesthesia and Critical Care* 16 (5): 231–241.

Southwell, M.T., Winstow, G.S. (1995) Sleep in hospital at night: are patients' needs being met? *Journal of Advanced Nursing* 21 (6): 1101–1109.

Spencer, L. (1994) How do nurses deal with their own grief when a patient dies on an intensive care unit, and what help can be given to enable them to overcome their grief effectively? *Journal of Advanced Nursing* 19 (6): 1141–1150.

Squadrone, E., Frigerio, P., Fogliati, C., Gregoretti, C., Conti, G., Antonelli, M., Costa, R., Baiardi, P., Navalesi, P. (2004) Noninvasive vs invasive ventilation in COPD patients with severe acute respiratory failure deemed to require ventilatory assistance. *Intensive Care Medicine* 30 (7): 1303–1310.

Steele, K., Hart, O., Nijentivis, E. (2001) Dependency in the treatment of complex post traumatic stress disorder and dissociative disorders. *Journal of Trauma and Dissociation* 2 (4): 79–116.

St George's Healthcare Trust (2006) *Guidelines for the Care of Patients with Tracheostomy Tubes*. London. Smiths-Medical Ltd.

Stanley, A.J., Hayes, P.C. (1997) Portal hypertension and variceal haemorrhage. *Lancet* 350 (9036): 1235–1239.

Steggall, M.J. (2007) Urine samples and urinalysis. *Nursing Standard* 22 (14–16): 42–45.

Steinberg, W., Tenner, S. (1994) Acute pancreatitis. *NEJM* 330 (17): 1198–1209.

Sternbach, R.A. (1968) *Pain: A Psychophysiological Analysis*. New York. Academic Press.

Stevens, M.S. (2008) Normal sleep, sleep physiology, and sleep deprivation: general principles. *emedicine*. www.emedicine.com/neuro/topic444.htm (accessed 27 November 2008).

Stevens, P. (2007) Assessment of patients presenting with acute renal failure (acute kidney injury). *Medicine* 35 (8): 429–433.

Stewart, D. (2001) The percussion technique for restoring patency to central venous catheters. *Care of the Critically Ill* 17 (3): 106–107.

Stewart, S., Blue, L. (eds) (2004) *Improving Outcomes in Chronic Heart Failure*. 2nd edition. London. BMJ Books.

Stocklmann, H.B.A.C., Hiemstra, C.A., Marquet, R.L., Jzermans, J.N.M. (2000) Extracorporeal perfusion for the treatment of acute liver failure. *Annals of Surgery* 231 (4): 460–470.

Stokes, T., Shaw, E.J., Juarez-Garcia, A., Camosso-Stefinovic, J., Baker, R. (2004) *Clinical Guidelines and Evidence Review for the Epilepsies: Diagnosis and Management in Adults and Children in Primary and Secondary Care*. London. Royal College of General Practitioners.

Stone, K.S., Preusser, B., Groch, K., Karl, J., Gonyon, D. (1991) The effect of lung hyperinflation and endotracheal suctioning on cardiopulmonary haemo-dynamics. *Nursing Research* 40 (2): 76–80.

Stoner, G. (2005) Hyperosmolar hyperglycaemic state. *American Family Physician* 17: 1723–1730.

Storr, J., Topley, K., Privett, S. (2005) The ward nurse's role in infection control. *Nursing Standard* 19 (41): 56–64.

Strahan, E.H., Brown, R.F. (2005) A qualitative study of the experiences of patients following transfer from intensive care. *Intensive and Critical Care Nursing* 21 (3): 160–171.

Straus, S.M.J.M., Kors, J.A., de Bruin, M.L., van der Hooft, C.S., Hofman, A., Heeringa, J., Deckers, J.W., Kingma, J.H., Sturkenboom, M.C.J.M., Stricker, B.M.C., Witteman, J.C.M. (2006) Prolonged QTC interval and risk of sudden cardiac death in a population of older adults. *Journal of the American College of Cardiology* 47 (2): 362–367.

Stringer, S. (2007) Quality of death: humanisation versus medicalisation. *Cancer Nursing Practice* 6 (3): 23–28.

Strunin, L., Rowbotham, D., Miles, A. (1999) *The Effective Management of Post-Operative Nausea and Vomiting*. London. Aesculapius Medical Press.

Sullivan, B. (2008) Nursing management of patients with a chest drain. *British Journal of Nursing* 17 (6): 388–393.

Swick, H.M. (2007) Professionalism and humanism beyond the academic health center. *Academic Medicine* 82 (11): 1022–1028.

Swift, C., Calcutawalla, S., Elliot, R. (2007) Nursing attitudes towards recording of religious and spiritual data. *British Journal of Nursing* 16 (20): 1279–1282.

Sykes, E., Cosgrove, J.F. (2007) Acute renal failure and the critically ill surgical patient. *Annals of the Royal College of Surgeons of England* 89 (1): 22–29.

Symonds, E.M., Symonds, I.M. (2004) *Essential Obstetrics and Gynaecology*. 4th edition. London. Churchill Livingstone/Elsevier Science Ltd.

Taher, A. (2007) Anemia, sickle cell. *emedicine*. www.emedicine.com/emerg/topic26.htm.

Taylor, V., Ashelford, S. (2008) Understanding depression in palliative and end-of-life care. *Nursing Standard* 23 (12): 48–57.

Teasdale, G., Jennett, B. (1974) Assessment of coma and impaired consciousness. *Lancet* ii (7872): 81–83.

Telfer, M., Lewin, A., Jenkins, P. (2007) Assisted ventilation in acute exacerbation of chronic obstructive pulmonary disease. *Journal of the Royal College of Physicians of Edinburgh* 37 (1): 44–48.

Teoh, L.S.G., Gowardman, J.R., Larsen, P.D., Green, R., Galletly, D.C. (2000) Glasgow Coma Scale: variation in mortality among permutations of specific total scores. *Intensive Care Medicine* 26 (2): 157–161.

Terman, M., Lewy, A.J., Dijk, D., Boulous, Z., Eastman, C., Campbell, S.S. (1995) Light treatment for sleep disorders: consensus report. *Journal of Biological Rhythms* 10 (2): 135–147.

Tham, T.C.K, Collins, J.S.A. (2000) *Gastrointestinal Emergencies*. London. BMJ Books.

The PLUS decision-making model (2008) www.ethics.org/resources/decision-making model.asp (accessed 1 July 2008).

Therapondos, G., Hayes, O.C. (2002) Management of gastro-oesophageal varices. *Clinical Medicine* 2 (4): 297–302.

Thomas, B., Bishop, J. (2007) *Manual of Dietetic Practice*. Oxford. Blackwell Publishing Ltd.

Thomas, G., Hirsch, N. (2003) Generalized convulsive status epilepticus. *Anaesthesia and Intensive Care* 4 (4): 120–122.

Thomas, H.C. (1999) Hepatitis B and D. *Surgery* 27 (1): 34–36.

Thomason, J.W., Shintani, A., Peterson, J.F., Pun, B.T., Jackson, J.C., Ely, E.W. (2005) Intensive care unit delirium is an independent predictor of longer hospital stay: a prospective analysis of 261 non-ventilated patients. *Critical Care* 9 (4): 335–336.

Thompson, L. (2000) Suctioning adults with an artificial airway. The Josanna Briggs Institute for Evidence Based Nursing and Midwifery. *Systemic Review* (9).

Thuong, M., Arvaniti, K., Ruimy, R., de la Salmonière, P., Scanvic-Hameg, A., Lucet, J.C., Régnier, B. (2003) Epidemiology of *Pseudomonas aeruginosa* and risk factors for carriage acquisition in an intensive care unit. *Journal of Hospital Infection* 53 (4): 274–282.

Thygesen, K., Alpert, J.S., White, H.D., on behalf of the Joint ESC/ACCF/AHA/WHF Task Force for the Redefinition of Myocardial Infarction (2007) Universal definition of myocardial infarction. *Circulation* 116 (116): 2634–2653.

Tilki, M. (2003) A study of the health of Irish born people in London: the relevance of social and economic factors, health beliefs and behaviour. Unpublished PhD thesis. London. Middlesex University.

Tingle, J. (2002) The role of the advanced scrub practitioner. *British Journal of Nursing* 11 (19): 1267–1269.

Tingle, J., Cribb, A. (2002) *Nursing Law and Ethics.* 2nd edition. Oxford. Blackwell Science.

Tobin, A., Santamaria, J. (2006) After-hours discharges from intensive care are associated with increased mortality. *Medical Journal of Australia* 184 (7): 334–337.

Todd, N. (1997) The physiological knowledge required by nurses caring for patients with unstable angina. *Nursing in Critical Care* 2 (4): 17–24.

Tones, K. (1991) Health promotion, empowerment and the psychology of control. *Journal of the Institute of Health Education* 29 (1): 17–26.

Tonkin, A. (2004) The metabolic syndrome: a growing problem. *European Heart Journal* 6 (supplement A): A37–A42.

Topf, M., Thompson, S. (2001) Interactive relationships between hospital patients, noise-induced stress and other stress with sleep. *Heart and Lung* 30 (4): 237–243.

Treasure, T. (2007) Minimally invasive surgery for pneumothorax: the evidence, changing practice and current opinion. *JRSM* 100 (9): 419–422.

Trew, G. (2007) Assisted reproduction. In Edmonds, D.K. (ed.) *Dewhurst's Textbook of Obstetrics and Gynaecology.* 7th edition. Oxford. Blackwell Science, pp. 461–478).

Tuncay, T., Musabak, I., Gok, D.E., Kutlu, M. (2008) The relationship between anxiety, coping strategies and characteristics of patients with diabetes. *Health and Quality of Life Outcomes* 6 (1): 79–84.

Turner, B. (2003) Acute pancreatitis: symptoms, diagnosis and management. *Nursing Times* 99 (46): 38–40.

Tvedt, C., Bukholm, G. (2005) Alcohol-based hand disinfection: a more robust hand-hygiene method in an intensive care unit. *Journal of Hospital Infection* 59 (3): 229–234.

Twycross, A. (2002) Educating nurses about pain management: the way forward. *Journal of Clinical Nursing* 11 (6): 705–714.

Uhl, W., Isenmann, R., Buchler, W. (1998) Infections complicating pancreatitis: diagnosing, treating, preventing. *New Horizons* 6 (supplement 2): S72–S79.

Uhl, W., Buchler, M.W., Malfertheiner, P., Beger, H.G., Adler, G., Gaus, W., German Pancreatitis Study Group (1999) A randomised, double-blind, multicentre trial of octreotide in moderate to severe acute pancreatitis. *Gut* 45 (1): 97–104.

UK Working Party on Acute Pancreatitis (2005) UK guidelines for the management of acute pancreatitis. *Gut* 54 (5 supplement), iii1–iii9.

Urden, L.D., Stacy, K.M., Lough, M.E. (2006) *Thelan's Critical Care Nursing*. 5th edition. San Francisco. Mosby.

Uusaro, A., Kari, A., Ruokonen, E. (2003) The effects of ICU admission and discharge times on mortality in Finland. *Intensive Care Medicine* 29 (12): 2144–2148.

van den Berghe, G. (2000) Euthyroid sick syndrome. *Current Opinion in Anaesthesiology* 13 (2): 89–92.

van den Berghe, G., Wouters, P., Weekers, F., Verwaest, C., Bruyninckx, F., Schetz, M., Vlasslelaers, D., Ferdinande, P., Lauwers, P., Bouillon, R. (2001) Intensive insulin therapy in critically ill patients. *NEJM* 345 (19): 1359–1367.

Van de Leur, J.P., Zwaveling, J.H., Loef, B.G., Van der Schans, C.P. (2003) Endotracheal suctioning versus minimally invasive airway suctioning in intubated patients: a prospective randomised controlled trial. *Intensive Care Medicine* 29 (3): 426–432.

Vargas, H.E., Gerber, D., Abu-Elmagd, K. (1999) Management of portal hypertension-related bleeding. *Surgical Clinics of North America* 79 (1): 1–22.

Vassallo, M. (2008) Heart failure survey. *Geriatric Medicine* 38 (supplement 01): 43–58.

Verhaegh, S., Defloor, T., Van Zuuren, F., Duijnstee, M., Grypdonck, M. (2005) The needs and experiences of family members of adult patients in an intensive care unit: a review of the literature. *Journal of Clinical Nursing* 14 (4): 501–509.

Vincent, J.-L. (2000) Microbial resistance: lessons from the EPIC study. *Intensive Care Medicine* 26 (supplement 1): S3–S8.

Viscusi, E.R., Siccardi, M., Damaraju, C.V., Hewitt, D.J., Kershaw, P. (2007) The safety and efficacy of fentanyl iontrophoretic transdermal system compared with morphine intravenous patient-controlled analgesia for postoperative pain management: an analysis of pooled data from three randomized, active-controlled clinical studies. *Anesthesia and Analgesia* 105 (5): 1428–1436.

Visser, E., Schug, S.A. (2006) The role of ketamine in pain management. *Biomedicine and Pharmacology* 60 (7): 341–348.

von Klemperer, K., Bunce, N.H. (2007) Chronic heart failure. *Care of the Critically Ill* 23 (95): 134–144.

Voth, D.E., Ballard, J.D. (2005) *Clostridium difficile* toxins: mechanism of action and role in disease. *Clinical Microbiology Reviews* 18 (2): 2247–2263.

Wainright, S.P., Gould, D. (1996) Endotracheal suctioning: an example of the problems of relevance and rigour in clinical research. *Journal of Clinical Nursing* 5 (6): 389–398.

Waldo, A.L. (2008) Anticoagulation: stroke prevention in patients with atrial fibrillation. *Medical Clinics of America* 92 (1): 143–159.

Walker, M. (2005) Status epilepticus: an evidence based review. *BMJ* 331 (7518): 673–677.

Wall, R.J., Curtis, R., Cooke, C.R., Engelberg, R.A. (2007) Families dissatisfaction in the ICU: differences between families of survivors and non-survivors. *Chest* 132 (5): 1425–1433.

Walsh, S.B., Tang, T., Wijewardena, C., Yarham, S.I., Boyle, J.R., Gaunt, M.E. (2007) Postoperative arrythmias in general surgical patients. *Annals of the Royal College of Surgeons of England* 89 (2): 91–95.

Ward, J.P., Ward, J., Leach, R.M., Wiener, C.M. (2006) *The Respiratory System at a Glance*. Oxford. Blackwell Publishing.

Waterhouse, C. (2005) The Glasgow Coma Scale and other neurological observations. *Nursing Standard* 19 (33): 56–64.

Watson, J. (1999) *Post Modern Nursing and Beyond*. New York. Churchill Livingstone.

Watson, J. (2007) Theoretical questions and concerns: response from a caring science framework. *Nursing Science Quarterly* 20 (1): 13–15.

Watson, R.D.S., Chin, B., Lip, G.Y.H. (2002) Antithrombotic therapy in acute coronary syndromes. *BMJ* 325 (7376): 1348–1351.

Watt, A. (2001) Caring for patients with phantom limb sensation. *Professional Nurse* 16 (9): 1350–1353.

Weetman, C., Allison, W. (2006) Use of epidural analgesia in post-operative pain management. *Nursing Standard* 20 (44): 54–64.

Weiltz, B. (2007) *Pocket Guide for Health Assessment*. 6th edition. St Louis. Mosby/Elsevier Inc.

Weir, R.A.P., McMurray, J.J.V., Taylor, J., Brady, A.J.B. (2005) Heart failure in older patients. *British Journal of Cardiology* 13 (4): 257–266.

Welie, J., Welie, S. (2001) Patient decision-making competence: outlines of a conceptual analysis. *Medicine, Health Care and Philosophy* 4 (2): 127–138.

Wellington, K., Wagstaff, A.J. (2003) Tranexamic acid: a review of its use in the management of hemorrhagic. *Drugs* 63 (13): 1417–1433.

Wendell, F., Mohandas, N., Petz, D., Steinberg, M. (2000) New views of sickle cell disease pathophysiology and treatment. *American Society of Hematology.* http://asheducationbook.hematologylibrary.org/cgi/content/full/2000/1/2.

Werner, C., Engelhard, K. (2007) Pathophysiology of traumatic brain injury. *BJA* 99 (1): 4–9.

Westerdale, N. (2004) Managing the problem of pain in adolescents with sickle cell disease. *Professional Nurse* 19 (7): 402–405.

Weston, D. (2008) *Infection Prevention and Control*. Chichester. John Wiley & Sons.

Wheeler, A.P., Marini, J.J. (2006) *Critical Care Medicine: The Essentials*. Philadelphia. Lippincott, Williams & Wilkins.

Whitehead, M., Dahlgren, G. (2006) Levelling up I: A discussion paper on concepts and principles for tackling inequalities in health. Denmark. World Health Organisation Regional Office for Europe.

WHO (1986) *Ottowa Charter for Health Promotion*. Geneva. World Health Organisation.

WHO (1996) *Cancer Pain Relief*. 2nd edition. Geneva. World Health Organisation.

WHO (2005) *Global Patient Safety Challenge: 2005–2006*. Geneva. World Health Organisation.

WHO (2006) *Genes and Human Disease*. World Health Organisation. www.who.int/genomics/public/geneticdiseases/en/indix.html (accessed 25 June 2008).

Whyte, D.A. (1997) *Explorations in Family Nursing*. London. Routledge.

Wigfull, J., Welchew, E. (2001) Survey of 1057 patients receiving postoperative patient-controlled epidural analgesia. *Anaesthesia* 56 (1): 70–75.

Wilkinson, R. (2000) Organ donation: the debate. *Nursing Standard* 14 (28): 41–42.

Willard, C., Luker, K. (2006) Challenges to end of life care in the acute hospital setting. *Palliative Medicine* 20 (6): 611–615.

Williams, B., Poulter, N.R., Brown, M.J., Davis, M., McInnes, G.T., Potter, J.F., Sever, P.S., Thom, S.McG. (2004) Guidelines for management of hypertension. *Journal of Human Hypertension* 18: 139–185.

Wilson, L.A. (2005) Urinalysis. *Nursing Standard* 19 (35): 51–54.

Winer, J.B. (2008) Guillain–Barré syndrome. *BMJ* 337 (7663): 227–231.

Winter, B., Knight, D. (2005) Spinal cord injury. *Anaesthesia and Intensive Care* 6 (9): 315–317.

Winter, G. (2005) A bug's life. *Nursing Standard* 19 (33): 16–18.

Wiseman, S. (2006) Prevention and control of healthcare-associated infection. *Nursing Standard* 20 (38): 41–45.

Wolfe, W.G. (2003) Pulmonary emboli. *Annals of Surgery* 238 (6 supplement): S6–S71.

Wolfsdorf, J., Craig, M.E., Daneman, D., Dunger, D., Edge, J., Lee, D. (2006) Diabetic ketoacidosis: SPAD, Clinical practice consensus guidelines 2006–2007. *Paediatric Diabetes* 8 (1): 28–43.

Wong, C.-K., Gao, W., Refel, C., French, J.K., Stewart, R.A., White, H.D., HERO-2 Investigators (2006) Initial Q waves accompanying ST-segment elevation at presentation of acute myocardial infarction and 30-day mortality in patients given streptokinase therapy: an analysis from HERO-2. *Lancet* 367 (9528): 2061–2067.

Wood, C. (1998) Endotracheal suctioning: a literature review. *Intensive and Critical Care Nursing* 14 (3): 124–136.

Wood, D., Wray, R., Poulter, N., Williams, B., Kirby, M.P.V., for British Cardiac Society, Diabetes UK, HEART UK, Primary Care Cardiovascular Society, Stroke Association (2005) Joint British societies' guidelines on the prevention of cardiovascular disease in clinical practice. *Heart* 91 (supplement 5): v1–v52.

Woodrow, P. (2006) *Intensive Care Nursing*. 2nd edition. London. Routledge.

Worrel, J. (1977) *Nursing Implications in the Care of the Patient Experiencing Sensory Deprivation*. Philadelphia. J.B. Lippincott.

Wort, S.J. (2003) The management of acute severe asthma in adults. *Current Anaesthesia and Critical Care* 14 (2): 81–89.

Wright, B. (1991) *Sudden Death. Intervention Skills for the Caring Professionals*. Edinburgh. Churchill Livingstone.

Wright, B. (1996) *Sudden Death. A Research Base for Practice*. 2nd edition. Edinburgh. Churchill Livingstone.

Writing Committee of the Second World Health Organization Consultation on Clinical aspects of Human Infection with Avian Influenza A (H5N1) Virus (2008) Update on Avian Influenza A (H5N1) virus infection in humans. *NEJM* 358 (3): 261–273.

Wyncoll, D.L.A. (2003) Management of acute poisoning. In Bersten, A.D., Soni, N. (eds) *Intensive Care Manual*. 5th edition. Edinburgh. Butterworth-Heinemann, pp. 823–832.

Yale, S., Nagib, N., Guthrie, T. (2000) Approach to vaso-occlusive crisis in adults with sickle cell disease. *American Family Physician* 61 (5): 1349–1356.

Yates, D.W., Elison, G., McGuiness, S. (1990) Care of the suddenly bereaved. *BMJ* 301 (6742): 29–31.

Yin, A.T., Bradley, T.D., Liu, P.P. (2001) The role of continuous positive airway pressure in the treatment of congestive heart failure. *Chest* 120 (5): 1675–1685.

Ympa, Y.P., Sakr, Y., Reinhart, K., Vincent, J.-L. (2005) Has mortality from acute renal failure decreased? A systematic review of the literature. *American Journal of Medicine* 118 (8): 827–832.

Younes, R.N., Gross, J.L., Aguiar, S., Haddad, F.J., Deheinzelin, D. (2002) When to remove a chest tube? A randomized study with subsequent prospective consecutive validation. *Journal of the American College of Surgeons* 195 (5): 658–662.

Young, J., Stiffleet, J., Nikoletti, S., Shaw, T. (2006) Use of a behavioural pain scale to assess pain in ventilated, unconscious and/or sedated patients. *Intensive and Critical Care Nursing* 22 (1): 32–39.

Yu, N., Nardella, A., Pechet, L. (2000) Screening tests for disseminated intravascular coagulation: guidelines for rapid and specific laboratory diagnosis. *Critical Care Medicine* 28 (6): 1777–1780.

Zacharisen, M.C. (2002) Occupational asthma. *Medical Clinics of North America* 86 (5): 951–972.

Zarich, S.W., Nesto, R.W (2007) Implications and treatment of acute hyperglycaemia in the setting of acute myocardial infarction. *Circulation* 115: 436–439.

Zarzaur, B.L., Fukatsu, K., Kudsk, K.A. (2000) The influence of nutrition on mucosal immunology and endothelial cell adhesion molecules. In Vincent, J.-L. (ed.) *Yearbook of Intensive Care and Emergency Medicine*. Berlin. Springer, pp. 63–71.

Zimetbaum, P. (2007) Amiodarone for atrial fibrillation. *NEJM* 356 (9): 935–941.

Zirakzadeh, A., Patel, R. (2006) Vancomycin-resistant *Enterococci*: colonization, infection, detection, and treatment. *Mayo Clinical Proceedings* 81 (4): 529–536.

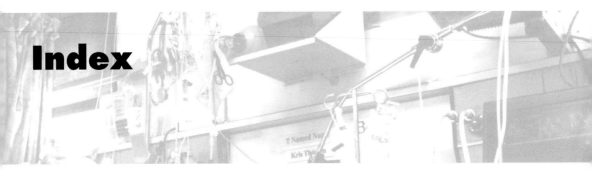

Index